Advanced Biomaterials and Biotechnology: Applications in Dental Medicine

Advanced Biomaterials and Biotechnology: Applications in Dental Medicine

Editors

Lavinia Cosmina Ardelean
Laura-Cristina Rusu

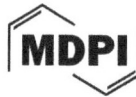

Basel • Beijing • Wuhan • Barcelona • Belgrade • Novi Sad • Cluj • Manchester

Editors

Lavinia Cosmina Ardelean
Department of Technology of
Materials and Devices in
Dental Medicine
"Victor Babes" University of
Medicine and Pharmacy
Timisoara
Romania

Laura-Cristina Rusu
Department of Oral
Pathology
"Victor Babes" University of
Medicine and Pharmacy
Timisoara
Romania

Editorial Office
MDPI AG
Grosspeteranlage 5
4052 Basel, Switzerland

This is a reprint of articles from the Special Issue published online in the open access journal *Journal of Functional Biomaterials* (ISSN 2079-4983) (available at: www.mdpi.com/journal/jfb/special_issues/MKBY06M08Z).

For citation purposes, cite each article independently as indicated on the article page online and as indicated below:

Lastname, A.A.; Lastname, B.B. Article Title. *Journal Name* **Year**, *Volume Number*, Page Range.

ISBN 978-3-7258-2006-1 (Hbk)
ISBN 978-3-7258-2005-4 (PDF)
doi.org/10.3390/books978-3-7258-2005-4

© 2024 by the authors. Articles in this book are Open Access and distributed under the Creative Commons Attribution (CC BY) license. The book as a whole is distributed by MDPI under the terms and conditions of the Creative Commons Attribution-NonCommercial-NoDerivs (CC BY-NC-ND) license. (https://creativecommons.org/licenses/by-nc-nd/4.0/).

Contents

About the Editors vii

Preface ix

Maryam Soleimani, Jarosław Żmudzki, Wojciech Pakieła, Anna Jaśkowska and Kornel Krasny
Dental Implant Abutment Screw Loss: Presentation of 10 Cases
Reprinted from: *J. Funct. Biomater.* **2024**, *15*, 96, doi:10.3390/jfb15040096 1

Anna Woźniak, Weronika Smok, Janusz Szewczenko, Marcin Staszuk and Grzegorz Chladek
Influence of Hybrid Surface Modification on Biocompatibility and Physicochemical Properties of Ti-6Al-4V ELI Titanium
Reprinted from: *J. Funct. Biomater.* **2024**, *15*, 52, doi:10.3390/jfb15030052 16

Ignacio Barbero-Navarro, Diego Velázquez-González, María Esther Irigoyen-Camacho, Marco Antonio Zepeda-Zepeda, Paulo Mauricio, David Ribas-Perez, et al.
Assessment of the Penetration of an Endodontic Sealer into Dentinal Tubules with Three Different Compaction Techniques Using Confocal Laser Scanning Microscopy
Reprinted from: *J. Funct. Biomater.* **2023**, *14*, 542, doi:10.3390/jfb14110542 40

Joanna Rygas, Jacek Matys, Magdalena Wawrzyńska, Maria Szymonowicz and Maciej Dobrzyński
The Use of Graphene Oxide in Orthodontics—A Systematic Review
Reprinted from: *J. Funct. Biomater.* **2023**, *14*, 500, doi:10.3390/jfb14100500 58

Maria Saridou, Alexandros K. Nikolaidis, Elisabeth A. Koulaouzidou and Dimitris S. Achilias
Synthesis and Characterization of Dental Nanocomposite Resins Reinforced with Dual Organomodified Silica/Clay Nanofiller Systems
Reprinted from: *J. Funct. Biomater.* **2023**, *14*, 405, doi:10.3390/jfb14080405 75

Perla Alejandra Hernández-Venegas, Rita Elizabeth Martínez-Martínez, Erasto Armando Zaragoza-Contreras, Rubén Abraham Domínguez-Pérez, Simón Yobanny Reyes-López, Alejandro Donohue-Cornejo, et al.
Bactericidal Activity of Silver Nanoparticles on Oral Biofilms Related to Patients with and without Periodontal Disease
Reprinted from: *J. Funct. Biomater.* **2023**, *14*, 311, doi:10.3390/jfb14060311 94

Anna Paradowska-Stolarz, Joanna Wezgowiec, Andrzej Malysa and Mieszko Wieckiewicz
Effects of Polishing and Artificial Aging on Mechanical Properties of Dental LT Clear® Resin
Reprinted from: *J. Funct. Biomater.* **2023**, *14*, 295, doi:10.3390/jfb14060295 111

Angelo Michele Inchingolo, Giuseppina Malcangi, Laura Ferrante, Gaetano Del Vecchio, Fabio Viapiano, Alessio Danilo Inchingolo, et al.
Surface Coatings of Dental Implants: A Review
Reprinted from: *J. Funct. Biomater.* **2023**, *14*, 287, doi:10.3390/jfb14050287 122

Zbigniew Raszewski, Katarzyna Chojnacka and Marcin Mikulewicz
Effects of Surface Preparation Methods on the Color Stability of 3D-Printed Dental Restorations
Reprinted from: *J. Funct. Biomater.* **2023**, *14*, 257, doi:10.3390/jfb14050257 140

Anna Paradowska-Stolarz, Marcin Mikulewicz, Mieszko Wieckiewicz and Joanna Wezgowiec
The Influence of Polishing and Artificial Aging on BioMed Amber® Resin's Mechanical Properties
Reprinted from: *J. Funct. Biomater.* **2023**, *14*, 254, doi:10.3390/jfb14050254 . . . . **154**

Ruth Betsabe Zamudio-Ceja, Rene Garcia-Contreras, Patricia Alejandra Chavez-Granados, Benjamin Aranda-Herrera, Hugo Alvarado-Garnica, Carlos A. Jurado, et al.
Decellularized Scaffolds of Nopal (*Opuntia Ficus-indica*) for Bioengineering in Regenerative Dentistry
Reprinted from: *J. Funct. Biomater.* **2023**, *14*, 252, doi:10.3390/ jfb14050252 . . . . **165**

Busra Kumrular, Orhan Cicek, İlker Emin Dağ, Baris Avar and Hande Erener
Evaluation of the Corrosion Resistance of Different Types of Orthodontic Fixed Retention Appliances: A Preliminary Laboratory Study
Reprinted from: *J. Funct. Biomater.* **2023**, *14*, 81, doi:10.3390/jfb14020081 . . . . **177**

Marco Roy, Alessandro Corti, Barbara Dorocka-Bobkowska and Alfonso Pompella
Positive Effects of UV-Photofunctionalization of Titanium Oxide Surfaces on the Survival and Differentiation of Osteogenic Precursor Cells—An In Vitro Study
Reprinted from: *J. Funct. Biomater.* **2022**, *13*, 265, doi:10.3390/ jfb13040265 . . . . **192**

About the Editors

Lavinia Cosmina Ardelean

Professor Lavinia Cosmina Ardelean, DMD, PhD, is a professor and head of the Department of Technology of Materials and Devices in Dental Medicine, "Victor Babes" University of Medicine and Pharmacy, Timisoara, Romania. She has authored/co-authored 19 books, 15 book chapters, and over 120 peer-reviewed papers. With a current H-index of 13, she is an Editorial Board Member and a member of the reviewer/topic boards of multiple journals, including *Scientific Reports*, *Materials*, *Prosthesis*, *Metals*, *Coatings*, *Polymers*, and the *Journal of Functional Biomaterials*. She has guest-edited ten Special Issues in different journals and six books. Being an active reviewer, with more than 270 reviews to her credit so far, she was awarded with the Top Reviewers in Cross-Field Award 2019 and the Top Reviewers in Materials Science Award 2019. She currently holds two patents. Her research interest includes most areas of dentistry, with a focus on dental materials/biomaterials, dental alloys, resins, ceramics/bioceramics, CAD/CAM milling, 3D printing/bioprinting in dentistry, welding, scanning, prosthodontics, and oral healthcare.

Laura-Cristina Rusu

Professor Laura Cristina Rusu, DMD, PhD, is a professor and head of the Oral Pathology Department, Faculty of Dental Medicine, "Victor Babes" University of Medicine and Pharmacy, Timisoara, Romania. Her PhD thesis was centered on allergens in dental materials. In 2017, she obtained a Dr. Habil and was confirmed as a PhD coordinator in the field of dental medicine. She took part in 11 research projects, including FP7 COST Action MP 1005, and authored over 140 peer-reviewed papers. She has published 10 books and book chapters as an author and co-author. She has guest-edited seven Special Issues in different journals and edited or co-edited six books. She currently holds three patents. With a current H-index of 15, she is a member of the Editorial Board of the *Journal of Science and Arts* and *Medicine in Evolution* and a topic editor for the journal *Materials*. Her main scientific interests are oral pathology and oral diagnosis in dental medicine, focusing on oral cancer.

Preface

"Advanced Biomaterials and Biotechnology: Applications in Dental Medicine" is a reprint of the Special Issue in the *Journal of Functional Biomaterials*, and consists of 13 articles, providing an updated outlook on the applications of advanced biomaterials and biotechnologies in dentistry and addresses to scholars and researchers in the field.

Biotechnology aims at the application of biological knowledge and techniques to enhance human health. From a healthcare perspective, a biomaterial is defined as a natural or synthetic material that can be placed into living tissues without developing an immune reaction.

Biomaterials and biotechnology applications in dentistry are currently on an upward trend and are leading dental research. As dentistry implies rehabilitation of damaged tissues and function restoration, tissue engineering applications in dentistry have advanced over the last few years in order to recreate functional, healthy tissues and thus replace diseased ones. Dental biomaterials play an important role in the reconstruction of damaged oral hard and soft tissues, encompassing the fields of periodontology, endodontics, oral surgery, implantology, and ultimately attempting the replacement of the whole tooth organ. Biomaterials have evolved from simply replacing the damaged tissue to allowing the 3D development of a structurally complex regenerated tissue. The development of biotechnology applications in dentistry has achieved its goal regarding the implementation of biomaterials in order to replace oral tissue, including various novel approaches such as biomimetics and nano-biotechnology.

The Guest Editors would like to thank all contributing authors for the success of this Special Issue. This Special Issue would not have been of such quality without the constructive criticism of the reviewers.

We also extend our sincere appreciation to the MDPI Section Managing Editor.

Lavinia Cosmina Ardelean and Laura-Cristina Rusu
Editors

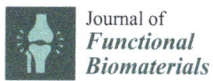

Article

Dental Implant Abutment Screw Loss: Presentation of 10 Cases

Maryam Soleimani [1,2], Jarosław Żmudzki [1,*], Wojciech Pakieła [1], Anna Jaśkowska [3] and Kornel Krasny [3]

[1] Department of Engineering Materials and Biomaterials, Faculty of Mechanical Engineering, Silesian University of Technology, 18a Konarskiego Str., 41-100 Gliwice, Poland; maryam.soleimani@polsl.pl (M.S.); wojciech.pakiela@polsl.pl (W.P.)

[2] Doctoral School, Silesian University of Technology, 2A Akademicka Str., 44-100 Gliwice, Poland

[3] Anident Dental Clinic, 12 Belgradzka Str., 02-793 Warszawa, Poland; poczta@anident.pl (A.J.); kornel.krasny@op.pl (K.K.)

* Correspondence: jaroslaw.zmudzki@polsl.pl

Abstract: Re-tightening the loosened dental implant abutment screw is an accepted procedure, however the evidence that such screw will hold sufficiently is weak. The purpose of this study was material analysis of lost dental implant abutment screws made of the TiAlV alloy from various manufacturers, which became lost due to unscrewing or damaged when checking if unscrewed; undamaged screws could be safely re-tightened. Among 13 failed screws retrieved from 10 cases, 10 screws were removed due to untightening and 3 were broken but without mechanical damage at the threads. Advanced corrosion was found on nine screws after 2 years of working time on all surfaces, also not mechanically loaded. Sediments observed especially in the thread area did not affect the corrosion process because of no pit densification around sediments. Pitting corrosion visible in all long-used screws raises the question of whether the screws should be replaced after a certain period during service, even if they are well-tightened. This requires further research on the influence of the degree of corrosion on the loss of the load-bearing ability of the screw.

Keywords: dental implant abutment screw; titanium alloy; titanium nitride coating; failure; fracture; loosening; unscrewing; pitting corrosion

1. Introduction

In dental implants, various types of failures may occur at the implant–abutment connection [1,2]. The abutment and screw are mainly made with titanium-vanadium-aluminum alloy (Ti6Al4V). There are many studies on load transfer onto abutment and implant–abutment connection, and the abutment screw itself between the head and screw thread [3–5]. Tests of contact stresses between the abutment and the implant reveal fretting and wear phenomena of the less harder pure titanium implant surface, but also tribochemical processes in the alloy [6–8].

Pitting corrosion is suggested to be the mechanism of the alloy degradation [9]. However, there is weak clinical study evidence for this, especially in the case of abutment screws which are not in direct contact with tissues and the oral environment. Available literature shows that re-tightening the mounting screw is an accepted procedure [10]. Routine screw replacement is not recommended, but routine screw-tightening assessment is recommended to minimize more serious complications. It seems reasonable to ask whether the unscrewed abutment screw is still a valid screw and can be reused to mount a prosthetic work.

The aim of this work was a material analysis of dental implant abutment screws made of the TiAlV alloy from various manufacturers which became lost due to unscrewing or damage.

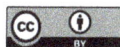

2. Materials

2.1. Clinical Study

On average, 300 implants are implanted annually at the ANIDENT Dental Clinic, and 645 implants were inspected from the period between 1 January 2023 and 1 June 2023. These were cases of our own and external patients. Among them, there were 45 loosened screws, including 7 broken ones. Among the 45 screws removed, 36 were single crowns and 9 were screws in prosthetic bridges (implants connected by a superstructure). Only 3 screws were from the anterior segment, but all of them were connected by a bridge to the posterior teeth, and 42 screws were from posterior crowns. Patients reported feeling the mobility of a single or multi-point denture. Patients who presented with a loose crown reported biting, for example, an eggshell, nut, bone, or salt crystal. They claimed that they felt this event, but without any consequences, and only after a few weeks did they notice the crown loosening. Interestingly, they claimed that they felt the loosening on soft foods such as a roll. In cases where the screws broke, it was easy to unscrew them. In other cases, the loose screws were removed also without any problems, disinfected, and sent for material assessment. A total of 13 screws from 10 cases (CsNo) were selected as representative for material investigation. Table 1 shows the characteristics of these clinical cases.

Table 1. Implant identification.

Case No.	Implant Side Anterior/Lateral	Denture Type	Implant Type/Abutment Dimensions and Manufacturer	Case Description
1	lateral	single crown 46	IRES 4.1 mm × 8 mm	The tested screw was used to attach a single crown in the lateral section 46 (mandibular first molar, right side) to an implant with a diameter of 4.1 × length of 8 mm. The implant was implanted in 2018, the crown was made in 2019, and the screw worked for four years. The patient did not come for regular check-ups and only came to the emergency room due to loosening of the crown.
2	anterior + lateral	bridge 6 pts. 21–26	ZIMMER 3.7 mm × 13 mm ZIMMER 4.1 mm × 11.5 mm ZIMMER 4.1 mm × 10 mm ZIMMER 4.1 mm × 10 mm	The four screws tested attached a six-point bridge to implants in sections 21–26 (front and lateral sections of the maxilla, left side). Implant in the incisor area with a diameter of 3.7 mm and a length of 13 mm, implant in the canine area with a diameter of 4.1 mm and a length of 11.5 mm, in the area of the first premolar with a diameter of 4.1 mm and a length of 10 mm, and last implant in the area of the molar tooth with a diameter 4 and 10 mm long. Implant placement in 2016. The prosthetic work was installed in 2020, the screws lasted for three years. The patient did not come for regular check-ups and started treatment in another office, which resulted in overloading the bridge on implants 21–26 and breaking two of the four implant-fixing screws in the premolar and molar area.
3	lateral	bridge 3 pts. 15–17	ZIMMER 3.7 mm × 11.5 mm ZIMMER 4.7 mm × 8 mm	The loosened screw came from a 3-point bridge based on two implants in the lateral part of the maxilla, right side 15–17. Implants in the area of the first premolar (14) with a diameter of 3.7 mm and a length of 11.5 mm (implanted in 2017) and the second one in the area of the first molar of the maxilla, right side (16) with a diameter of 4.7 mm and a length of 8 mm (implanted in 2018). The bridge was constructed in 2021, the screw operated for two years. The patient came for follow-up visits and the screw was tightened once.
4	lateral	single crown 14	ZIMMER 4.1 mm × 10 mm	The tested screw attached a single crown placed on the right side of the maxillary first premolar (14), lateral section. Implant with a diameter of 4.1 mm and a length of 10 mm. It was implanted in 2014. The prosthetic work was installed in 2015. The screw functioned for eight years. The patient did not attend regular follow-up visits. The screw did not come loose before.

Table 1. Cont.

Case No.	Implant Side Anterior/Lateral	Denture Type	Implant Type/Abutment Dimensions and Manufacturer	Case Description
5	lateral	single crown 37	ZIMMER 3.7 mm × 8 mm	The screw comes from a single crown on an implant placed near the second molar of the mandible on the left side (37), lateral section. The 3.7 mm diameter and 8 mm long implant was placed in 2015, and the single crown was placed in 2016. The screw lasted for six years. The patient came for follow-up visits sporadically and irregularly, and the screw was tightened twice.
6	lateral	single crown 36	ZIMMER 3.7 mm × 10 mm	The screw comes from a single crown on an implant placed near the first molar of the mandible, left side (36), lateral section. An implant with a diameter of 3.7 mm and a length of 10 mm was implanted in 2015. A single crown on the implant was placed in 2016. The screw functioned for six years. The patient came for follow-up visits sporadically, irregularly. The screw was tightened once.
7	lateral	bridge 3 pts. 44–46	IRES 3.75 mm × 11.5 mm IRES 3.75 mm × 10 mm	The screw tested comes from a 3-point bridge in the lateral section 44–46 mounted on two implants. Implants in the area of the mandibular first premolar (44) with a diameter of 3.75 mm and a length of 11.5 mm. And the second one in the area of the first molar of the mandible, right side (46), with a diameter of 3.75 and a length of 10 mm were implanted in 2018. The prosthetic work was installed in 2019. The tested screw functioned for four years. The patient did not come for regular check-ups, and the screws did not loosen earlier. The examination revealed, in addition to the loose screw, a fracture of the implant 46.
8	lateral	single crown 24	IRES 4.1 mm × 11.5 mm	The tested screw was used to attach a single crown to the implant in the area of the maxillary first premolar, left side (24), lateral section. Implant with a diameter of 4.1 mm and a length of 11.5 mm was implanted in 2019. The crown was installed in 2021. The screw worked for two years. The patient came for follow-up visits and the screw was tightened once.
9	lateral	single crown 46	IDI 3.7 mm × 12 mm	The broken screw attached a single crown to the implant in the area of the first mandibular premolar, right side (46) in the lateral section. Implant with a diameter of 3.7 mm and a length of 12 mm was implanted in 2009. The screw worked for one year. The patient did not come for follow-up visits.
10	lateral	single crown 36	ZIMMER 4.1 mm × 10 mm	Patient 10. The broken screw attached a single crown to the implant in the area of the first molar of the mandible, left side (36), lateral section. Implant with a diameter of 4.1 mm and a length of 10 mm was implanted in 2020. The crown was attached in 2020. The screw lasted three years and was tightened twice. The patient did not attend regular follow-up visits.

2.2. SEM

Analysis of the implant screw surfaces were made using a Supra 35 scanning electron microscope from Zeiss (Jena, Germany). Observations were made in both SE and InLens modes. The analysis of the chemical composition in micro-areas and the element distribution maps were performed using an EDS scattered X-ray detector from Thermo Fisher Scientific (Waltham, MA, USA) at an accelerating voltage in the range from 10 to 20 keV and the required work distance of 14 mm.

2.3. Light Microscopy

A digital microscope (Leica DVM6 A, Wetzlar, Germany) with image sensor 1/2.3″ CMOS 3664 × 2748 pixel and LED light source software-controlled was used. Images with resolution from 2MP (1600 × 1200) to 10MP (3648 × 2736) were snaped with LAS X software 5.0.3. Automated motorized focus drive allows 3D imaging with resolution of

0.25 µm in vertical direction. Screws were investigated with two lenses (PlanAPO FOV 43.75, working distance: 60 mm, max. magnification: 190:1, max. resolution: 415 lp/mm; PlanAPO FOV 12.55, working distance: 33 mm, max. magnification: 675:1, max. resolution: 1073 lp/mm)

Metallographic examinations of the specimens were performed on the implant using 2 broken screws, CsNo2 and CsNo10, using a light microscope (Zeiss Axio VertA1 MET Brightfield/Darkfield Metallurgical Microscope, Oberkochen, Germany). Cross-sections were standardly ground, polished, and etched with Kroll's reagent (Sigma Aldrich, Darmstadt, Germany). Grinding and pit searching were repeated, and the deepest pits were documented.

2.4. Surface Roughness

The roughness measurement was made with using mechanical contact profilometer (Taylor Hobson, Leicester, United Kingdom) on the shank along the screw axis. Due to the impossibility of measuring perfectly on the axis, the curvature of the cylinder was superimposed on the roughness measurement.

3. Results

3.1. Clinical Observations

Figure 1 shows an example of a broken screw, while Figure 2 shows X-ray exemplary images of the failures. The case histories were known and the duration of screw use is given in Table 2.

The analysis showed that single crowns were more likely to unscrew than those connected in prosthetic bridges. This seems logical, as when biting, there will be an additional rotational force on the chewing surface of the tooth. So far, we have not observed any unscrewing of the crown or bridge installed in the anterior section. The problem most often concerned the posterior section—the molar area. Screws regardless of diameter became loose. The sets we use included implants with a diameter of 2.7 mm—used only in the anterior section due to very narrow ridges and small interdental space—we have not observed any breakage or unscrewing of them. All other available diameters, i.e., 3.7, 4.1, and 4.7 were loosened or broken in the side sections. The doctor performing the procedure has no influence on the type, shape, or method of screwing/stabilizing the prosthetic superstructure. All these features depend on the implant socket, the shape of the hex, the depth of the hex, the type of screw stabilizing the superstructure, and the shape, depth, and type of hex of the prosthetic superstructure/connector. All these elements are specified and prepared by the implant manufacturer and were the same in all these cases.

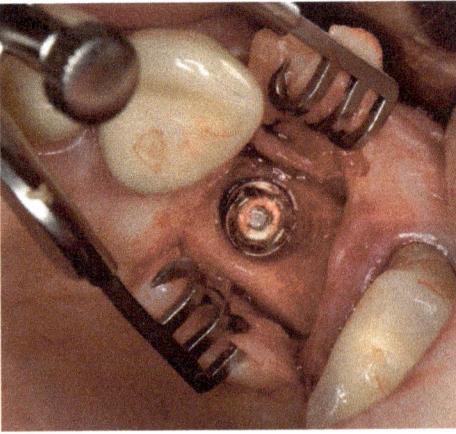

Figure 1. Service of broken screw exemplary case.

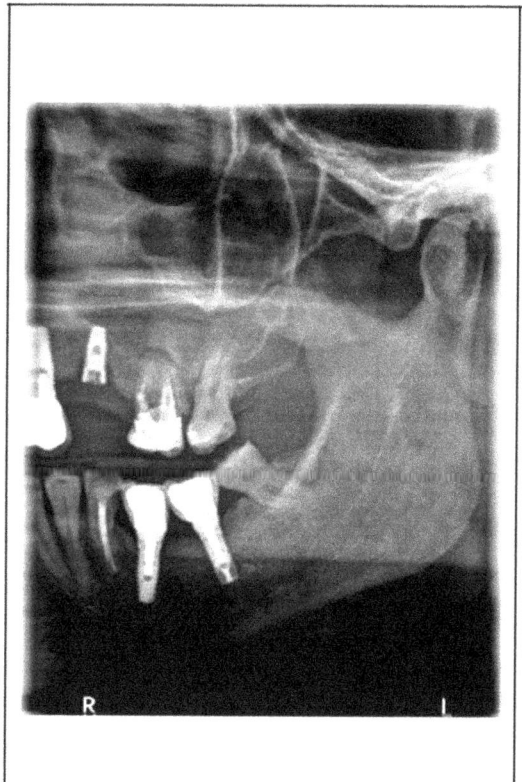 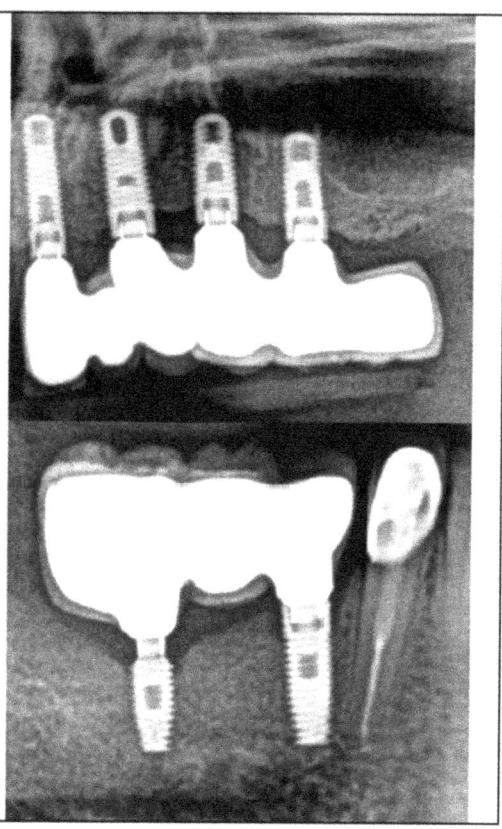

Figure 2. X-ray exemplary imaging of the screw failures: left X-ray, loose/broken screw in the upper left premolar CsNo8; upper-right X-ray, broken screws in implants 21 and 23 and loosened screws in implants 24 and 25 CsNo2; lower-right X-ray, broken hex in implant 46, both screws in 44 and 46 were loose in CSNo7.

Table 2. Results of retrieved abutment screw investigation.

Case No.	Clinical Inspection	Optical/SEM Inspection	Lifetime Years
1	1 screws loosening	extremely numerous deep pits	4
2	2 fractured screws 2 screws loosening	extremely numerous deep pits	3
3	1 screws loosening	less numerous deep pits	2
4	1 screws loosening	numerous deep pits brownish sediment	8
5	1 screws loosening	numerous deep pits	7
6	1 screws loosening	moderately numerous deep pits	7
7	1 screws loosening	numerous deep pits white sediment	4
8	1 screws loosening	crack on the shank below head extremely numerous deep pits	2
9	1 fractured screw	few initial shallow pits difficult to see	1
10	1 fractured screw	numerous deep pits	3

3.2. Material Analysis

Light microscopy revealed pitting corrosion in all screws, although in the one that had been in use for 1 year, initial pits were few and difficult to find. Figures 3 and 4 show sample selected images for the cases: CsNo1, CsNo2, CsNo4, CsNo8. Pits were revealed on all surfaces and were not concentrated on the thread or screw head contact surfaces. There was also no density of pits around the sediments. No signs of wear or tribo-corrosion were revealed on the threads and screw heads. The threads showed no signs of plastic deformation, and the traces of mechanical machining were intact. Minor scratches and mechanical damage that were clearly caused by screwing and removing screws were not considered. Screw CsNo8 with a gold-colored titanium nitride coating (TiNc) was corroded after 2 years to at least the same extent as screws with a standard oxide coating that lasted in the oral cavity much longer. A screw with TiN coating had an extensive crack (but not a fracture) on the shank in the stress concentration area around the notch under the head.

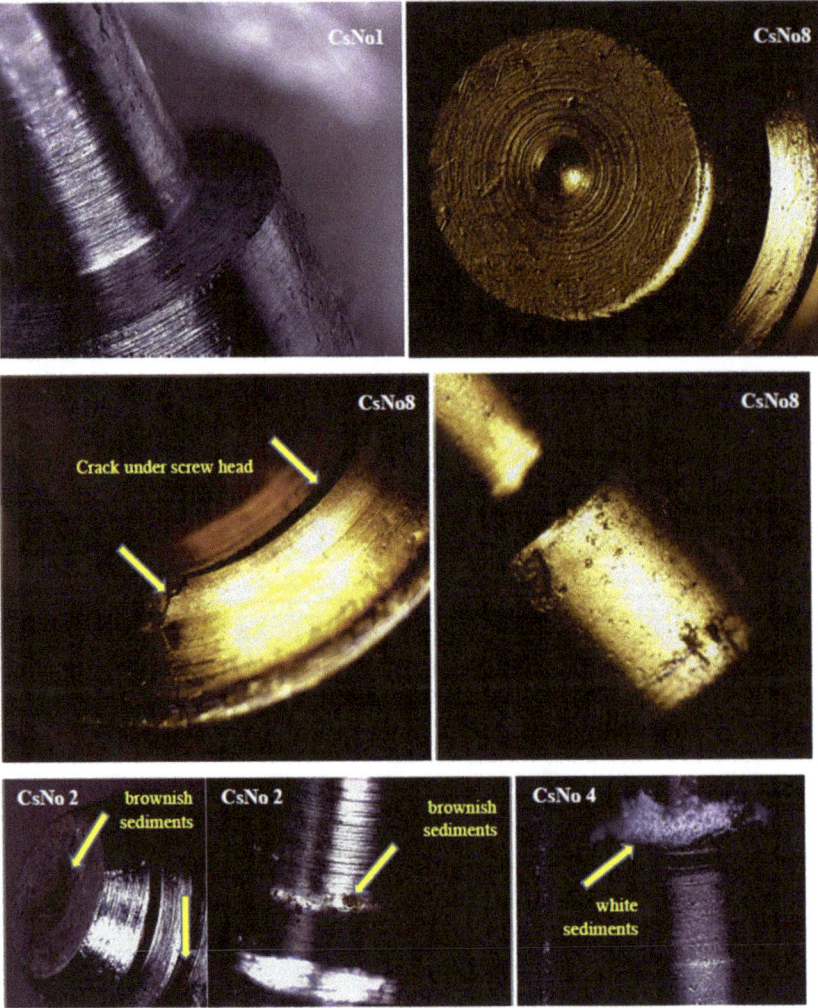

Figure 3. Pitting corrosion, crack on the shank below screw head, and brownish/white sediments shown in order: CsNo1, CsNo8 (TiNc), CsNo2, CsNo4.

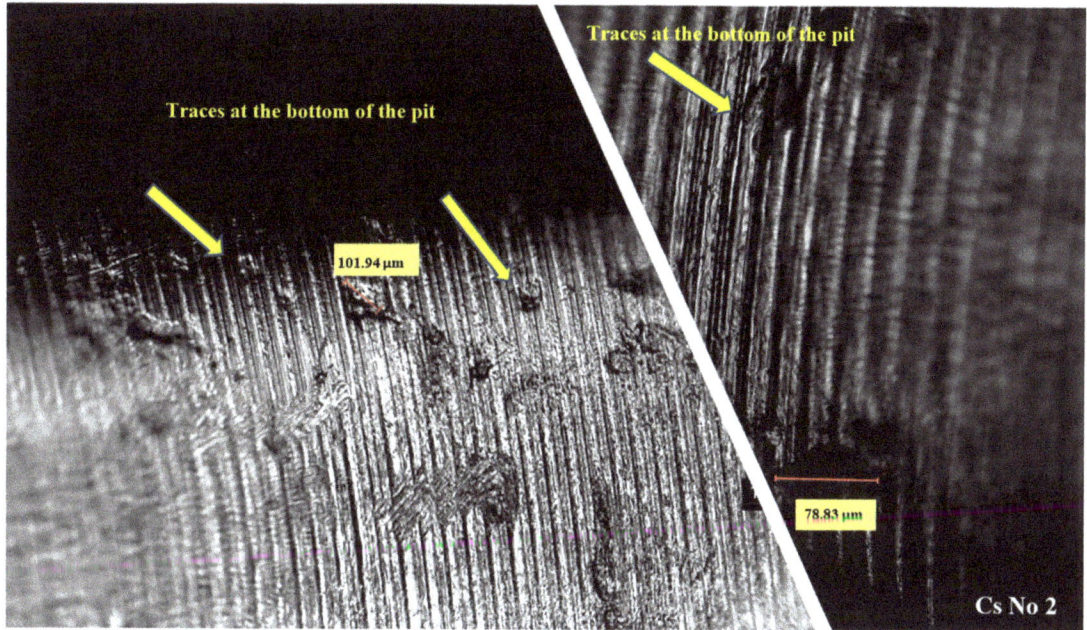

Figure 4. Pits on the shank of CsNo2 implant abutment screw and visible traces at the bottom of the pit.

The selected screws for cross-sectional study had the most pits that appeared to be the deepest, however, repeated grinding and cross-sectional study allowed us to find the deepest pits as shown in Figure 5. In thread root, an example was found at the beginning of the dissolution of tips remaining after machining. The Figure 6 profile shows the roughness for the CsNo2 implant screw with visible uniform machining traces. Sediment heights were revealed, which are difficult to measure reliably on a microscope. An example of wide pitting corrosion was shown along with its depth, which turned out to be relatively shallow, as the depth relative to the adjacent tip only exceeded 2 microns. Due to the surprisingly shallow dimensions of the pits, we additionally looked at them under a microscope and, in fact, most of them were visible at the bottom of the remains of the machining grooves. The 3D measurement on the microscope also did not exceed a few microns, but due to the lower quantitative reliability of this technique, we chose a contact profilometer for presentation.

The fractures in the broken screws in case CsNo2 as shown in Figure 7 were kneaded, which proves that still compression loads were transferred on the two remaining unbroken screws in the denture supported on 4 implants. At one of the fractures were visible sediments grouped along a line that appears to be a fatigue fracture. Fracture type was hard to estimate due to the destroyed fracture surface during kneading. Primarily, plastically deformed zones during fracture were mixed with those plastically destroyed during kneading, and the zone of fatigue initiation was not distinct. Numerous cracks were also visible in the areas of plastic rupture and ran parallel to the lines of the sediment cluster. The front of the fracture was indicated only on the basis of general shape and clear direction of cracks.

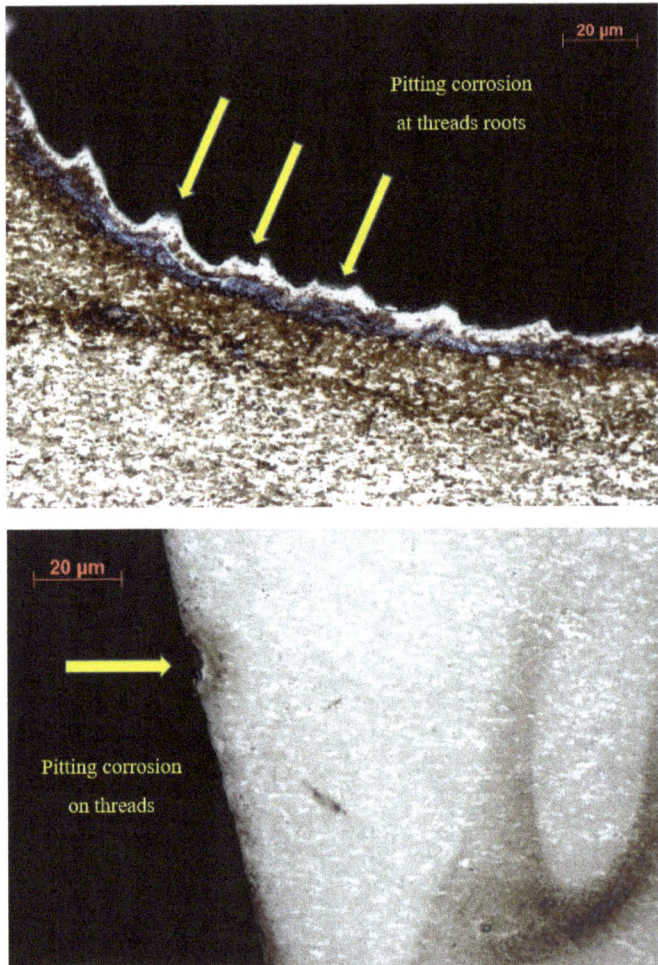

Figure 5. Examples of the deepest pitting corrosion found on the thread and the beginnings of dissolution of machining tips at thread root in cross-sectional micrographs of a CsNo2 implant screw.

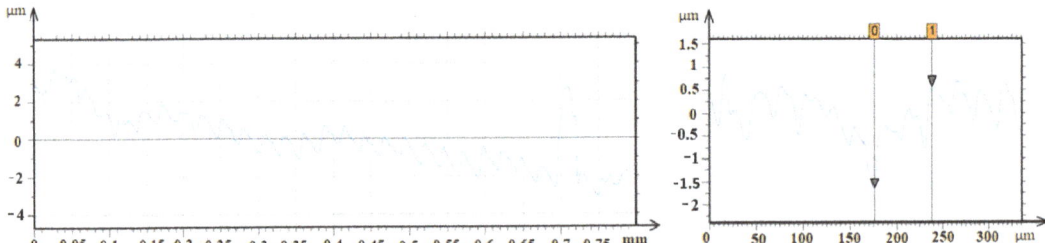

Figure 6. Roughness profile for implant screw CsNo2 with visible uniform traces of machining and clear dimensions of deposits, and an example of wide pitting corrosion with its depth. Region between 0 and 1 related to bottom and the edge of the pits respectively.

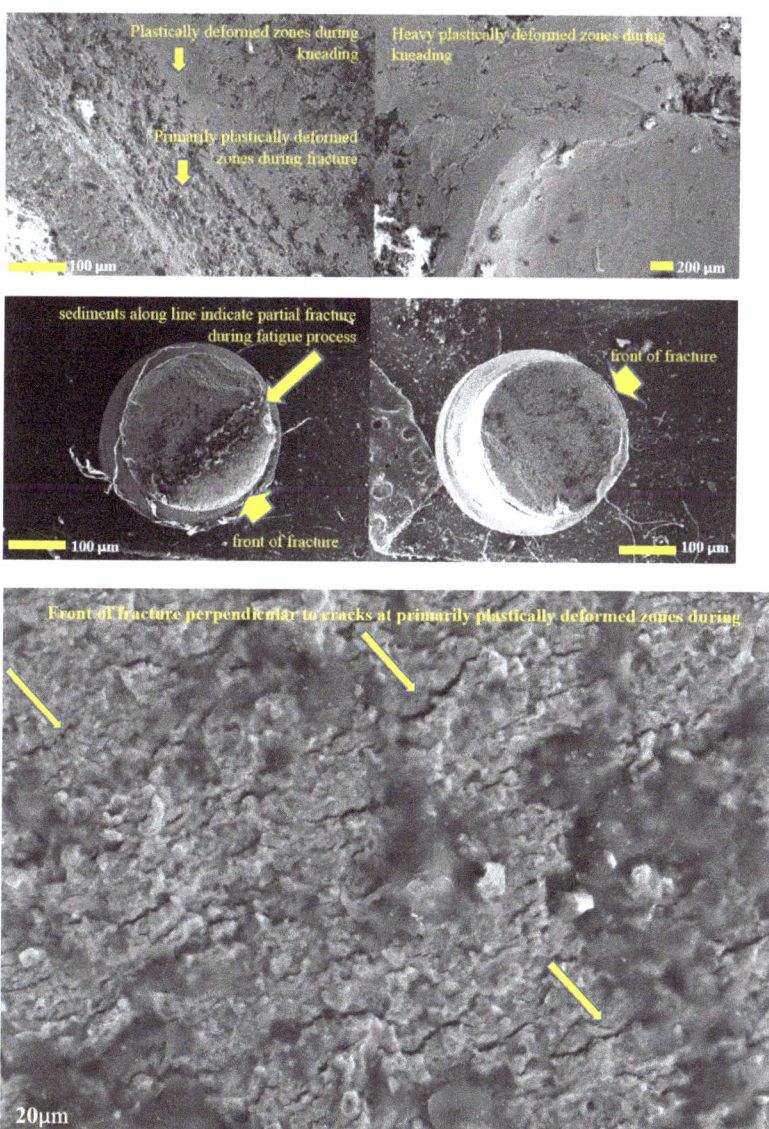

Figure 7. Fractures in the two broken screws among four implants which supported denture in case CsNo2.

The SEM EDS analysis of sediments presented in Figure 8 in places of signal, where different elements overlapped, were those that were least likely to be arbitrarily eliminated. Analysis showed that a brownish sediment mainly contained elements from food or toothpastes. The white sediment was rich in zinc.

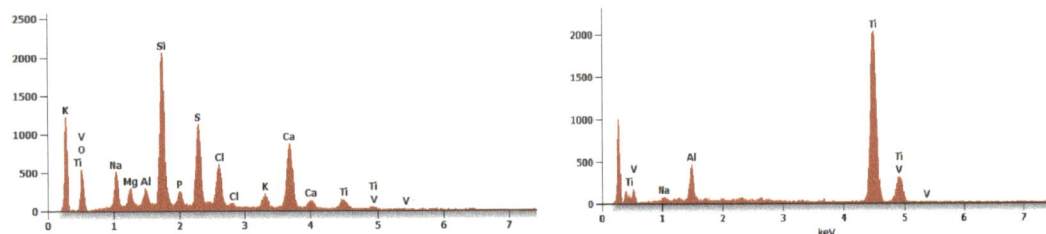

Figure 8. SEM EDS of brownish and white sediments.

Figure 9 shows an EDS map for a TiNc screw around a corrosion pit. The distribution of nitrogen shows its loss inside the pit, while more oxygen appears, which comes from the spontaneously formed titanium oxide. The exposure of the alloy substrate resulted in the appearance of a strong aluminum and vanadium signal, as well as a significant increase in the titanium signal.

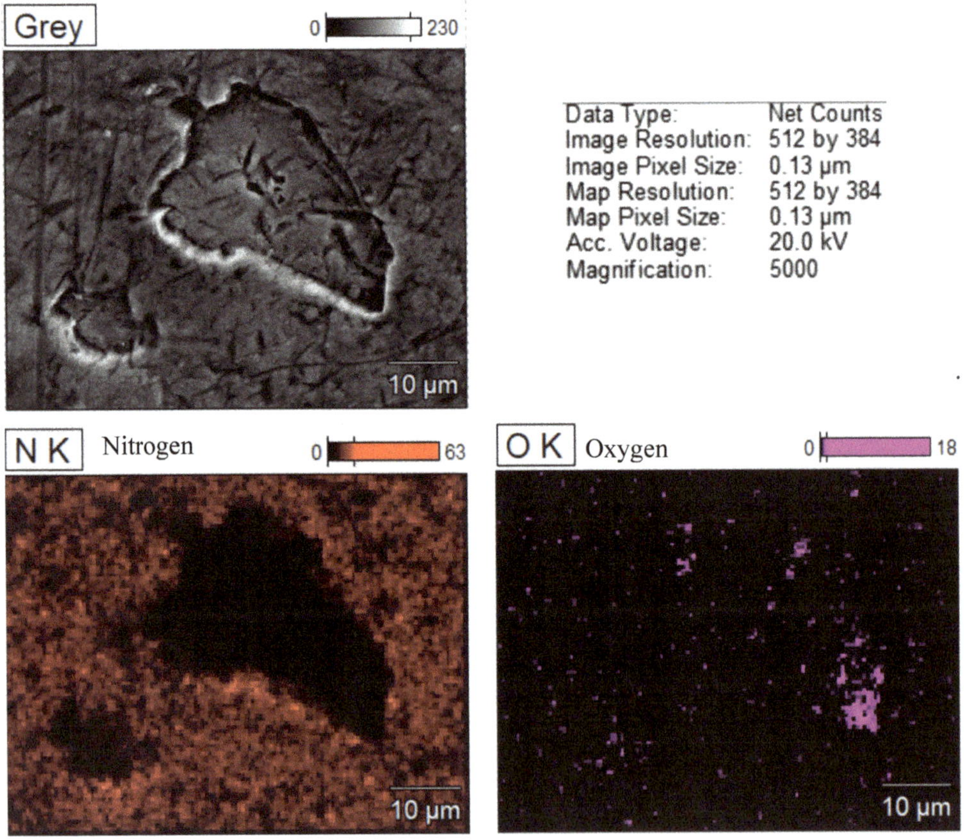

Figure 9. *Cont.*

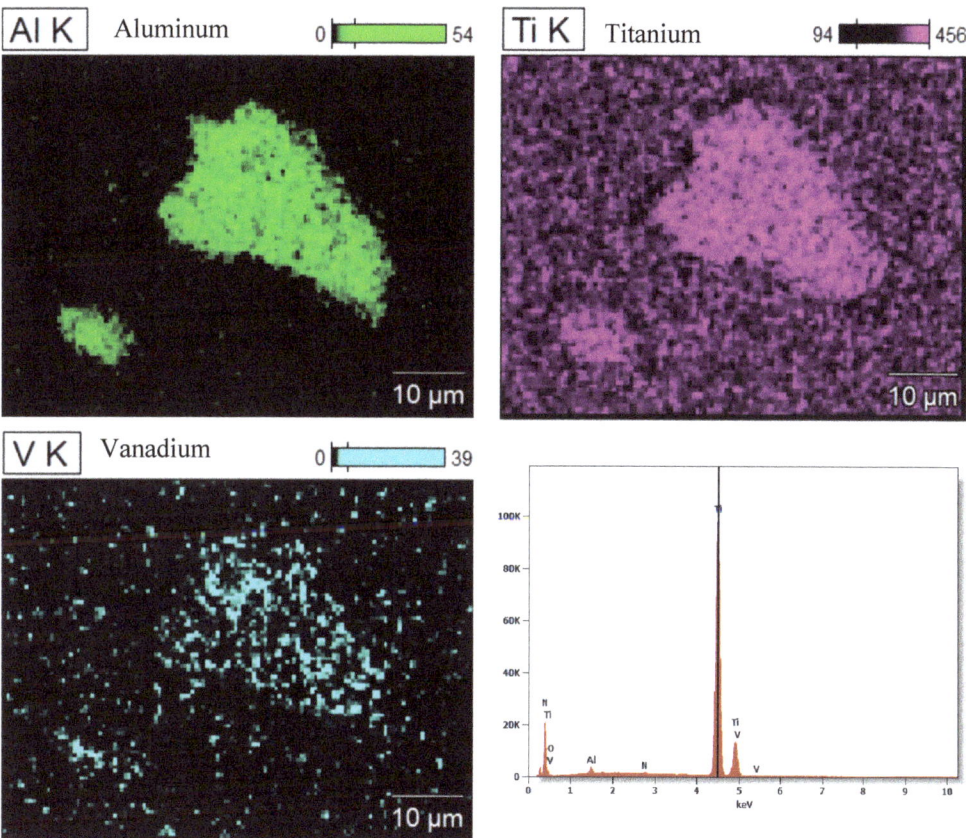

Figure 9. SEM EDS map around a corrosion pit on the CsNo8 implant screw with TiN coating.

4. Discussion

The analysis showed that among inspected implants all types of crowns are subject to unscrewing regardless of the implant diameter (3.7, 4.1, and 4.7 mm), implant abutment diameter, and used abutment screw. Analysis led to the conclusion that the implantation area (usually the lateral/distal section) had a greater impact on crown unscrewing rather than the implant diameter.

In threaded connections, failure under cyclic loading is often caused by screw loosening and loss of preload due to micro-movements on the contacting thread surfaces. Especially with simultaneous activation of corrosion processes, micro-damages, fretting and wear, and plastic deformations of the thread will appear in heavily loaded areas, which result in the loss of preload. Among ten failed screws, seven screws were removed due to untightening and three were broken albeit without mechanical damage at the threads. Advanced corrosion was found on nine screws after 2 years of working time on all surfaces, also not mechanically loaded. A long crack on the one non-fractured screw was found located close to the notch on the shank under the screw head. Among three fractured screws, there was the one with the shortest working time of 1 year and there were difficulties in seeing a few initial shallow corrosion pits. The summary of our finding is that the existence of mechanical deformations or micro-damages on the threads has not been confirmed.

The outcome observed in the in vivo result was unexpected, particularly because we anticipated the mechanical effects identified in in-vitro studies which were suggested as the mechanism for the decrease in screw preload and unscrewing [8,9,11–13]. However, our results were consistent with those showing pitting corrosion in this titanium alloy. In the work [9], on the basis of X-ray spectroscopy (EDS) of the Ti6Al4V implant removed from the patient due to inflammation, after one year it showed that the titanium and vanadium decreased on the surface and the content of aluminum slightly increased. The study is based on one implant and it is not known how it can be personally dependent. In the work, the initiation of micro cracks and the destruction of the implant under the influence of mechanical loads are suggested, however, there is no confirmation of the hypothesis.

In the work [14], pitting attacks were observed in the five clinically retrieved implants, albeit pits, located mostly in the abutment surfaces over the implant edge. A crack nucleating inside a pit about 20 μm in size is documented. The implant bone interface discoloration is justified with oxidation of unprotected bulk titanium to the violet-colored trivalent ions (Ti 3+) and also in SEM/EDS analysis metal ion dissolution with depletion of the Ti oxide film. In the work, it is suggested that degradation is the combining effect of corrosion and mechanical loadings, because scratches, fretting, cracks, and surface delamination are observed. The discovery of pitting on many screws in mechanically weakly loaded and free from interfacial compression areas in our study shows that corrosion progresses inside the implant directly under the influence of the oral environment without contact with tissues or other materials. The screws came from different manufacturers, which allows us to conclude that this is not a material defect caused by the technological process of the selected manufacturer. We cannot confirm that the sediment was rich in elements of screw alloy. The signal from substrate metals may be an artifact and a thorough examination of the composition of the sediment requires its removal from the surface and examination separately from the substrate. We were able to evaluate signals from elements that are not present on the alloy substrate. The brownish sediment gave a signal of many elements that are commonly found in foods or toothpaste, while the white sediment gave a Zn-rich signal.

Corrosion of Ti6Al4V hip joint implants can occur in a tissue environment isolated from external factors present in the oral cavity [13]. However, some in vitro investigations [15–18] indicate that factors of the oral cavity may influence corrosion. Our observations lack a concentration of pits around the deposits, but this does not prove that there is no acceleration of corrosion by oral environmental factors that are found in saliva or biofilm.

Measurements of the depth of the pits showed that they are very shallow and do not reach such depths as in in vitro tests. Our results also differ from the in vivo results of work [17] in which depth is assessed based on microscopic images from three hip implants. Based on our surface images, we were convinced of the great depth of the pits, but neither profilometer measurements nor cross-sectional imaging showed a depth greater than several microns. However, our samples were not exposed to friction, as in works [13,17], and did not show wear, cracks, or mechanical damages, which lead to failures in the oxide layer and a different mechanism of pitting corrosion. These depths were slightly greater than the roughness after the machining process, so their influence as a notch on fatigue strength seems to be very limited, although it cannot be ruled out, especially in the context of hydrogen corrosion demonstrated in the work [13], which we were unable to investigate due to our hardware limitations. However, in vivo pitting corrosion depth results indicate that in vitro corrosion simulation conditions may differ significantly from actual conditions for surfaces exposed only to corrosion without mechanical loads.

The limitation of the study was three manufacturers, and among the cases we had only one screw coated with TiN. The time-consuming statistical analysis of the number and dimensions of pits was abandoned, although determining the relationship between the growth of pits and the material working period may be useful in comparative studies between variable materials in the future.

Our cases were limited to one similar design of implant–abutment connection. Incidence of screw loosening is related to many factors albeit among them only several factors depend on system design. Initial torque and clamped force loss are affected by torque magnitude, screw diameter, head and thread design, and implant–abutment connection design [17]. The compressive force that shortens the shank of a screw when it is greater than the preload in the shank can activate unscrewing. Hence, theoretically, the more flexible implant–abutment connection promotes screw loosening. The phenomena become complicated and compliance is not a clear determinant due to bending. On the tension side, the compliance prevents shortening of the screw. However, at the same time, the additional tension of the preloaded screw may cause it to break. In practice, screw loosening is a common mechanical complication with an incidence of 4.3–10% during the first year [17,18] and 12.7% in single crowns and 6.7% in fixed partial dentures [17]. In vitro, an overloading study suggests that the internal and external connection systems could not prevent screw loosening [19]. In the in vitro studies, on the basis of reverse torque value, this shows that the ITI system is the most stable and resistant to screw loosening compared to others [20,21]. In turn, according to work [22], one-piece abutments are more resistant to screw loosening than the two-piece. The use of compatible components with original implants showed significant micromovements when compared with the use of the same manufacturer part [23]. Other works present opposite results in that the non-original components are interchangeable and do not lead to screw loosening if manufacturing discrepancies are lower than 10 microns [5,24–26]. Manufacturers are not able to guarantee failure-free screws, so for each system, it is worth having proprietary tools for removing broken screws and, above all, using radiographic detection of the gap at the implant–abutment interface [27,28].

The limitation of these in vivo tests was the lack of an implant for testing, which, being softer with pure titanium, may be subject to wear and deformation, and we did not find any traces of this on the screws. Although ideal thread surfaces do not indicate such a scenario, it cannot be ruled out without testing the implants also at the implant–abutment interface, where wear leads to changes in the forces existing on the screw.

5. Conclusions

No clear signs of "fretting", wear, or tribo-corrosion were found at the screw head and thread contact interfaces. However, numerous corrosion pits were found in many areas, including those not subject to mechanical loadings. Sediments observed especially in the thread area did not affect the corrosion process because of no pit densification around sediments.

The pitting corrosion visible in all long-used screws raises the question of whether the screws should be replaced after a certain period during service, even if they are well tightened. This requires further research on the influence of the degree of corrosion in in vivo conditions on the loss of fatigue strength of the screw.

Author Contributions: Conceptualization, J.Ż., A.J. and K.K.; Methodology, J.Ż., W.P., A.J. and K.K.; Validation, M.S., A.J. and K.K.; Formal analysis, K.K.; Investigation, M.S., J.Ż., W.P., A.J. and K.K.; Data curation, M.S., W.P., A.J. and K.K.; Writing—original draft, J.Ż., A.J. and K.K.; Writing—review and editing, M.S. and J.Ż.; Visualization, W.P.; Supervision, K.K.; Project administration, A.J. and K.K.; Funding acquisition, A.J. All authors have read and agreed to the published version of the manuscript.

Funding: This research received no external funding.

Institutional Review Board Statement: Ethical review and approval were waived for this study due to the origin of the screws used for testing as they were waste from the implantological procedure.

Informed Consent Statement: Informed consent was obtained from all subjects involved in the study.

Data Availability Statement: The original contributions presented in the study are included in the article, further inquiries can be directed to the corresponding author.

Conflicts of Interest: The authors declare no conflicts of interest.

References

1. Lee, K.Y.; Shin, K.S.; Jung, J.H.; Cho, H.W.; Kwon, K.H.; Kim, Y.L. Clinical Study on Screw Loosening in Dental Implant Prostheses: A 6-Year Retrospective Study. *J. Korean Assoc. Oral Maxillofac. Surg.* **2020**, *46*, 133. [CrossRef] [PubMed]
2. Alsubaiy, E.F. Abutment Screw Loosening in Implants: A Literature Review. *J. Fam. Med. Prim. Care* **2020**, *9*, 5490. [CrossRef] [PubMed]
3. Tribst, J.P.M.; de Piva, A.M.O.D.; da Silva-Concílio, L.R.; Ausiello, P.; Kalman, L. Influence of Implant-Abutment Contact Surfaces and Prosthetic Screw Tightening on the Stress Concentration, Fatigue Life and Microgap Formation: A Finite Element Analysis. *Oral* **2021**, *1*, 88–101. [CrossRef]
4. Epifania, E.; di Lauro, A.E.; Ausiello, P.; Mancone, A.; Garcia-Godoy, F.; Tribst, J.P.M. Effect of Crown Stiffness and Prosthetic Screw Absence on the Stress Distribution in Implant-Supported Restoration: A 3D Finite Element Analysis. *PLoS ONE* **2023**, *18*, e0285421. [CrossRef] [PubMed]
5. Honório Tonin, B.S.; He, Y.; Ye, N.; Chew, H.P.; Fok, A. Effects of Tightening Torque on Screw Stress and Formation of Implant-Abutment Microgaps: A Finite Element Analysis. *J. Prosthet. Dent.* **2022**, *127*, 882–889. [CrossRef] [PubMed]
6. Kheder, W.; Al Kawas, S.; Khalaf, K.; Samsudin, A.R. Impact of Tribocorrosion and Titanium Particles Release on Dental Implant Complications—A Narrative Review. *Jpn. Dent. Sci. Rev.* **2021**, *57*, 182. [CrossRef] [PubMed]
7. Souza, J.C.M.; Henriques, M.; Teughels, W.; Ponthiaux, P.; Celis, J.P.; Rocha, L.A. Wear and Corrosion Interactions on Titanium in Oral Environment: Literature Review. *J. Bio-Tribo-Corros.* **2015**, *1*, 13. [CrossRef]
8. Corne, P.; De March, P.; Cleymand, F.; Geringer, J. Fretting-Corrosion Behavior on Dental Implant Connection in Human Saliva. *J. Mech. Behav. Biomed. Mater.* **2019**, *94*, 86–92. [CrossRef] [PubMed]
9. Tepla, T.; Pleshakov, E.; Sieniawski, J.; Bohun, L. Causes of Degradation of Titanium Dental Implants. *Ukr. J. Mech. Eng. Mater. Sci.* **2022**, *8*, 31–40. [CrossRef]
10. Revathi, A.; Borrás, A.D.; Muñoz, A.I.; Richard, C.; Manivasagam, G. Degradation Mechanisms and Future Challenges of Titanium and Its Alloys for Dental Implant Applications in Oral Environment. *Mater. Sci. Eng. C* **2017**, *76*, 1354–1368. [CrossRef]
11. Sun, F.; Cheng, W.; Zhao, B.H.; Song, G.Q.; Lin, Z. Evaluation the Loosening of Abutment Screws in Fluid Contamination: An in Vitro Study. *Sci. Rep.* **2022**, *12*, 10797. [CrossRef] [PubMed]
12. Gao, J.; Min, J.; Chen, X.; Yu, P.; Tan, X.; Zhang, Q.; Yu, H. Effects of Two Fretting Damage Modes on the Dental Implant–Abutment Interface and the Generation of Metal Wear Debris: An in Vitro Study. *Fatigue Fract. Eng. Mater. Struct.* **2021**, *44*, 847–858. [CrossRef]
13. Rodrigues, D.C.; Urban, R.M.; Jacobs, J.J.; Gilbert, J.L. In Vivo Severe Corrosion and Hydrogen Embrittlement of Retrieved Modular Body Titanium Alloy Hip-Implants. *J. Biomed. Mater. Res. B Appl. Biomater.* **2009**, *88*, 206–219. [CrossRef] [PubMed]
14. Chin, M.Y.H.; Sandham, A.; de Vries, J.; van der Mei, H.C.; Busscher, H.J. Biofilm Formation on Surface Characterized Micro-Implants for Skeletal Anchorage in Orthodontics. *Biomaterials* **2007**, *28*, 2032–2040. [CrossRef] [PubMed]
15. Ossowska, A.; Zieliński, A. The Mechanisms of Degradation of Titanium Dental Implants. *Coatings* **2020**, *10*, 836. [CrossRef]
16. Prestat, M.; Thierry, D. Corrosion of Titanium under Simulated Inflammation Conditions: Clinical Context and in Vitro Investigations. *Acta Biomater.* **2021**, *136*, 72–87. [CrossRef] [PubMed]
17. El-Sheikh, M.A.Y.; Mostafa, T.M.N.; El-Sheikh, M.M. Effect of Different Angulations and Collar Lengths of Conical Hybrid Implant Abutment on Screw Loosening after Dynamic Cyclic Loading. *Int. J. Implant Dent.* **2018**, *4*, 39. [CrossRef]
18. Fokas, G.; Ma, L.; Chronopoulos, V.; Janda, M.; Mattheos, N. Differences in Micromorphology of the Implant-Abutment Junction for Original and Third-Party Abutments on a Representative Dental Implant. *J. Prosthet. Dent.* **2019**, *121*, 143–150. [CrossRef]
19. Michalakis, K.X.; Lino, P.; Muftu, S.; Pissiotis, A.; Hirayama, H. The Effect of Different Implant-Abutment Connections on Screw Joint Stability. *J. Oral Implantol.* **2014**, *40*, 146–152. [CrossRef] [PubMed]
20. Cashman, P.M.; Schneider, R.L.; Schneider, G.B.; Stanford, C.M.; Clancy, J.M.; Qian, F. In Vitro Analysis of Post-Fatigue Reverse-Torque Values at the Dental Abutment/Implant Interface for a Unitarian Abutment Design. *J. Prosthodont.* **2011**, *20*, 503–509. [CrossRef] [PubMed]
21. Kim, E.S.; Shin, S.Y. Influence of the Implant Abutment Types and the Dynamic Loading on Initial Screw Loosening. *J. Adv. Prosthodont.* **2013**, *5*, 21–28. [CrossRef] [PubMed]
22. Ghanbarzadeh, J.; Dashti, H.; Abbasi, M.; Nakhaei, M. Torque Removal Evaluation of One-Piece and Two-Piece Abutment Screws under Dry and Wet Conditions. *J. Mashhad Dent. Sch.* **2015**, *39*, 89–98. [CrossRef]
23. Berberi, A.; Maroun, D.; Kanj, W.; Amine, E.Z.; Philippe, A. Micromovement Evaluation of Original and Compatible Abutments at the Implant-Abutment Interface. *J. Contemp. Dent. Pract.* **2016**, *17*, 907–913. [CrossRef] [PubMed]
24. Pournasiri, I.; Farid, F.; Zaker Jafari, H.; Simdar, N.; Maleki, D. Screw Loosening of Original and Non-Original Abutments in Implant Dentistry: An in Vitro Study. *J. Osseointegration* **2022**, *14*, 155–158. [CrossRef]
25. Alonso-Pérez, R.; Bartolomé, J.; Ferreiroa, A.; Salido, M.; Pradíes, G. Evaluation of the Mechanical Behavior and Marginal Accuracy of Stock and Laser-Sintered Implant Abutments. *Int. J. Prosthodont.* **2017**, *30*, 136–138. [CrossRef] [PubMed]
26. Solá-Ruíz, M.F.; Selva-Otaolaurruchi, E.; Senent-Vicente, G.; González-de-Cossio, I.; Amigó-Borrás, V. Accuracy Combining Different Brands of Implants and Abutments. *Med. Oral Patol. Oral Cir. Buccal* **2013**, *18*, e332. [CrossRef] [PubMed]

27. Cameron, S.M.; Joyce, A.; Brousseau, J.S.; Parker, M.H. Radiographic Verification of Implant Abutment Seating. *J. Prosthet. Dent.* **1998**, *79*, 298–303. [CrossRef] [PubMed]
28. de Oliveira Mota, V.P.; Braga, M.S.; Loss, A.A.; Mello, H.N.; Rosetti, E.P.; de-Azevedo-Vaz, S.L. Detection of Misfits at the Abutment-Prosthesis Interface in the Esthetic Zone: Implications of the Radiographic Technique and the Magnitude of the Misfit. *J. Prosthet. Dent.* **2023**, *130*, 239.e1–239.e9. [CrossRef] [PubMed]

Disclaimer/Publisher's Note: The statements, opinions and data contained in all publications are solely those of the individual author(s) and contributor(s) and not of MDPI and/or the editor(s). MDPI and/or the editor(s) disclaim responsibility for any injury to people or property resulting from any ideas, methods, instructions or products referred to in the content.

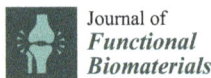

Article

Influence of Hybrid Surface Modification on Biocompatibility and Physicochemical Properties of Ti-6Al-4V ELI Titanium

Anna Woźniak [1,*], Weronika Smok [2], Janusz Szewczenko [3], Marcin Staszuk [2] and Grzegorz Chladek [1,*]

1. Materials Research Laboratory, Faculty of Mechanical Engineering, Silesian University of Technology, Konarskiego 18A Street, 44-100 Gliwice, Poland
2. Department of Engineering Materials and Biomaterials, Silesian University of Technology, Konarskiego 18A Street, 44-100 Gliwice, Poland; weronika.smok@polsl.pl (W.S.); marcin.staszuk@polsl.pl (M.S.)
3. Department of Biomaterials and Medical Devices Engineering, Faculty of Biomedical Engineering, Silesian University of Technology, Franklina Roosevelta 40 Street, 41-800 Zabrze, Poland; janusz.szewczenko@polsl.pl
* Correspondence: anna.wozniak@polsl.pl (A.W.); grzegorz.chladek@polsl.pl (G.C.)

Citation: Woźniak, A.; Smok, W.; Szewczenko, J.; Staszuk, M.; Chladek, G. Influence of Hybrid Surface Modification on Biocompatibility and Physicochemical Properties of Ti-6Al-4V ELI Titanium. *J. Funct. Biomater.* **2024**, *15*, 52. https://doi.org/10.3390/jfb15030052

Academic Editors: Lavinia Cosmina Ardelean and Laura-Cristina Rusu

Received: 24 January 2024
Revised: 14 February 2024
Accepted: 18 February 2024
Published: 20 February 2024

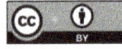

Copyright: © 2024 by the authors. Licensee MDPI, Basel, Switzerland. This article is an open access article distributed under the terms and conditions of the Creative Commons Attribution (CC BY) license (https://creativecommons.org/licenses/by/4.0/).

Abstract: Titanium-based materials are the most widely used materials in biomedical applications. However, according to literature findings, the degradation products of titanium have been associated with potential allergic reactions, inflammation, and bone resorption. The corrosion process of Ti-6Al-4V in the human body environment may be exacerbated by factors such as reduced pH levels and elevated concentrations of chloride compounds. Coatings made of biopolymers are gaining attention as they offer numerous advantages for enhancing implant functionality, including improved biocompatibility, bioactivity, wettability, drug release, and antibacterial activity. This study analyzes the physicochemical and electrochemical behavior of the Ti-6Al-4V ELI alloy subjected to PCL and PCL/TiO$_2$ deposition by the electrospinning method. To characterize the polymer-based layer, tests of chemical and phase composition, as well as surface morphology investigations, were performed. Wetting angle tests were conducted as part of assessing the physicochemical properties. The samples were subjected to corrosion behavior analysis, which included open circuit potential measurements, potentiodynamic tests, and the electrochemical impedance spectroscopy method. Additionally, the quantification of released ions post the potentiodynamic test was carried out using the inductively coupled plasma atomic emission spectrometry (ICP–AES) method. Cytotoxicity tests were also performed. It was found that surface modification by depositing a polymer-based layer on the titanium substrate material using the electrospinning method provides improved corrosion behavior, and the samples exhibit non-toxic properties.

Keywords: Ti-6Al-4V; corrosion; EIS; SEM; electrospinning; nanofibers; PCL

1. Introduction

In medical applications, stainless steel, cobalt-based alloys, and titanium and its alloys are often used for long-term implants. Each is characterized by distinct properties and applications. Stainless steel, especially type 316 L, is used in orthopedic applications such as joint replacements, bone plates, and screws. However, corrosion-resistant stainless steel may exhibit wear and tear over time. Additionally, stainless steel is characterized by the lowest corrosion resistance in the metal biomaterials group. Its magnetic properties can interfere with medical imaging [1,2]. In turn, cobalt-based alloys, known for their high strength, corrosion resistance, and biocompatibility, find application in orthopedic implants, dental prosthetics, and cardiovascular devices. Despite their advantages, the density of cobalt-based alloys can be high, resulting in increased weight in implants. Moreover, some individuals may experience allergic reactions to cobalt [1,3]. While stainless steel and cobalt-based alloys have their applications, titanium alloys, despite potential cost considerations and a challenging fabrication process, stand out due to their superior biocompatibility, mechanical properties, corrosion resistance, and ability to promote osseointegration [4,5]. Ti6-Al-4V is characterized by the best biocompatibility in the metal biomaterials group, thereby reducing the likelihood of negative reactions within the human system. Its surface properties facilitate the formation of a biologically inert oxide layer, promoting favorable interactions with the surrounding tissues [6]. In addition, titanium-based materials exhibit good corrosion resistance due to their ability to spontaneously form a thin and stable protective oxide layer, which constitutes a compact and dense kinetic barrier for extensive corrosion [7]. Additionally, titanium alloys exhibit an excellent strength-to-weight ratio and their low density results in lightweight implants, and they actively promote osseointegration, ensuring long-term stability. These attributes collectively position titanium, especially Ti-6Al-4V, as the preferred material for medical implants where long-term stability and success are paramount. Despite its numerous advantages, Ti-6Al-4V does pose certain challenges in biomedical applications. Iwabuchi et al. [8] and Beake et al. [9] pointed to the poor wear resistance of Ti-6Al-4V, which was lower than that of most metallic biomaterials. Wear debris generated during the abrasion process can lead to the release of particles into the surrounding biological environment. While the biological response to these particles varies, the potential for adverse reactions and inflammation exists [10]. In addition, abrasion or frictional forces may compromise the integrity of the protective passive layer, exposing the biomaterial to corrosion. Moreover, in aggressive biological environments, such as those with high chloride concentrations, the passive film may become susceptible to breakdown. Corrosive attack can compromise the structural integrity of implants, potentially leading to mechanical failure [11].

Presently, surface laser texturing is acknowledged as a highly effective method for improving material performance [12,13]. Laser texturing proves to be a precise, accurate, reproducible, and environmentally friendly technique for modifying surfaces. Literature findings reveal that the laser-texturing process not only results in an enhancement of tribological behavior attributed to improved lubrication [14–21], but also leads to superior microbiological properties owing to the contact guide effect [22,23].

It is worth paying attention to coatings made of biopolymers, because they offer many benefits for increasing the functionality of the implant, including improved biocompatibility, bioactivity, wettability, drug release, and antibacterial activity [24,25]. The most commonly used methods for applying polymer coatings on biomedical alloys include dip-coating [26,27], spin-coating [28], electrochemical assembly [29], and electrospinning from solution [30]. Electrospinning is a simple, low-cost, and repeatable method of manufacturing homogeneous, porous nanofiber networks that mimic the extracellular matrix (ECM) of the cell with their morphology, which additionally improves their bioactivity [31,32]. Previous research indicates that this technique is successfully used to coat biomedical alloys with fibrous layers [33–35]. Karthega et al. [36] showed that polycaprolactone/titanium dioxide (PCL/TiO_2) nanofibers deposited by electrospinning on the surface of the AM50 Mg alloy not only improve the corrosion resistance of the alloy, but are also beneficial for cell proliferation. Kim et al. [37] significantly improved the biocompatibility of MC3T3-E1 osteoblasts (an osteoblast precursor cell line derived from mouse calvaria) on the AZ31 Mg alloy by covering its surface with polycaprolactone/zinc oxide (PCL/ZnO) nanofibers via electrospinning. The electrospinning method also allows for the deposition of nanofibers on the Ti-6Al-4V alloy, as reported by Rajabi et al. [38] and Camargo et al. [39]. E.R. Camargo et al., on a previously prepared surface of a commercial Ti-6Al-4V alloy, built a network of poly(methyl methacrylate) (PMMA) nanofibers and functionalized PMMA-OH nanofibers by electrospinning. It was observed that the use of a polymer coating significantly improved the adhesion and proliferation of fibroblasts. Rajabi et al. performed a two-stage modification of the surface of the Ti-6Al-4V alloy: first, the surface was modified with the Nd:YAG (neodymium-doped yttrium aluminum garnet) laser; then, drug-loaded poly(vinyl alcohol) (PVA) nanofibers with vancomycin were deposited on it.

The applied surface modifications improved biocompatibility, cell viability, and adhesion, as well as extended the drug release rate.

This study aims to investigate the influence of a hybrid surface modification through laser texturing and the deposition of a polycaprolactone-based (PCL) nanofiber layer using the electrospinning method on the physicochemical properties of the Ti-6Al-4V titanium alloy. The use of polycaprolactone (PCL) nanofiber layers shows significant promise for drug delivery post-implantation in the human body. Electrospinning enables the creation of nanofibrous structures with a high surface area, providing an optimal platform for controlled drug release. The potential impact of this approach on post-implantation therapeutics is substantial, offering controlled and sustained drug release, minimizing side effects, and improving overall treatment outcomes. Combining nanofiber layers deposited via the electrospinning method with a laser-texturing process may ensure the increased biocompatibility of biomaterials and overcome the primary usage limitations of the Ti-6Al-4V alloy. Nevertheless, the initial impact of this proposed hybrid surface modification on the physicochemical properties, especially the wettability and corrosion resistance, of the titanium alloy must be rigorously evaluated. This study represents the initial step in the development of new biomaterials for long-term implants, ensuring the potential for controlled drug release. The integration of PCL nanofibers and laser texturing offers a synergistic approach to addressing biocompatibility concerns and usage limitations, laying the foundation for advancements in the field of implantable medical devices.

In this work, surface morphology analysis was conducted using scanning electron microscopy and confocal microscopy. Particular attention was devoted to the assessment of the wettability and corrosion behavior of the modified biomaterials. Contact angle measurements and surface free energy calculation were performed to investigate the chemical character of the samples. The corrosion behavior was analyzed by a potentiodynamic test, supplemented by an electrochemical impedance spectroscopy test. In addition, biological (toxicity) properties were evaluated.

2. Materials and Methods

The Ti-6Al-4V samples in cubic shape (φ 14) were wet-ground (using silicon carbide SiC paper with grit of P500 to P4000), and then polished using a colloidal silica suspension (OP-U) with a particle size of 0.04 μm. The mean roughness of the samples was Ra = 0.52 μm.

Next, samples were subjected to surface modification. The surface texturing process was accomplished using an A-355 picosecond laser system (Oxford Lasers Ltd., Didcot, UK), utilizing a 355 nm wavelength diode-pumped solid-state picosecond laser which generates 5–10 ps pulse durations of 120 μJ average power at 400 Hz pulse frequency. The system of pulsed laser beams guarantees high energy densities and the ability to perform ablation (atoms evaporate layer by layer due to the strength of bonds being decreased between the particles). Micromachining system guarantees average power of 24 mW. The laser beam intensity distribution is Gaussian. The experiment was performed in air at atmospheric pressure. The path of laser texturing was a system of grooves, which formed a truss shape. The Cimita software (2013 version, Oxford laser, Didcot, UK), integrated into the micromachining system, was used to design the laser pattern and process parameters setup. The process parameters are as follows: number of the passes of the laser beam (N)—2, laser scan speed—1 mm/s, beam width—30 μm, and beam quality factor (M^2) < 1.2.

To prepare polymer and composite coatings on the Ti-6Al-4V alloy, the electrospinning form solution method was used. The first stage was the preparation of spinning solutions, for which the following reagents were used: polycaprolactone (PCL purity average Mw 45000, Sigma Aldrich, St. Louis, MO, USA), formic acid (purity 96%, Sigma Aldrich), acetic acid (purity 99%, Sigma Aldrich), and TiO_2 nanoparticles (purity 99.5%, Bionovo). To prepare PCL solution, acetic acid was mixed with formic acid in a 3:1 ratio; then, 3 g of PCL in the form of granules was added and left on a magnetic stirrer to mix for 24 h. The spinning solution of PCL/TiO_2 nanofibers was prepared by adding 0.06 g of TiO_2 to the above-mentioned acid mixture and sonicated for 15 min to break down the nanoparticle agglomerates. Then, 3 g of PCL were added and left on a magnetic stirrer for 24 h until a homogeneous solution was obtained. The next stage was to subject the solutions to the electrospinning process using the FLOW device—Nanotechnology Solutions Electrospinner 2.2.0–500 (Manufacturer Yflow Nanotechnology Solutions, Malaga, Spain) with these constant parameters for both samples: distance, voltage, and flow rate of 15 cm, 16 kV, and 0.2 mL/h, respectively. The deposition time of the fibrous layer for each sample was 15 min (Figure 1). These parameters were selected experimentally to ensure the stability of the electrospinning process.

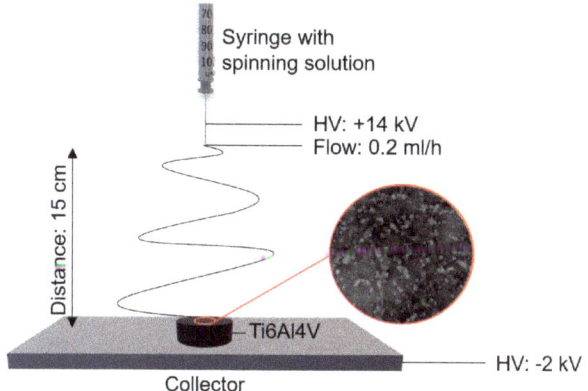

Figure 1. Scheme of electrospinning process.

The microstructure and morphology of the coatings obtained were examined using high-resolution scanning electron microscopy (SEM), the FEI Supra 35 (Zeiss) type, equipped with energy dispersive X-ray spectroscopy (EDX).

The wettability of tested samples was evaluated by contact angle (θ) measurements (sitting drop method), and surface free energy (γ) calculations using Owens–Wendt methods were performed. The test stand was equipped with a Surftens Universal goniometer (OEG, Frankfurt, Germany) and PC with Surftens 4.5. Distilled water $θ_w$ (POCH S.A., Gliwice, Poland) and diiodonomethane $θ_d$ (Merck, Warsaw, Poland) served as the measured liquids (drop volume of 1.0 µm³). The measurements were conducted at room temperature T = 23 ± 1 °C over time t = 60.

Pitting corrosion resistance tests were performed using the potentiodynamic method. The test stand comprised of an Atlas 0531 EU potentiostat (ATALS-SOLLICH, Rębiechowo, Poland) and three-electrode cell. A platinum rod (auxiliary electrode) and a silver chloride electrode Ag/AgCl electrode (reference electrode) were used for the tests. Corrosion testing commenced following 3600 s of open-circuit potential stabilization (E_{ocp}). The scan rate was configured at 0.175 mV/s.

Electrochemical impedance spectroscopy (EIS) tests were performed using an identical test stand to that of the corrosion resistance test. The test was conducted in the frequency range of 10^4 to 10^{-3} Hz. The amplitude of the sinusoidal voltage of the excitation signal was 10 mV. In the study, the impedance spectra in the form of the Nyquist and Bode diagrams were determined, and, next, obtained data were adjusted to the equivalent circuit using the least-squares method. All electrochemical analyses were carried out in a Ringer solution of the following chemical composition: NaCl—8.6 g/dm³, KCl—0.3 g/dm³, and $CaCl_2 \cdot 2H_2O$—0.33 g/dm³, at T = 37 ± 1 °C.

The content of the titanium, aluminum, and vanadium in Ringer solutions after the immersion test was determined using inductively coupled plasma atomic emission spectrometry (ICP-AES). A Varian 710-ES spectrometer, equipped with a OneNeb nebulizer and twister glass spray chamber, was used. The parameter is given in Table 1.

Table 1. Parameters of plasma atomic emission spectrometry parameters test.

Parameter		Value (u)
RF power		1.0 kW
Plasma flow		15 (L/min)
Auxiliary flow		1.5 (L/min)
Nebulizer pressure		210 (kPa)
Pump rate		15 (rpm)
Emission lines	Ti	λ = 334.188; 334.941 and 336.122 (nm)
	Al	λ = 237.312 and 396.152 (nm)
	V	λ = 268.796; 292.401; 309.310 and 311.837 (nm)

The cytotoxicity of the modified samples was examined with a 3-[4,5-dimethylthiazol-2-yl]-2,5 diphenyltetrazolium bromide (MTT) test. The HCT116 cancer cells (obtained from the American Type Culture Collection) were used for the test. The cell lines were treated with 10% fetal bovine serum (Eurx) supplemented with 1% antibiotic antifungal solution. The cells were seeded onto the tested samples and incubated for 72 h at 37 °C in a humidified atmosphere of 5% CO_2. Next, the culture medium was removed, and, after trypsin neutralization, the cell suspension was centrifuged (2000 rpm, t = 3 min, T = 23 $\pm$ 1 °C), and the cell pellet in MTT solution was resuspended. After incubation (t = 3 h), the MTT solution was removed. In effect, obtained formazan was dissolved in C_3H_7OH:HCl. After that, the optical density at 550 nm with a reference wavelength of 670 nm was measured using an ELISA reader. The mean absorbance in control wells was considered to be 100% viable cells.

The names of the samples subjected to the test are given in Table 2.

Table 2. List of tested samples with their names and surface conditions.

Name	Surface Condition
S_is	Samples in the initial state—after mechanical grinding and polishing
S_tex	Samples after laser-texturing process
S_PCL	Samples with PCL nanofiber layer de-posted by electrospinning method
S_PCL/TiO$_2$	Samples with PCL/TiO$_2$ nanofiber layer de-posted by electrospinning method
S_tex/PCL	Samples after laser-texturing process and with PCL nanofiber layer de-posted by electrospinning method
S_tex/PCL/TiO$_2$	Samples after laser-texturing process and with PCL/TiO$_2$ nanofiber layer de-posted by electrospinning method

3. Results

3.1. Surface Morphology Analysis

The surface morphology of the samples after the laser-texturing process was characterized using a scanning electron microscope and a confocal microscope, as depicted in Figure 2. For the S_tex sample groups, cross-like micro-groove patterns were observed, which are characteristic features of photothermal ablation. The average width between micro-grooves was 242 $\pm$ 4 µm, consistent with the designed laser texture pattern. Additionally, a small amount of deposition, called micro-bugle or micro-crown, was noted on the edge of the micro-grooves of the titanium alloy. The height of the micro-bugle measured from confocal microscopy observation was 5.2 $\pm$ 0.5 µm (Figure 2c). This phenomenon could be attributed to the formation of a remelting layer on the titanium alloy surface during the thermal effects of laser processing. Wang et al. [7] and Huerta-Murillo et al. [40] also reported the existence of micro-bugles along the laser texture pattern. The groove depth was 9.4 $\pm$ 0.4 µm (Figure 2b). Additionally, the roughness of the central area of the laser pattern (single square) was Sn = 270 nm.

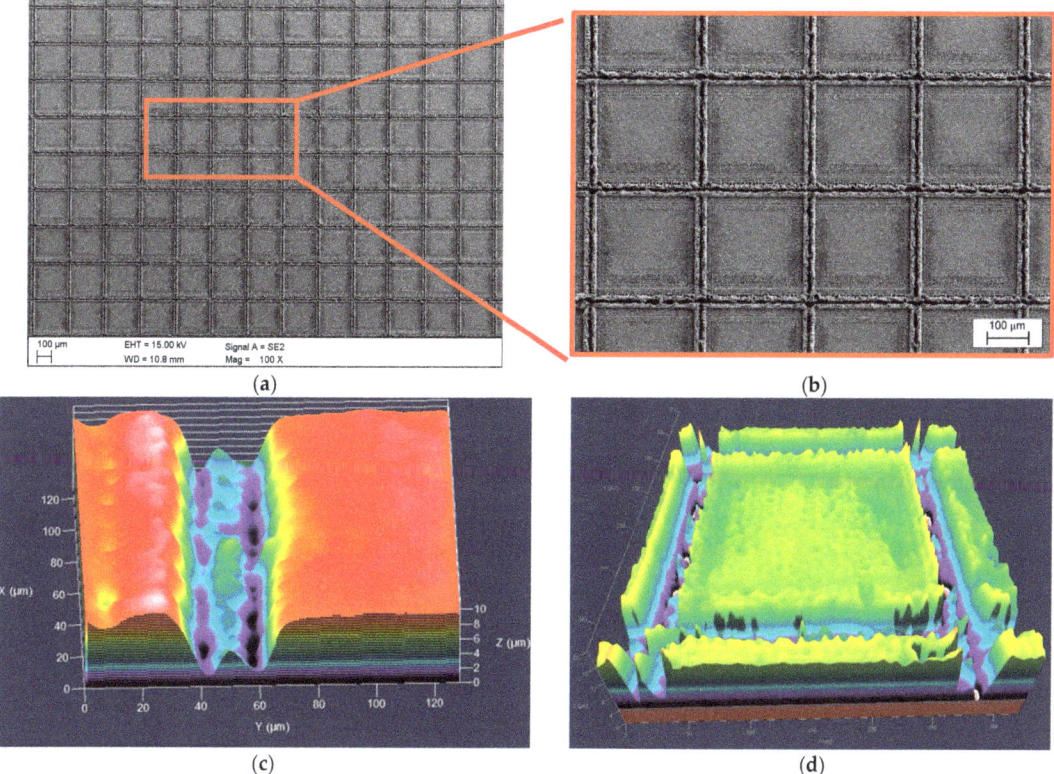

Figure 2. Results of microscopic observation for samples after laser-texturing process (S_tex): (**a**,**b**) SEM; and (**c**,**d**) confocal microscope.

The analysis of the morphology of electrospun PCL and PCL/TiO$_2$ nanofibers was performed based on SEM images (Figure 3). At first, to select the electrospinning process parameters, the PCL nanofibers were deposited on the aluminum foil. The PCL nanofibers deposited on the aluminum foil were homogeneous, had a smooth surface, and did not show any defects, e.g., beads and spindles, and their average diameter was 85 nm (Figure 3a,b). The absence of defects indicates that the parameters of the spinning solution were appropriate. The PCL nanofibers deposited on a Ti-6Al-4V substrate both before and after texturization were characterized by the presence of beads whose diameter ranged from 50 to several micrometers, while the diameter of the fibers themselves in both samples was approximately 60 nm (Figure 3c,d,g,h). Moreover, PCL/TiO$_2$ nanofibers deposited on Ti-6Al-4V substrates had visible beads with a diameter reaching several microns, while the average fiber diameter was 33 and 73 nm for the unmodified and textured substrates, respectively. Comparing Figures 3g and 3i, it was also found that the addition of TiO$_2$ to PCL had a positive effect on the uniform coverage of the textured substrate with nanofibers.

The presence of beads and spindles in nanofibers electrospun onto a Ti-6Al-4V substrate was also observed by Camargo et al. [39] and Santhosh et al. [41], who studied the PMMA and hydroxyapatite–polysulfone coating, respectively. This type of defect appears mainly as a result of a too-low polymer concentration in the spinning solution or a too-low molecular weight of the polymer; however, in this study, nanofibers deposited from the same spinning solution deposited on the aluminum foil showed no defects, which suggests that the morphology of the fibers was largely influenced by the substrate. As indicated by [42–44], electrospinning on a non-conductive substrate such as Ti-6Al-4V is difficult due to electric field distortion, which destabilizes the polymer jet, adversely affecting the morphology of the obtained fibers.

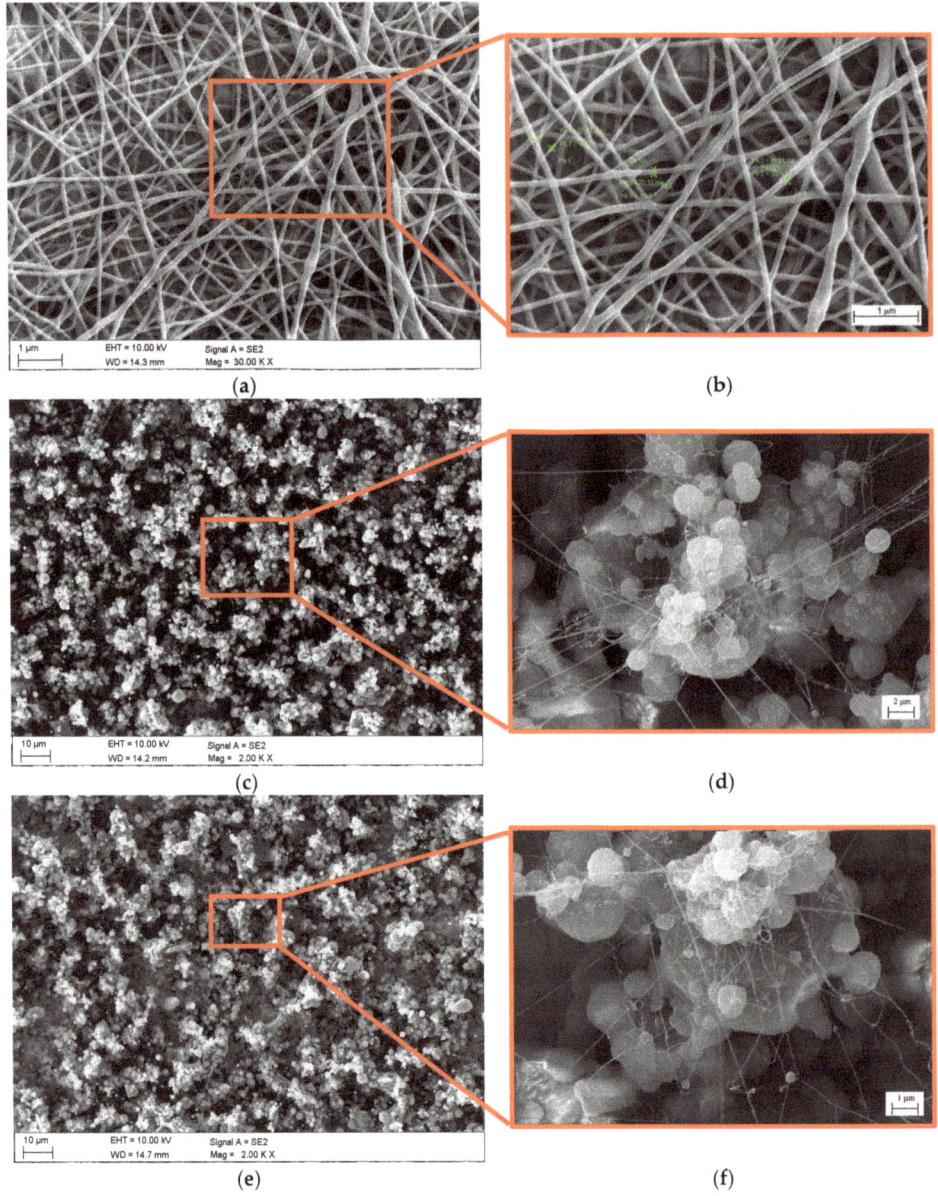

Figure 3. Cont.

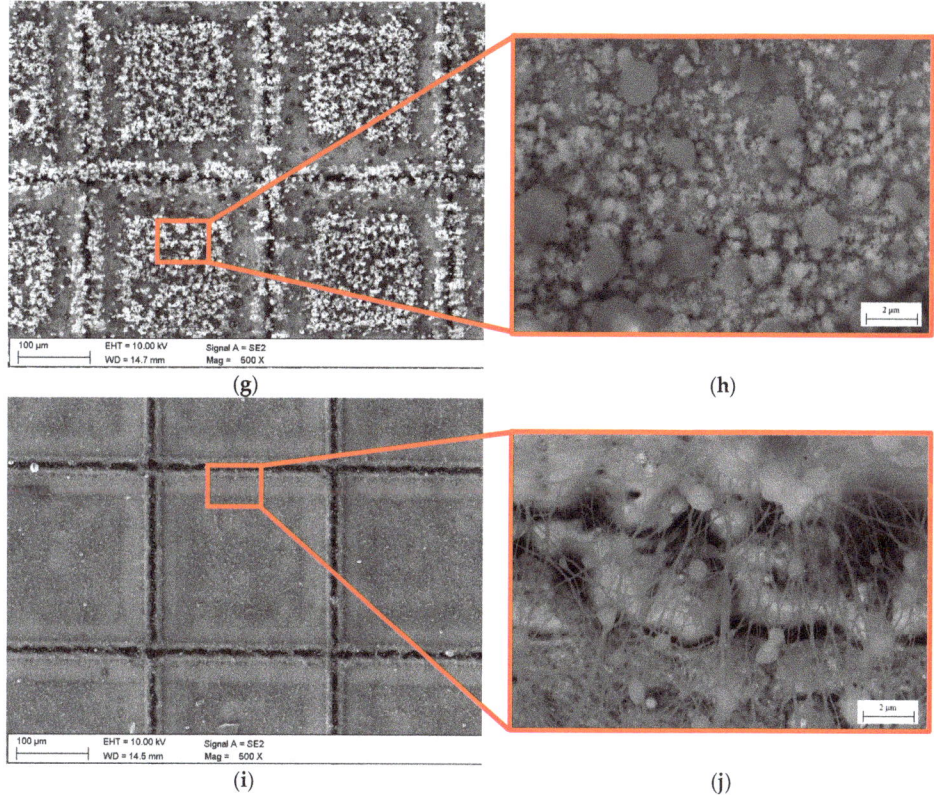

Figure 3. Results of samples surface morphology (SEM): (**a,b**) PCL nanofibers on aluminum foil, (**c,d**) samples with PCL nanofibers (S_PCL), (**e,f**) samples with PCL nanofibers with the addition of TiO$_2$ particles (S_PCL/TiO$_2$), (**g,h**) samples after laser-texturing process with PCL nanofibers (S_tex/PCL), and (**i,j**) samples after laser-texturing process with PCL nanofibers with the addition of TiO$_2$ particles (S_tex_PCL/TiO$_2$).

3.2. Wettability Test

The results of the wettability test are presented in Table 3. The diagram illustrating changes in the contact angle of distilled water over time and example images of drops placed on the tested sample surfaces are shown in Figure 4.

Table 3. Results of contact angle measurements.

Name	Contact Angle (°)		Surface Free Energy (mJ/m^2)		
	Distilled Water	Diiodomethane	γ_S	γ_S^d	γ_S^p
S_is	68.7 ± 2.9	47.0 ± 3.1	36.6	22.7	18.9
S_tex	95.4 ± 3.9	42.0 ± 2.8	39.4	38.1	1.7
S_PCL	128.2 ± 1.4	17.2 ± 1.1	106.6	85.7	20.9
S_PCL/TiO$_2$	137.8 ± 1.2	10.4 ± 0.7	116.4	91.1	25.3
S_tek/PCL	133.3 ± 2.1	13.5 ± 3.4	111.0	88.3	22.6
S_tex/PCL/TiO$_2$	137.9 ± 1.5	-	-	-	-

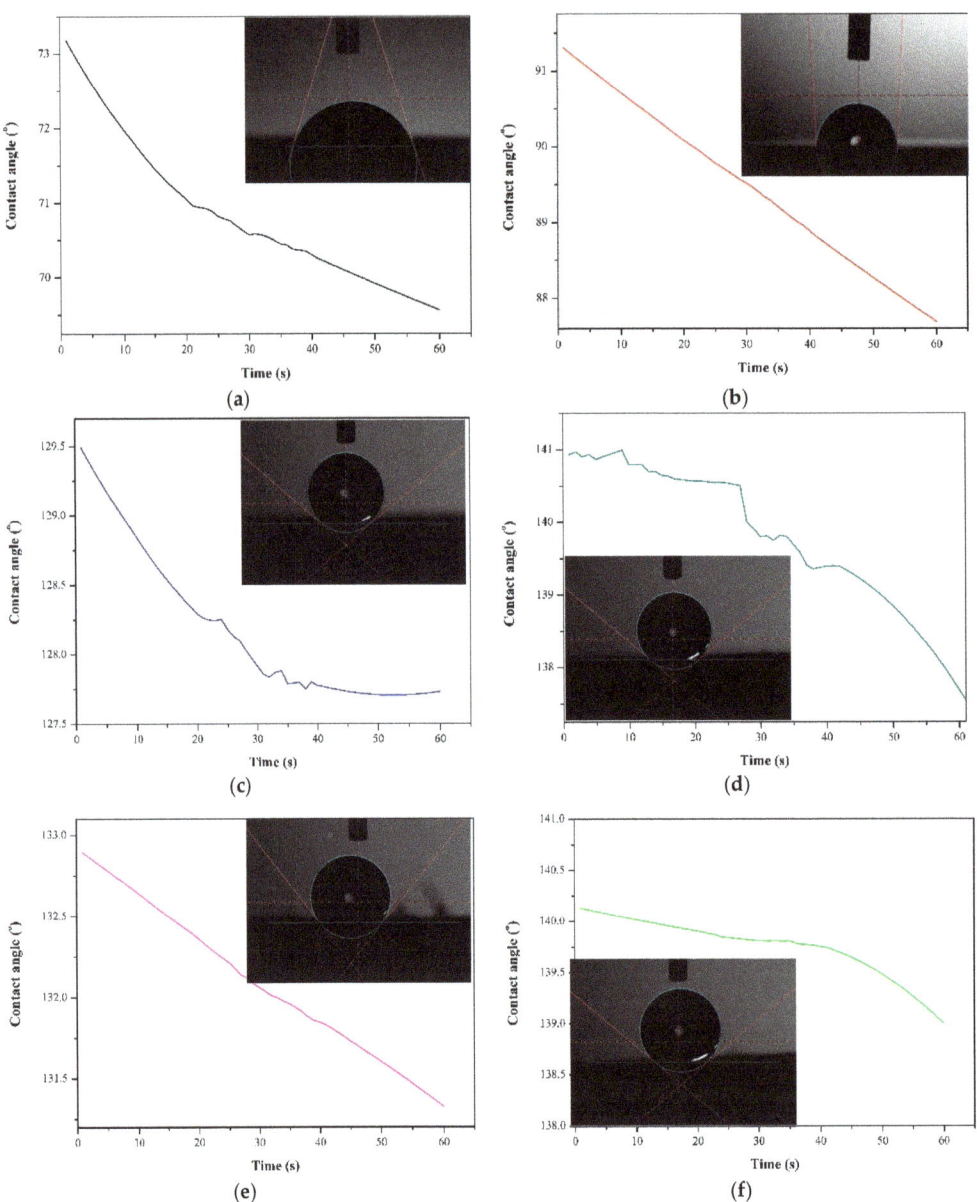

Figure 4. Results of wettability test: diagram of contact angle changes in time function and examples image of water drop on sample's surface: (**a**) S_is, (**b**) S_PCL, (**c**) S_tex, (**d**) S_PCL/TiO$_2$, (**e**) S_tex/PCL, and (**f**) S_tex/PCL/TiO$_2$.

Significant differences in the values of wettability were observed between the untreated samples and samples after surface modification. It was found that laser texturing and layer deposition by electrospinning have a significant effect on the contact angle of T Ti-6Al-4V-based biomaterial. For the untreated (S_is) samples group, the average water contact angle for the samples was approximately 68°, signifying a hydrophilic nature of the surface ($\Theta < 90°$). The observed wetting state is characteristic of titanium surfaces stored under atmospheric conditions (air) [45]. Moreover, Melo-Fonseca et al. [46] and Reggio et al. [47] reported the hydrophilic nature of mechanically polished Ti-6Al-4V alloy. In contrast, for the samples after surface modification, a switch from hydrophilic to hydrophobic behavior is evident. For the S_tex samples group, the average value of the water contact angle was 95°, reaching the threshold for the transition from the hydrophilic to the hydrophobic state (where the hydrophilic state is <90° < hydrophobic state). The highest values were obtained for the samples with PCL and composite PCL-TiO$_2$ layers, irrespective of the surface condition of the substrate material (polished or textured), with mean values falling within the range of 128–137°. According to the literature, electrospinning is a well-known method that enables the production of hydrophobic, ultrathin fibers with micrometer and sub-micrometer diameters from various polymeric materials. The electrospun fibers, due to their size, guarantee a single-length scale of roughness for superhydrophobicity. Sheela et al. [48] also indicated the hydrophobic nature of polycaprolactone electrospun membranes, reporting a mean value of 129°, which is similar to the values presented in our work. The addition of TiO$_2$ particles to the PCL fibers led to a slight increase in the water contact angle. Generally, TiO$_2$ particles exhibit hydrophilic behavior due to their polar nature. However, when introduced into a nanofiber matrix, they can influence the overall wetting properties. The inorganic TiO$_2$ was easily covered by airborne organic contaminations and, in effect, demonstrate hydrophobic surface properties. Moreover, incorporating TiO$_2$ particles into a nanofiber matrix can alter the composite material's wettability, and this transition may depend on factors such as particle concentration and dispersion. Sahoo et al. [49] demonstrated that, with an increase in the titanium content from 1 to 2wt.% in the polyvinylidene fluoride (PVDF) matrix, the contact angle increased from 124 to 129°. Additionally, they indicated that a titanium dioxide concentration of more than 2wt.% strongly affects increased wettability. This finding confirms our investigation, where the TiO$_2$ concentration in PCL fiber material was 2%.

The values of surface free energy of the S_is and S_tex samples were similar and fell within the range of 37–39 mJ/m^2. The calculated values for samples with a nanofiber layer were approximately three times higher compared to the S_is and S_tex sample groups. In addition, for the samples with a hybrid surface modification, the S_tex/PCL/TiO$_2$ SFE calculation was impossible, due to the extremely low value of the diiodomethane contact angle—close to 0°. Additionally, all tested samples demonstrated a greater affinity for apolar groups than polar ones, as evidenced by higher values of the apolar components of surface free energy (SFE). However, the apolar components of samples with PCL and PCL/TiO$_2$ layers were four and two times higher compared to those for samples in the initial state and after the laser-texturing process, respectively. Dispersive interactions are primarily driven by van der Waals forces and occur between nonpolar molecules or regions of molecules. Dispersion forces are generally weaker than polar forces but can be more prevalent across a surface.

The wettability of materials is regulated by their chemical composition and surface morphology, including surface roughness. This property is directly manifested in contact, as described by the Young formula:

$$\cos\Theta = r\frac{\gamma_{sg} - \gamma_{sl}}{\gamma_{lg}} = r \cdot \cos\Theta, \quad (1)$$

where:

γ—surface tension, s—solid state, g—gas, and l—liquid;
Θ—water contact angle (°);
r—roughness ratio (r = 1—smooth surface, and r > 1—rough surface).

From (1), it is observed that the contact angle increases with an increasing roughness ratio value if the contact angle on a smooth surface is more than 90°. The laser-texturing process leads to Ti-6Al-4V titanium alloy surface development at the micro- and nanoscale. Moreover, layers consisting of nanofibers of PCL and PCL/TiO$_2$ deposited by electrospinning drastically affect the overall surface.

According to the literature data, in general, three models that describe the wetting behavior on the rough or restored surface can be distinguished (Figure 5): (I) Wenzel, (II) Cassie–Baxter, and (III) the middle state, which is a transitional state between the Wenzel and Cassie–Baxter states. In the Wenzel state, a liquid completely wets a rough surface, filling the surface asperities. The liquid wets the roughness at a microscopic level, increasing the apparent contact area. In the Cassie–Baxter state, the liquid only partially wets the rough surface, with air trapped within the surface asperities. The air exhibits absolutely hydrophobic properties with a contact angle of 180° [50]. The apparent contact area is reduced, leading to a higher contact angle compared to the Wenzel state. In the middle state of wettability, the liquid partially occupies the surface features, creating a mixed wetting behavior. For the samples after surface modification, the wettability state probably occurs at the Cassie–Baxter state or the middle state of wettability. Moreover, external influences, such as the absorption of hydrocarbons from the atmosphere, may have impacted the results, as reported by Yamauch et al. [51] and Khan et al. [52].

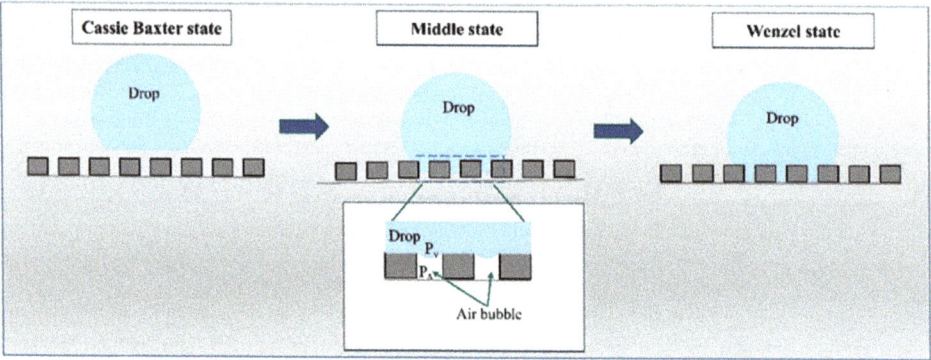

Figure 5. Scheme of wettability states.

3.3. EIS Test

Figure 6 shows the EIS spectra recorded for both sample groups in the form of Nyquist and Bode plots.

Based on the obtained results, it can be seen that the impedance response of the titanium alloy has remarkably changed after surface modification by laser texturing and PCL-based nanofiber layer deposition in the corrosive solution. The Nyquist plots (Figure 6a,c,e,g,i,k) presented fragments of semi-circles, which is a typical response of a thin layer. In addition, from Nyquist-impedance plots, it can be seen that only for the samples after the laser-texturing process was the radius of curvature lower than that of the untextured surface. For other samples, diagrams show a larger radius of the semicircle than that of the samples in the initial state. The diameter of the semicircle increases in the order of S_PCL < S_tex/PCL < S_PCL/TiO$_2$ < S_tex/PCL/TiO$_2$. According to the literature data [7,53,54], and our previous reports [6,55–57], the larger the radius of curvature in the Nyquist plots, the better the corrosion resistance of the sample surface. This suggests that surface modification by electrospinning provides superior corrosion resistance compared to the textured surface. Additionally, the results depicted in the Bode diagrams corroborate those of the Nyquist plots. The lowest value of the maximum phase displacement, over a broad range of frequencies, was observed for the S_is and S_tex sample group, with mean values of 65 and 50°, respectively. In contrast, for other samples, the phase displacement ranged from 70 to 95°, indicating that samples with PCL and PCL/TiO$_2$ layers exhibit a higher impedance and better corrosion resistance.

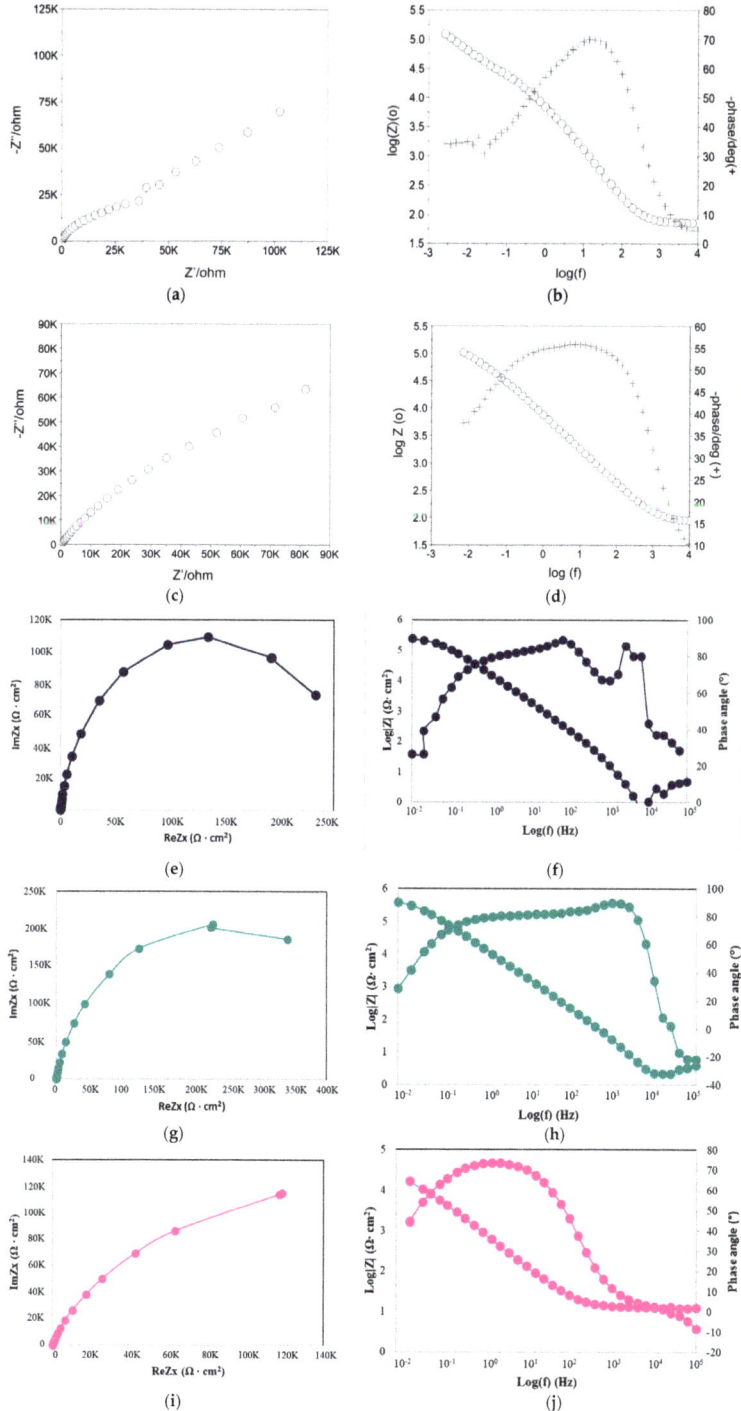

Figure 6. *Cont.*

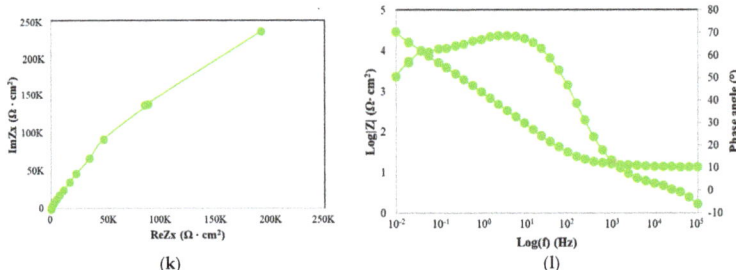

(k)   (l)

Figure 6. Results of EIS test in form of Nyquist and Bode diagram for the following: (**a**,**b**) S_is, (**c**,**d**) S_tex, (**e**,**f**) S_PCL, (**g**,**h**) S_PCL/TiO$_2$, (**i**,**j**) S_tex/PCL, and (**k**,**l**) S_tex/PCL/TiO$_2$.

The characterization of the interface impedance of the tested samples was performed by approximating the EIS experimental data using physical electrical models of the equivalent circuits. As shown in Figure 7, for the S_tex/PCL samples group, an equivalent circuit with single constants was used to analyze the EIS data, which indicates the occurrence of a single layer. The electrical equivalent circuit model of the textured surfaces with PCL nanofiber layers consists of solution resistance (R_s), the resistance of the conformal layer (R_{ct}), and the capacity of the layer (CPE_{dl}). For other samples, an equivalent circuit with two time constants was used to analyze the EIS data, which indicates the occurrence of two sub-layers. In this case, the equivalent circuit consists of C_{pore}/CPE_{pore} (capacity of the double-layer porous surface) and R_{pore} (resistance of double-layer porous surface), which are representatives of the electrical porous layer, whereas CPE_{dl} and R_{ct} represent the resistive and non-ideal capacitive behavior of the passive film. In particular, we have the following:

R_{pore}—the electrolyte resistance in the porous phase;
C_{pore}/CPE_{pore}—the capacity of the double-layer porous surface;
R_{ct}—the electric charge transfer resistance at the boundary of phases;
CPE_{dl}—the capacity used to describe the low-frequency region (11–0.001 Hz).

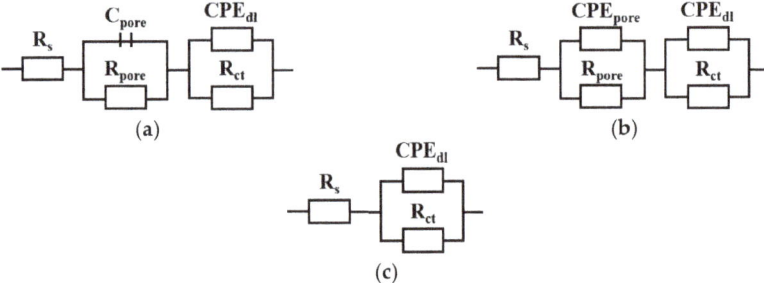

Figure 7. Electric substitute scheme: (**a**) S_is; S_tex; S_PCL/TiO$_2$, (**b**) S_PCL; S_tex/PCL/TiO$_2$, and (**c**) S_tex/PCL.

The mathematical impedance model of the above system is also presented in Equations (2)–(4).

$$Z = R_s + \frac{1}{\frac{1}{R_{pore}} + j\omega C_{pore}} + \frac{1}{\frac{1}{R_{ct}} + Y_l(j\omega)^{n_{dl}}} \quad (2)$$

$$Z = R_s + \frac{1}{\frac{1}{R_{pore}} + Y_1(j\omega)^{n_1}} + \frac{1}{\frac{1}{R_{ct}} + Y_{02}(j\omega)^{n_2}} \quad (3)$$

$$Z = R_s + \cfrac{1}{\cfrac{1}{R_{ct}} + Y_{01}(j\omega)^{n_2}} \qquad (4)$$

The parameters characterizing the electrochemical response of the surface of the tested samples are provided in Table 4. The samples with the PCL or PCL/TiO$_2$ layer exhibited the highest resistance values, affirming that the applied protective layers on the material played a role in enhancing its anticorrosive properties.

Table 4. Results of EIS test—values of resistances.

No	Name	R$_{pore}$ (Ω·cm^2)	R$_{ct}$ (kΩ·cm^2)
1	S_is	30	432
2	S_tex	48	393
3	S_PCL	10	885
4	S_PCL/TiO$_2$	650	244
5	S_tex/PCL	650	890
6	S_tex/PCL/TiO$_2$	-	890

3.4. Potentiodynamic Test

The open circuit potential curves recorded in t = 1 h are depicted in Figure 8. In the case of the samples in the initial state (S_is), the open circuit potential values consistently increased throughout the entire measurement time, reaching more electropositive values without attaining a stable or stabilized state. The positive shift in E$_{cop}$ values indicates an augmentation in the compactness of the passive layer or corrosion products on the samples with time. Samples after the laser-texturing process (S_tex) and samples with a deposited PCL layer (S_PCL) exhibit a similar progression of E$_{ocp}$ curves, showing almost no change over the measuring time. For the S_tex/PCL samples group, the E$_{ocp}$ values begin to increase, and then gradually stabilize. Additionally, up to 1650 s, some oscillation of E$_{ocp}$ was visible, which pointed to some instability of the surface layers, or was due to localized corrosions on the metal surface in the aqueous solution. An initial increase in E$_{cop}$ values with a gradual stabilization was also observed for the S_PCL/TiO$_2$ and S_tex/PCL/TiO$_2$. However, the steady-state for those samples was reached after approximately 200 s.

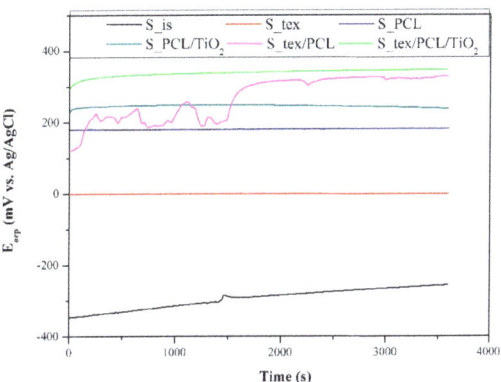

Figure 8. Results of E$_{ocp}$ in time function measurements.

The lowest values of E$_{ocp}$ were recorded for the S_is samples group, and the mean value was close to −242 mV vs. Ag/AgCl (corresponding to approximately −45 mV vs. NEH). The recorded values belong to the domains of the passive region of TiO$_2$ in the titanium Pourbaix diagram. This means that the alloys form a stable oxide layer of TiO_2, as we also recorded in our previous article [6,58]. The surface modification of Ti-6Al-4V substrate materials results in shifts in the E_{ocp} value towards more electropositive values, in the following order: S_tex/PCL/TiO_2 > S_tex/PCL > S_PCL/TiO_2 > S_PCL > S_tex. For the S_tex samples group, the E_{ocp} value was +10 mV vs. Ag/AgCl (+207 mV vs. NEH), which could fall within the domains of the $TiO_3 \cdot 2H_2O$ region in the titanium Pourbaix diagram. However, the increase in values compared to those obtained for the samples in the initial state can be associated with the head-build effect during the laser-texturing process, promoting oxidation and microstructural changes near the surface. Similar observations were reported by Annamala et al. [59], Yue et al. [60], and Bussoli et al. [61]. In effect, as a result of laser interaction, different titanium oxides could be formed.

To evaluate the effect of the surface modification on the corrosion resistance of the titanium alloy, potentiodynamic tests were carried out. The results of the potentiodynamic test for all tested samples are presented in the form of Tafel's plot and polarization curves in Figure 9. The characteristic corrosion parameters are given in Table 5.

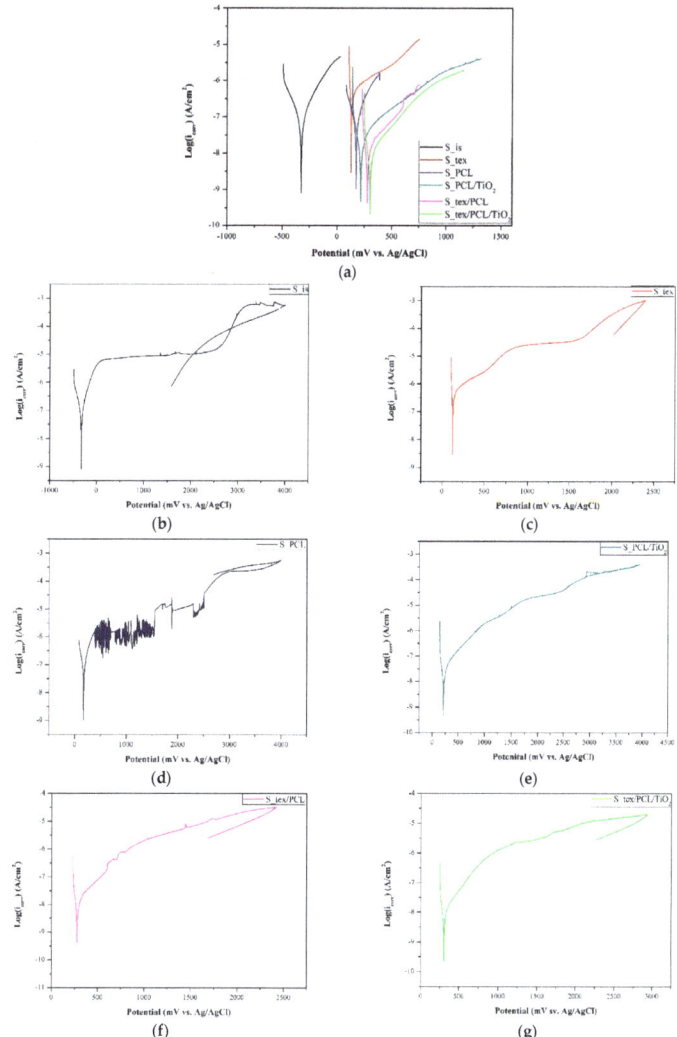

Figure 9. Results of potentiodynamic test: (**a**) Tafles plot for all tested samples, and example potentiodynamic curves for (**b**) S_is, (**c**) S_tex, (**d**) S_PCL, (**e**) S_PCL/TiO$_2$, (**f**) S_tex/PCL, and (**g**) S_tex/PCL/TiO$_2$.

Table 5. Results of potentiodynamic test—value of characteristic corrosion parameters.

No	Name	E_{corr} (mV vs. Ag/AgCl)	E_{tr} (mV vs. Ag/AgCl)	E_b (mV vs. Ag/AgCl)	i_{corr} (µA/cm^2)
1	S_is	−301 ± 27	1952 ± 35	-	0.033
2	S_tex	+110 ± 35	1794 ± 41	-	0.052
3	S_PCL	+172 ± 12	-	2290 ± 39	0.019
4	S_PCL/TiO$_2$	+220 ± 26	2392 ± 32	-	0.012
5	S_tex/PCL	+275 ± 52	2446 ± 57	-	0.015
6	S_tex/PCL/TiO$_2$	+296 ± 44	2652 ± 61	-	0.011

It was found that the registered values of the corrosion potential (E_{corr}) confirm the E_{ocp} behavior. The surface modification led to shifts in the values of the corrosion potential to more noble values. Additionally, it was observed that TiO_2 particles in the nanofiber PCL matrix provide higher values of E_{corr}. The most favorable values of E_{corr} were indicated for S_tex/PCL/TiO_2 and S_tex/PCL, while the lowest values were recorded for the S_tex and S_is samples groups. Analysis of the recorded curves revealed variations in the corrosion resistance based on the surface condition of the tested samples. For the S_is and S_tex samples, plateau regions were recorded from +200 to +2200 mV vs. Ag/AgCl and from +900 to +1600 mV vs. Ag/AgCl, respectively, followed by a steady increase in current densities. Voltammetric curves for both sample groups showed an active-to-passive transition with current densities of about −350 and 300 $\mu A/cm^2$, respectively. Other tested samples displayed a steady increase in the current density without a plateau region. For the S_PCL and S_PCL/TiO_2 samples, an active-to-passive transition occurred with current densities of about −330 $\mu A/cm^2$, and, for S_tex/PCL and S_tex/PCL/TiO_2, the transition was with current densities of about −450 $\mu A/cm^2$. In general, the active-to-passive transition refers to the change in the electrochemical behavior of the material. Negative current densities signify the cathodic current, which typically corresponds to reduction reactions and can be associated with the transition from an active to a passive state. Therefore, the more negative the current density is, the more effective the material is in transitioning to a more corrosion-resistant, passive state. The existence of breakdown potential (E_b) was recorded only for the S_PCL samples group, hysteresis loop. For the other tested samples, the existence of the transpassivation potential was recorded. For samples in the initial state, the transpassivation potential (E_{tr}) and corrosion current density (i_{corr}) were +1952 mV vs. Ag/AgCl, and 0.033 $\mu A/cm^2$, which correspond to our previous work [6] and literature data. It was found that the laser-texturing treatment worsened the corrosion resistance of the titanium alloy surface. The registered values of E_{tr} were lower than those in the initial state, and the i_{corr} was higher. According to the literature data, conflicting information about the influence of laser texturing on Ti-6Al-4V's corrosion resistance can be found. For some authors [7,19,62,63], the laser-texturing process leads to an improvement of the corrosion resistance of the Ti-6Al-4V titanium alloy, which can be directly correlated with an increase in the wetting angle, and the grain refinement of laser-textured surfaces. As indicated by Kumari et al. [64], grain refinement improves the passive film formation due to the increased grain boundary density. Contrarily, Grabowski et al. [65] showed a decrease in corrosion resistance after laser texturing Ti-6Al-4V alloy, contributing to increasing roughness. Moreover, Wang et al. [66] investigated the corrosion resistance of Ti-6Al-4V after the laser-texturing process with the micro-groove width in the range of 25 to 65 μm. Depending on texture patterns, different corrosion resistances of the substrate materials were found. Based on the potentiodynamic test only for the samples with a groove width of 35 and 45 μm, an increase in the corrosion resistance was observed. As mentioned above, the laser-texturing process can lead to microstructural changes and increase the passivation ability. However, in some cases, laser texturing can induce crystallography orientation changes, which may influence corrosion susceptibility, especially if the changes result in preferential corrosion along a specific path. In general, titanium exhibits the spontaneous ability to form a robust and uniform TiO_2 passive layer, which is critical for protecting the alloy against corrosion. A well-formed passivation layer acts as a barrier, hindering the penetration of corrosive agents. However, the laser-texturing process may alter the composition or characteristics of this oxide layer. Changes in the oxide layer can impact the overall corrosion resistance of the material. Additionally, laser texturing may not uniformly passivate the entire surface, leaving some areas more susceptible to corrosion. This corresponds to the E_{ocp} behavior examination, which shows the possible formation of a Ti_2O_3 passive layer on the laser-textured surface, which is less stable than a TiO_2 passive layer. The Ti_2O_3 is more prone to further oxidation and can be less protective as a passive layer under certain conditions [67]. The reduced protective capability of the Ti_2O_3 passive layer may lead to an increase in implant degradation and the release of metal ions from the implant into the surrounding tissues. Consequently, this may result in chronic inflammatory responses. A decrease in corrosion resistance after laser texturing can be attributed to residual stresses in the material, particularly at the textured regions. These stresses may create microcracks or defects in the surface, providing initiation sites for corrosion and compromising the overall resistance. For other samples after surface modification, an increase in the E_{tr}/E_b values and a decrease in the i_{corr} values were registered. This indicates an improvement in the corrosion resistance of the Ti-6Al-4V titanium alloy. The most favorable corrosion parameter was registered for the samples with a PCL/TiO$_2$ nanofiber layer—S_PCL/TiO$_2$ and S_tex/PCL/TiO$_2$. First, the better corrosion resistance of those sample groups can be attributed to the barrier effect. The electrospun nanofiber layers can act as a physical barrier, limiting the direct contact between the corrosive environment and the Ti-6Al-4V substrate. The barrier effect was also indicated as a reason for improving corrosion resistance in our previous work [56,57,68,69]. Moreover, according to the literature data [70–72], enhanced corrosion resistance has been observed by preventing the diffusion of corrosive ions into the substrate material through the deposition of a PCL-based layer. However, PCL, as a biocompatible polymer, can contribute to the overall biocompatibility of the modified surface. The interaction between the modified surface and biological environments may influence the corrosion behavior and the response of the surrounding tissues. Additionally, the incorporation of TiO$_2$ nanofibers in the layers can enhance the formation and stability of a protective oxide layer on the Ti-6Al-4V surface.

Moreover, an increase in the contact angle and hydrophobic surface properties can provide a better corrosion behavior. Generally, hydrophobic surfaces (higher contact angles) repel water, potentially minimizing the contact between the corrosive medium and the material. However, the influence of the micro- and nanoscale roughness on the wettability and the corrosion resistance must also be taken into account. The surface roughness can impact both the contact angle and corrosion resistance. That is why an analysis of the wettability state presented in Section 3.2 could be helpful in corrosion resistance analysis. Dănăilă et al. [73] showed that the passivation behavior of the Ti-6Al-4V alloy was affected by the surface's roughness. Researchers have also shown that samples with higher microroughness exhibit lower corrosion resistance. However, sub-microroughness or hierarchical roughness can be beneficial for corrosion resistance. Micro- and nanoscale features may affect the ability of corrosive agents to come into contact with the material, influencing the corrosion process. As was reported in [74–76], the air entrapped in surface roughness can prevent aggressive ions from attacking the substrate material surface. In effect, the presence of the hydrophobic surface leads to a shift in the anodic corrosion potential toward more noble values, and both the anodic and cathodic corrosion currents are significantly reduced [77]. Zhang et al. [78] explained that the deposition of a densely packed superhydrophobic layer on a titanium-based substrate material was enough to prevent oxygen from diffusing into the substrate. Moreover, capillarity is an important aspect to consider in order to improve the corrosion resistance of a hydrophobic surface. As indicated by Liu et al. [78], for high contact angle values, water transport against gravity is easy in the porous structure of superhydrophobic surfaces. In effect, as a result of the Laplace pressure, the corrosion solution can be pushed out from the pores. Additionally, in our work, the micro-grooves of the laser-textured samples could be filled with PCL and PCL/TiO$_2$ nanofiber layer deposition. Khoshanood et al. [79] indicated the better corrosion behavior of the AZ31 alloy as a result of the deposition hybrid PCL/chitosan scaffold coatings. Cataruo et al. [80] investigate the influence of surface modification by the deposition of an inorganic TiO$_2$ matrix with different percentages of PCL by the sol–gel method. The electrochemical results pointed to the notion that the coatings have a significant effect in terms of the corrosion potential, as also shown in our work. However, during the drying and curing stages, the sol–gel film may experience cracking and shrinkage. This can compromise the integrity of the coating and reduce its effectiveness, particularly in applications requiring a continuous and defect-free layer.

Moreover, coating complex shapes or intricate structures with sol–gel films can be difficult. The electrospinning process eliminates this limitation.

3.5. Inductively Coupled Plasma Atomic Emission Spectroscopy

According to the results obtained by ICP-AES it can be seen that laser surface texturing leads to an increase in the amount of titanium and aluminum ions released into the Ringer solution. Ions released from metal implants into a corrosive environment have the potential to trigger inflammatory responses in the surrounding tissues, compromising the overall biocompatibility of the implant. This immune reaction may manifest as localized inflammation and, in some cases, allergic responses, which can range from mild irritation to more severe reactions that may jeopardize the implant's functionality. Furthermore, the toxicity of certain metal ions could pose risks to tissues, affecting the health of the surrounding anatomical structures. Prolonged exposure to released ions, even at low concentrations, may contribute to chronic health issues and impact the normal healing process at the implant site [81–83]. For example, elevated aluminum levels could lead to neurotoxicity and neurological disorders. In addition, aluminum ions can interfere with bone mineralization. Excessive aluminum exposure has also been linked to renal impairment. As is well-known, the kidneys play a crucial role in filtering and excreting ions from the body. The release of aluminum ions may present challenges for renal function [84].

The concentration of titanium ions in the solution after the immersion test (t = 7 days) of the S_tex samples group was close to 60% higher compared to that for the S_is samples group, confirming the lower corrosion resistance of samples after laser texturing as indicated by the EIS and potentiodynamic tests (Table 6). Moreover, the deposition of PCL and PCL/TiO$_2$ nanofiber layers on the Ti-6Al-4V titanium alloy surface via the electrospinning method was observed to offer effective protection against the release of Ti-6Al-4V alloy elemental ions into the corrosive environment (human organism). The lowest amount of released ions was observed for the S_PCL/TiO$_2$ samples group. Moreover, the protective properties of the PCL or PCL/TiO$_2$ nanofiber layers on laser-textured surfaces were observed.

Table 6. Results of ICP-AES analysis.

No	Name	Release Ions (mg/L)		
		Ti	V	Al
1	S_is	1.03	0.06	0.07
2	S_tex	1.63	0.06	0.09
3	S_PCL	0.91	0.04	0.05
4	S_PCL/TiO$_2$	0.67	0.03	0.05
5	S_tex/PCL	0.80	0.04	0.05
6	S_tex/PCL/TiO$_2$	0.82	0.05	0.05

3.6. Cytotoxicity Tests

The results of the microbiological tests for all tested samples are presented in Figure 10. The objective of the test was to evaluate the toxicity of the examined materials intended for potential use as biomaterials. Toxicity is characterized by the ability of a material to disrupt the functioning or cause the death of body cells. Initial signs of these changes manifest in abnormal cell metabolism, and the extent of this phenomenon can be assessed using the MTT test. The results are depicted in graphs illustrating the correlation between the average viability (expressed in %) and the incubation time of cells with the tested material.

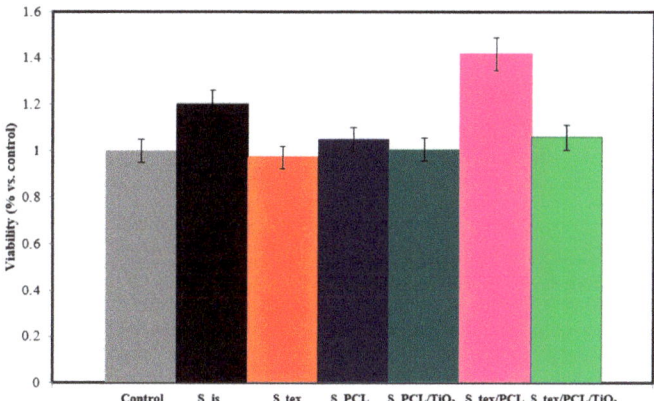

Figure 10. Results of microbiological test t = 72 h.

After 72 h, for the S_is, S_tex, S_PCL, S_PCL/TiO$_2$, S_tex/PCL, and S_tex/PCL/TiO$_2$ samples group, the average cell viability of HCT116 cells was 120, 97, 104, 101, 141, and 105%, respectively, compared to the control sample (100%). The obtained results indicate that all samples except S_is and S_tex/PCL do not affect the proliferation of cancer cells. The percentage viability fraction for these materials was approximately 5% of the difference compared to the control sample. This change is too low to suggest that the mentioned materials may have features that stimulate the growth of cancer cells. Any observed changes are likely caused by environmental factors and the accuracy of the test equipment. The only result that differs significantly from the others is the survival fraction of HCT116 cells for the S_tex/PCL sample groups. In this case, an increase in cell proliferation by over 41% was observed compared to the control sample. The duration of the experiment is also important. In the initial period of culture (first 24 h), a decrease in cell viability is often observed. This can be elucidated by the cellular stress induced by the introduction of a foreign element into the medium, such as the tested sample, along with the partial mechanical damage incurred by a specific number of cells during the sample implementation in the culture. After 72 h, the cell count in the culture rises, which can be attributed to the alleviation of cellular stress and the proliferation of cells under favorable conditions in the laboratory. The analysis of the microbiological results after 72 h showed that none of the tested samples exhibited cytotoxicity. It can be stated that the smallest number of cells multiplied after t = 72 h occurred in the case of the S_tex and S_PCL samples group. It can be assumed that the deposition of a layer of PCL and TiO$_2$ has a better effect on cell proliferation compared to the deposition of a layer with only PCL.

4. Conclusions

Based on the obtained results, it was found that the hybrid surface modification of the Ti-6Al-4V titanium alloy by laser texturing and PCL or PCL/TiO$_2$ nanofiber layer deposition using the electrospinning method improves the biofunctional properties of the proposed biomaterial. An increase in the wetting angle and corrosion resistance was observed. Additionally, non-toxic properties of the tested surface conditions were recorded. Future research is planned, to continue exploring these promising findings.

Author Contributions: Conceptualization, A.W. and W.S.; methodology, A.W. and W.S.; software, A.W., W.S. and M.S.; validation, A.W., J.S. and G.C.; formal analysis, J.S.; investigation, A.W., W.S. and M.S.; writing—original draft preparation, A.W., W.S. and G.C.; writing—review and editing, A.W. and J.S.; visualization, A.W., W.S. and M.S.; supervision, A.W., W.S., J.S. and M.S.; project administration, A.W.; funding acquisition, A.W. and G.C. All authors have read and agreed to the published version of the manuscript.

Funding: This research received no external funding.

Institutional Review Board Statement: Not applicable.

Informed Consent Statement: Not applicable.

Data Availability Statement: The data presented in this study are available upon request from the appropriate author. The research results are presented in the article, and the data obtained during the tests are private.

Conflicts of Interest: The authors declare no conflicts of interest.

References

1. Hamidi, M.F.F.A.; Harun, W.S.W.; Samykano, M.; Ghani, S.A.C.; Ghazalli, Z.; Ahmad, F.; Sulong, A.B. A review of biocompatible metal injection moulding process parameters for biomedical applications. *Mater. Sci. Eng. C* **2017**, *78*, 1263–1276. [CrossRef]
2. Li, K.; Yao, W.; Xie, Y.; Zhang, J.; Li, B.; Wan, Z.; Zhang, Z.; Lu, L.; Tang, Y. A strongly hydrophobic and serum-repelling surface composed of CrN films deposited on laser-patterned microstructures that was optimized with an orthogonal experiment. *Surf. Coat. Technol.* **2020**, *391*, 125708. [CrossRef]
3. Hedberg, Y.S. Role of proteins in the degradation of relatively inert alloys in the human body. *npj Mater. Degrad.* **2018**, *2*, 26. [CrossRef]
4. Ionescu, F.; Reclaru, L.; Ardelean, L.C.; Blatter, A. Comparative analysis of the corrosion resistance of titanium alloys intended to come into direct or prolonged contact with live tissues. *Materials* **2019**, *12*, 2841. [CrossRef] [PubMed]
5. Yu, F.; Addison, O.; Davenport, A.J. A synergistic effect of albumin and H_2O_2 accelerates corrosion of Ti6Al4V. *Acta Biomater.* **2015**, *26*, 355–365. [CrossRef] [PubMed]
6. Woźniak, A.; Walke, W.; Jakóbik-Kolon, A.; Ziębowicz, B.; Brytan, Z.; Adamiak, M. The Influence of ZnO Oxide Layer on the Physicochemical Behavior of Ti6Al4V Titanium Alloy. *Materials* **2021**, *14*, 230. [CrossRef] [PubMed]
7. Wang, C.; Tian, P.; Cao, H.; Sun, B.; Yan, J.; Xue, Y.; Lin, T.; Ren, T.; Han, S.; Zhao, X. Enhanced Biotribological and Anticorrosion Properties and Bioactivity of Ti6Al4V Alloys with Laser Texturing. *ACS Omega* **2022**, *7*, 31081–31097. [CrossRef] [PubMed]
8. Iwabuchi, A.; Lee, J.W.; Uchidate, M. Synergistic effect of fretting wear and sliding wear of Co-alloy and Ti-alloy in Hanks' solution. *Wear* **2007**, *263*, 492–500. [CrossRef]
9. Beake, B.D.; Liskiewicz, T.W. Comparison of nano-frètting and nano-scratch tests on biomedical materials. *Tribol. Int.* **2013**, *63*, 123–131. [CrossRef]
10. Babis, G.C.; Stavropoulos, N.A.; Sasalos, G.; Ochsenkuehn-Petropoulou, M.; Megas, P. Metallosis and elevated serum levels of tantalum following failed revision hip arthroplasty—A case report. *Acta Orthop.* **2014**, *85*, 677–680. [CrossRef]
11. Kao, W.H.; Su, Y.L.; Horng, J.H.; Chang, C.Y. Tribological, electrochemical and biocompatibility properties of Ti6Al4V alloy produced by selective laser melting method and then processed using gas nitriding, CN or Ti-C:H coating treatments. *Surf. Coat. Technol.* **2018**, *350*, 172–187. [CrossRef]
12. Conradi, M.; Kocijan, A.; Klobčar, D.; Podgornik, B. Tribological response of laser-textured Ti6Al4V alloy under dry conditions and lubricated with Hank's solution. *Tribol. Int.* **2021**, *160*, 107049. [CrossRef]
13. Ye, Y.; Wang, C.; Chen, H.; Wang, Y.; Zhao, W.; Mu, Y. Micro/Nanotexture Design for Improving Tribological Properties of Cr/GLC Films in Seawater. *Tribol. Trans.* **2017**, *60*, 95–105. [CrossRef]
14. Tewelde, F.B.; Zhou, T.; Zhou, J.; Guo, W.; Zhao, B.; Ge, X.; Wang, W.; Wang, X.; Wang, X. Asymmetric surface texturing for directional friction control under dry sliding condition. *Tribol. Int.* **2023**, *181*, 108321. [CrossRef]
15. Song, S.; Xiao, G.; Liu, Y.; Zhou, K.; Liu, S.; Huang, J. Tribological response of groove-textured surface with compressive stress on Ti6Al4V processed by laser and abrasive belt. *Tribol. Int.* **2023**, *180*, 108265. [CrossRef]
16. Wang, C.; Hong, J.; Cui, M.; Huang, H.; Zhang, L.; Yan, J. The effects of simultaneous laser nitriding and texturing on surface hardness and tribological properties of Ti6Al4V. *Surf. Coat. Technol.* **2022**, *437*, 128358. [CrossRef]
17. Huang, J.; Guan, Y.; Ramakrishna, S. Tribological behavior of femtosecond laser-textured leaded brass. *Tribol. Int.* **2021**, *162*, 107115. [CrossRef]
18. Dinesh Babu, P.; Vignesh, S.; Vignesh, M.; Balamurugan, C. Enhancement of wear resistance of Ti—6Al—4V alloy by picosecond laser surface micro texturing process. *J. Cent. South Univ.* **2018**, *25*, 1836–1848. [CrossRef]
19. Conradi, M.; Kocijan, A.; Klobčar, D.; Godec, M. Influence of Laser Texturing on Microstructure, Surface and Corrosion Properties of Ti-6Al-4V. *Metals* **2020**, *10*, 1504. [CrossRef]
20. Sadeghi, M.; Kharaziha, M.; Salimijazi, H.R.; Tabesh, E. Role of micro-dimple array geometry on the biological and tribological performance of Ti6Al4V for biomedical applications. *Surf. Coat. Technol.* **2019**, *362*, 282–292. [CrossRef]
21. Erdemir, A. Review of engineered tribological interfaces for improved boundary lubrication. *Tribol. Int.* **2005**, *38*, 249–256. [CrossRef]
22. Chebolu, A.; Laha, B.; Ghosh, M.; Nagahanumaiah. Investigation on bacterial adhesion and colonisation resistance over laser-machined micro patterned surfaces. *Micro Nano Lett.* **2013**, *8*, 280–283. [CrossRef]

23. Veiko, V.; Karlagina, Y.; Zernitckaia, E.; Egorova, E.; Radaev, M.; Yaremenko, A.; Chernenko, G.; Romanov, V.; Shchedrina, N.; Ivanova, E.; et al. Laser-Induced μ-Rooms for Osteocytes on Implant Surface: An In Vivo Study. *Nanomaterials* **2022**, *12*, 4229. [CrossRef] [PubMed]
24. Nathanael, A.J.; Oh, T.H. Biopolymer Coatings for Biomedical Applications. *Polymers* **2020**, *12*, 3061. [CrossRef] [PubMed]
25. Pallickal Babu, S.; Sam, S.; Joseph, B.; Kalarikkal, N.; Radhakrishnan, E.K.; Nair, R.; Thomas, S. Nanoscale polymer coatings for biomedical implants. In *Polymer-Based Nanoscale Materials for Surface Coatings*; Elsevier: Amsterdam, The Netherlands, 2023; pp. 435–457. [CrossRef]
26. Wang, T.; Xu, Y.; Liu, Z.; Li, G.; Guo, Y.; Lian, J.; Zhang, Z.; Ren, L. A chitosan/polylactic acid composite coating enhancing the corrosion resistance of the bio-degradable magnesium alloy. *Prog. Org. Coat.* **2023**, *178*, 107469. [CrossRef]
27. Ghanbari, A.; Bordbar-Khiabani, A.; Warchomicka, F.; Sommitsch, C.; Yarmand, B.; Zamanian, A. PEO/Polymer hybrid coatings on magnesium alloy to improve biodegradation and biocompatibility properties. *Surf. Interfaces* **2023**, *36*, 102495. [CrossRef]
28. Alabbasi, A.; Liyanaarachchi, S.; Kannan, M.B. Polylactic acid coating on a biodegradable magnesium alloy: An in vitro degradation study by electrochemical impedance spectroscopy. *Thin Solid Film.* **2012**, *520*, 6841–6844. [CrossRef]
29. Liu, S.; Chen, C.; Chen, L.; Zhu, H.; Zhang, C.; Wang, Y. Pseudopeptide polymer coating for improving biocompatibility and corrosion resistance of 316L stainless steel. *RSC Adv.* **2015**, *5*, 98456–98466. [CrossRef]
30. Zhu, Y.; Liu, W.; Ngai, T. Polymer coatings on magnesium-based implants for orthopedic applications. *J. Polym. Sci.* **2022**, *60*, 32–51. [CrossRef]
31. Huang, Z.M.; Zhang, Y.Z.; Kotaki, M.; Ramakrishna, S. A review on polymer nanofibers by electrospinning and their applications in nanocomposites. *Compos. Sci. Technol.* **2003**, *63*, 2223–2253. [CrossRef]
32. Matysiak, W.; Tanski, T.; Smok, W. Electrospinning as a Versatile Method of Composite Thin Films Fabrication for Selected Applications. *Solid State Phenom.* **2019**, *293*, 35–49. [CrossRef]
33. Chen, Z.; Zhang, Z.; Ouyang, Y.; Chen, Y.; Yin, X.; Liu, Y.; Ying, H.; Yang, W. Electrospinning polycaprolactone/collagen fiber coatings for enhancing the corrosion resistance and biocompatibility of AZ31 Mg alloys. *Colloids Surf. A Physicochem. Eng. Asp.* **2023**, *662*, 131041. [CrossRef]
34. Abdal-hay, A.; Barakat, N.A.M.; Lim, J.K. Influence of electrospinning and dip-coating techniques on the degradation and cytocompatibility of Mg-based alloy. *Colloids Surf. A Physicochem. Eng. Asp.* **2013**, *420*, 37–45. [CrossRef]
35. Vurat, M.T.; Elçin, A.E.; Elçin, Y.M. Osteogenic composite nanocoating based on nanohydroxyapatite, strontium ranelate and polycaprolactone for titanium implants. *Trans. Nonferrous Met. Soc. China* **2018**, *28*, 1763–1773. [CrossRef]
36. Karthega, M.; Pranesh, M.; Poongothai, C.; Srinivasan, N. Poly caprolactone/titanium dioxide nanofiber coating on AM50 alloy for biomedical application. *J. Magnes. Alloys* **2021**, *9*, 532–547. [CrossRef]
37. Kim, J.; Mousa, H.M.; Park, C.H.; Kim, C.S. Enhanced corrosion resistance and biocompatibility of AZ31 Mg alloy using PCL/ZnO NPs via electrospinning. *Appl. Surf. Sci.* **2017**, *396*, 249–258. [CrossRef]
38. Rajabi, T.; Naffakh-Moosavy, H.; Bagheri, F.; Sadrnezhaad, S.K.; Pour, H.M. Tailoring metallurgical and biological characteristics of Ti–6Al–4V alloy by synergetic application of Nd:YAG laser and drug-loaded electrospun PVA. *J. Mater. Res. Technol.* **2023**, *24*, 3759–3771. [CrossRef]
39. Camargo, E.R.; Serafim, B.M.; da Cruz, A.F.; Soares, P.; de Oliveira, C.C.; Saul, C.K.; Marino, C.E.B. Bioactive response of PMMA coating obtained by electrospinning on ISO5832-9 and Ti6Al4V biomaterials. *Surf. Coat. Technol.* **2021**, *412*, 127033. [CrossRef]
40. Huerta-Murillo, D.; García-Girón, A.; Romano, J.M.; Cardoso, J.T.; Cordovilla, F.; Walker, M.; Dimov, S.S.; Ocaña, J.L. Wettability modification of laser-fabricated hierarchical surface structures in Ti-6Al-4V titanium alloy. *Appl. Surf. Sci.* **2019**, *463*, 838–846. [CrossRef]
41. Santhosh, S.; Balasivanandha Prabu, S. Nano hydroxyapatite-polysulfone coating on Ti-6Al-4V substrate by electrospinning. *Int. J. Mater. Res.* **2013**, *104*, 1254–1262. [CrossRef]
42. Cho, S.J.; Kim, B.; An, T.; Lim, G. Replicable multilayered nanofibrous patterns on a flexible film. *Langmuir* **2010**, *26*, 14395–14399. [CrossRef] [PubMed]
43. Martinez-Prieto, N.; Ehmann, K.; Cao, J. Near-field electrospinning on nonconductive substrates using AC fields. *Procedia CIRP* **2020**, *93*, 120–124. [CrossRef]
44. Choi, W.S.; Kim, G.H.; Shin, J.H.; Lim, G.; An, T. Electrospinning onto Insulating Substrates by Controlling Surface Wettability and Humidity. *Nanoscale Res. Lett.* **2017**, *12*, 610. [CrossRef]
45. Gittens, R.A.; Scheideler, L.; Rupp, F.; Hyzy, S.L.; Geis-Gerstorfer, J.; Schwartz, Z.; Boyan, B.D. A review on the wettability of dental implant surfaces II: Biological and clinical aspects. *Acta Biomater.* **2014**, *10*, 2907–2918. [CrossRef] [PubMed]
46. Melo-Fonseca, F.; Guimarães, B.; Gasik, M.; Silva, F.S.; Miranda, G. Experimental analysis and predictive modelling of Ti6Al4V laser surface texturing for biomedical applications. *Surf. Interfaces* **2022**, *35*, 102466. [CrossRef]
47. Reggio, C.; Barberi, J.; Ferraris, S.; Spriano, S. Functionalization of Ti6Al4V Alloy with Polyphenols: The Role of the Titanium Surface Features and the Addition of Calcium Ions on the Adsorption Mechanism. *Metals* **2023**, *13*, 1347. [CrossRef]
48. Sheela, S.; AlGhalban, F.M.; Khalil, K.A.; Laoui, T.; Gopinath, V.K. Synthesis and Biocompatibility Evaluation of PCL Electrospun Membranes Coated with MTA/HA for Potential Application in Dental Pulp Capping. *Polymers* **2022**, *14*, 4862. [CrossRef]
49. Sahoo, B.N.; Kandasubramanian, B.; Thomas, A. Effect of TiO_2 Powder on the Surface Morphology of Micro/Nanoporous Structured Hydrophobic Fluoropolymer Based Composite Material. *J. Polym.* **2013**, *2013*, 615045. [CrossRef]

50. Ogihara, H.; Xie, J.; Saji, T. Factors determining wettability of superhydrophobic paper prepared by spraying nanoparticle suspensions. *Colloids Surf. A Physicochem. Eng. Asp.* **2013**, *434*, 35–41. [CrossRef]
51. Yamauchi, R.; Itabashi, T.; Wada, K.; Tanaka, T.; Kumagai, G.; Ishibashi, Y. Photofunctionalised Ti6Al4V implants enhance early phase osseointegration. *Bone Jt. Res.* **2017**, *6*, 331–336. [CrossRef]
52. Khan, S.; Azimi, G.; Yildiz, B.; Varanasi, K.K. Role of surface oxygen-to-metal ratio on the wettability of rare-earth oxides. *Appl. Phys. Lett.* **2015**, *106*, 061601. [CrossRef]
53. Oliveira, V.M.C.A.; Aguiar, C.; Vazquez, A.M.; Robin, A.; Barboza, M.J.R. Improving corrosion resistance of Ti–6Al–4V alloy through plasma-assisted PVD deposited nitride coatings. *Corros. Sci.* **2014**, *88*, 317–327. [CrossRef]
54. Dai, N.; Zhang, L.C.; Zhang, J.; Zhang, X.; Ni, Q.; Chen, Y.; Wu, M.; Yang, C. Distinction in corrosion resistance of selective laser melted Ti-6Al-4V alloy on different planes. *Corros. Sci.* **2016**, *111*, 703–710. [CrossRef]
55. Woźniak, A.; Adamiak, M.; Ziębowicz, B. The Surface Morphology and Electrochemical Properties of Pure Titanium Obtained by Selective Laser Melting Method. *Solid State Phenom.* **2020**, *308*, 21–32. [CrossRef]
56. Woźniak, A.; Staszuk, M.; Reimann, Ł.; Bialas, O.; Brytan, Z.; Voinarovych, S.; Kyslytsia, O.; Kaliuzhnyi, S.; Basiaga, M.; Admiak, M. The influence of plasma-sprayed coatings on surface properties and corrosion resistance of 316L stainless steel for possible implant application. *Arch. Civ. Mech. Eng.* **2021**, *21*, 148. [CrossRef]
57. Woźniak, A.; Adamiak, M.; Chladek, G.; Bonek, M.; Walke, W.; Bialas, O. The Influence of Hybrid Surface Modification on the Selected Properties of CP Titanium Grade II Manufactured by Selective Laser Melting. *Materials* **2020**, *13*, 2829. [CrossRef] [PubMed]
58. Kadowaki, N.T.; Martinez, G.A.S.; Robin, A. Electrochemical behavior of three CP titanium dental implants in artificial saliva. *Mater. Res.* **2009**, *12*, 363–366. [CrossRef]
59. Annamalai, M.; Gopinadhan, K.; Han, S.A.; Saha, S.; Park, H.J.; Cho, E.B.; Kumar, B.; Patra, A.; Kim, S.W.; Venkatesan, T. Surface energy and wettability of van der Waals structures. *Nanoscale* **2016**, *8*, 5764–5770. [CrossRef]
60. Yue, L.; Wang, Z.; Li, L. Material morphological characteristics in laser ablation of alpha case from titanium alloy. *Appl. Surf. Sci.* **2012**, *258*, 8065–8071. [CrossRef]
61. Bussoli, M.; Desai, T.; Batani, D.; Gakovic, B.; Trtica, M. Nd:YAG laser interaction with titanium implant surfaces for medical applications. *Radiat. Eff. Defects Solids* **2008**, *163*, 349–356. [CrossRef]
62. Kosec, T.; Legat, A.; Kovač, J.; Klobčar, D. Influence of Laser Colour Marking on the Corrosion Properties of Low Alloyed Ti. *Coatings* **2019**, *9*, 375. [CrossRef]
63. Xu, Y.; Li, Z.; Zhang, G.; Wang, G.; Zeng, Z.; Wang, C.; Wang, C.; Zhao, S.; Zhang, Y.; Ren, T. Electrochemical corrosion and anisotropic tribological properties of bioinspired hierarchical morphologies on Ti-6Al-4V fabricated by laser texturing. *Tribol. Int.* **2019**, *134*, 352–364. [CrossRef]
64. Pfleging, W.; Kumari, R.; Besser, H.; Scharnweber, T.; Majumdar, J.D. Laser surface textured titanium alloy (Ti–6Al–4V): Part 1—Surface characterization. *Appl. Surf. Sci.* **2015**, *355*, 104–111. [CrossRef]
65. Grabowski, A.; Sozańska, M.; Adamiak, M.; Kępińska, M.; Florian, T. Laser surface texturing of Ti6Al4V alloy, stainless steel and aluminium silicon alloy. *Appl. Surf. Sci.* **2018**, *461*, 117–123. [CrossRef]
66. Wang, C.; Li, Z.; Zhao, H.; Zhang, G.; Ren, T.; Zhang, Y. Enhanced anticorrosion and antiwear properties of Ti–6Al–4V alloys with laser texture and graphene oxide coatings. *Tribol. Int.* **2020**, *152*, 106475. [CrossRef]
67. Brittain, H.G.; Barbera, G.; DeVincentis, J.; Newman, A.W. Titanium Dioxide. *Anal. Profiles Drug Subst. Excip.* **1992**, *21*, 659–691. [CrossRef]
68. Ziębowicz, A.; Woźniak, A.; Ziębowicz, B.; Kosiel, K.; Chladek, G. The Effect of Atomic Layer Deposition of ZrO_2 on the Physicochemical Properties of Cobalt based Alloys Intended for Prosthetic Dentistry. *Arch. Metall. Mater.* **2018**, *63*, 1077–1082. [CrossRef] [PubMed]
69. Woźniak, A.; Bialas, O.; Adamiak, M. Improvement of the properties of Ti6Al7Nb titanium alloy in terms of the type of surface modification. *Arch. Metall. Mater.* **2020**, *65*, 735–741. [CrossRef]
70. Palanisamy, M.S.; Kulandaivelu, R.; Nellaiappan, S.N.T.S. Improving the corrosion resistance and bioactivity of magnesium by a carbonate conversion-polycaprolactone duplex coating approach. *New J. Chem.* **2020**, *44*, 4772–4785. [CrossRef]
71. Mojarad Shafiee, B.; Torkaman, R.; Mahmoudi, M.; Emadi, R.; Karamian, E. An improvement in corrosion resistance of 316L AISI coated using PCL-gelatin composite by dip-coating method. *Prog. Org. Coat.* **2019**, *130*, 200–205. [CrossRef]
72. Singh, N.; Batra, U.; Kumar, K.; Mahapatro, A. Investigating TiO_2–HA–PCL hybrid coating as an efficient corrosion resistant barrier of ZM21 Mg alloy. *J. Magnes. Alloys* **2021**, *9*, 627–646. [CrossRef]
73. Dǎnǎilǎ, E.; Benea, L. The effect of surface roughness on corrosion behavior of Ti-6Al-4V alloy in saliva solution. In Proceedings of the 2015 E-Health and Bioengineering Conference (EHB), Iasi, Romania, 19–21 November 2015. [CrossRef]
74. Jeong, C.; Choi, C.-H.; Sheppard, K. Nano-Engineering of Superhydrophobic Aluminum Surfaces for Anti-Corrosion. Ph.D. Thesis, Stevens Institute of Technology, Hoboken, NJ, USA, 2013. Volume 115.
75. Zhang, F.; Zhao, L.; Chen, H.; Xu, S.; Evans, D.G.; Duan, X.; Zhang, F.; Zhao, L.L.; Chen, H.Y.; Xu, S.L.; et al. Corrosion Resistance of Superhydrophobic Layered Double Hydroxide Films on Aluminum. *Angew. Chem.* **2008**, *120*, 2500–2503. [CrossRef]
76. Acatay, K.; Simsek, E.; Ow-Yang, C.; Menceloglu, Y.Z.; Acatay, K.; Simsek, E.; Ow-Yang, C.; Menceloglu, Y.Z. Tunable, Superhydrophobically Stable Polymeric Surfaces by Electrospinning. *Angew. Chem.* **2004**, *116*, 5322–5325. [CrossRef]

77. Ning, T.; Xu, W.; Lu, S. Fabrication of superhydrophobic surfaces on zinc substrates and their application as effective corrosion barriers. *Appl. Surf. Sci.* **2011**, *258*, 1359–1365. [CrossRef]
78. Zhang, F.; Chen, S.; Dong, L.; Lei, Y.; Liu, T.; Yin, Y. Preparation of superhydrophobic films on titanium as effective corrosion barriers. *Appl. Surf. Sci.* **2011**, *257*, 2587–2591. [CrossRef]
79. Khoshnood, N.; Frampton, J.P.; Alavi Zaree, S.R.; Jahanpanah, M.; Heydari, P.; Zamanian, A. The corrosion and biological behavior of 3D-printed polycaprolactone/chitosan scaffolds as protective coating for Mg alloy implants. *Surf. Coat. Technol.* **2024**, *477*, 130368. [CrossRef]
80. Catauro, M.; Bollino, F.; Giovanardi, R.; Veronesi, P. Modification of Ti_6Al_4V implant surfaces by biocompatible TiO_2/PCL hybrid layers prepared via sol-gel dip coating: Structural characterization, mechanical and corrosion behavior. *Mater. Sci. Eng. C* **2017**, *74*, 501–507. [CrossRef] [PubMed]
81. Asri, R.I.M.; Harun, W.S.W.; Samykano, M.; Lah, N.A.C.; Ghani, S.A.C.; Tarlochan, F.; Raza, M.R. Corrosion and surface modification on biocompatible metals: A review. *Mater. Sci. Eng. C* **2017**, *77*, 1261–1274. [CrossRef] [PubMed]
82. Chen, Q.; Thouas, G.A. Metallic implant biomaterials. *Mater. Sci. Eng. R Rep.* **2015**, *87*, 1–57. [CrossRef]
83. Rautray, T.R.; Narayanan, R.; Kim, K.H. Ion implantation of titanium based biomaterials. *Prog. Mater. Sci.* **2011**, *56*, 1137–1177. [CrossRef]
84. Tsai, W.T.; Lin, C.L.; Pan, S.J. Susceptibility of Ti-6Al-4V alloy to stress corrosion cracking in a Lewis-neutral aluminium chloride-1-ethyl-3-methylimidazolium chloride ionic liquid. *Corros. Sci.* **2013**, *76*, 494–497. [CrossRef]

Disclaimer/Publisher's Note: The statements, opinions and data contained in all publications are solely those of the individual author(s) and contributor(s) and not of MDPI and/or the editor(s). MDPI and/or the editor(s) disclaim responsibility for any injury to people or property resulting from any ideas, methods, instructions or products referred to in the content.

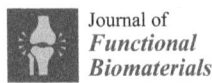

Journal of *Functional Biomaterials*

Article

Assessment of the Penetration of an Endodontic Sealer into Dentinal Tubules with Three Different Compaction Techniques Using Confocal Laser Scanning Microscopy

Ignacio Barbero-Navarro [1,2], Diego Velázquez-González [1], María Esther Irigoyen-Camacho [3,*], Marco Antonio Zepeda-Zepeda [3], Paulo Mauricio [4], David Ribas-Perez [2,*] and Antonio Castano-Seiquer [2]

1. Dental School, University Institute Egas Moniz (IUEM), 2800-064 Almada, Portugal; ibarbero2@us.es (I.B.-N.)
2. Dental School, University of Seville, 41009 Seville, Spain; acastano@us.es
3. Health Care Department, Autonomous Metropolitan University-Xochimilco, Mexico City 04960, Mexico; mzepeda@correo.xoc.uam.mx
4. Interdisciplinary Research Centre, University Institute Egas Moniz (IUEM), 2800-064 Almada, Portugal
* Correspondence: meirigo@correo.xoc.uam.mx (M.E.I.-C.); dribas@us.es (D.R.-P.)

Abstract: Adequate root canal sealing is essential for the success of endodontic treatment. There are numerous techniques available; identifying simple and efficient techniques is important to provide good patient care. The purpose of the study was to compare the maximum penetration depth and the percentage of sealant penetration of an endodontic sealer into dentine tubules using cold lateral condensation, continuous wave, and hybrid techniques, and to contrast the effectiveness of two different tapered gutta-percha master cones (0.02 and 0.04). A sample of sixty single root teeth was used. Six experimental groups were formed from the three filling techniques and the two tapered master cones. Images were acquired using a confocal laser scanning microscope. In the apical root third, the penetration percentage was higher in the hybrid compared with the continuous wave technique. The results indicated a higher penetration depth of hybrid compared with cold lateral condensation in the middle and coronal thirds, and in the apical third, a higher penetration was identified in the hybrid group compared with the continuous wave group. No significant differences in penetration were found comparing 0.02 with 0.04 taper gutta-percha groups. The coronal cross-sections presented a higher penetration than the apical third sections. In conclusion, the hybrid technique a had higher maximum sealer penetration than the continuous wave in the apical third, and the coronal third hybrid and continuous wave had a higher penetration than cold lateral condensation.

Keywords: endodontic obturation; obturation technique; sealers' penetration depth; dentin tubule penetration; confocal laser scanning microscope

Citation: Barbero-Navarro, I.; Velázquez-González, D.; Irigoyen-Camacho, M.E.; Zepeda-Zepeda, M.A.; Mauricio, P.; Ribas-Perez, D.; Castano-Seiquer, A. Assessment of the Penetration of an Endodontic Sealer into Dentinal Tubules with Three Different Compaction Techniques Using Confocal Laser Scanning Microscopy. *J. Funct. Biomater.* **2023**, *14*, 542. https://doi.org/10.3390/jfb14110542

Academic Editors: Lavinia Cosmina Ardelean and Laura-Cristina Rusu

Received: 11 October 2023
Revised: 31 October 2023
Accepted: 3 November 2023
Published: 7 November 2023

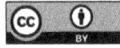

Copyright: © 2023 by the authors. Licensee MDPI, Basel, Switzerland. This article is an open access article distributed under the terms and conditions of the Creative Commons Attribution (CC BY) license (https://creativecommons.org/licenses/by/4.0/).

1. Introduction

Successful root canal treatment requires an impermeable tridimensional seal along the root canal's length, thereby ensuring the healing of periapical tissues and preventing intracanal recontamination from coronal leakage [1]. The techniques for root canal filling have improved; however, there are still challenges, such as inadequately prepared areas affecting the adaptation of obturation material [2], apical extrusion of gutta-percha and sealer, difficulty in performing the technique, the lack of hermetic sealing leading to favorable environments for bacterial colonization, and the challenge of addressing obturations in the face of different anatomical variations within endodontic spaces, ranging from oval and curved canals to lateral canals, isthmuses, and other issues, resulting in obturation failure.

The cold lateral condensation technique remains the most accepted approach for root canal filling, being a reliable technique that may be used in most cases [3]. An important advantage of cold lateral condensation is the controlled placement of the gutta-percha in the canal [4]. Additionally, it is frequently used for comparison with other compaction techniques [5]. However, cold lateral condensation has some limitations, such as potential deficiencies in gutta-percha mass homogeneity, partial filling in certain hard-to-reach areas of the root canal system, and, in the case of fragile teeth, there is a risk of root fractures [6–8].

Techniques based on gutta-percha heating were introduced to improve the three-dimensional filling of root canal systems. Schilder [9] developed a technique using heat and vertical condensation. This was modified, and the continuous wave condensation technique was introduced [10]. Root canal obturation with injected thermoplasticized gutta-percha was presented by Yee et al. [11] Subsequently, Tagger [12] developed a hybrid technique combining mechanical and thermal obturation with cold lateral condensation.

Thermoplastic methods offer the benefit of achieving good adaptation to the root canal walls and require less treatment time when compared to cold lateral condensation. Nevertheless, there is a possibility of gutta-percha undergoing physicochemical changes with the use of this technique. Thermomechanical compaction has demonstrated commendable adaptation, especially within the middle and coronal thirds of the root. Although there is limited supporting evidence regarding the effectiveness of a hybrid approach combining cold lateral condensation in the apical third and thermoplastic techniques in the middle and coronal thirds of the root canal, it has the potential to harness the advantages of both techniques. Yet, the assessment of filling quality in hybrid condensation techniques has yielded inconclusive findings [13,14].

The introduction of the nickel-titanium (Ni-Ti) rotary instruments in root canal preparation can improve the results and reduce the time required during the canal's instrumentation. Rotary instruments may help maintain the root canals' original curvature, shape, and patency [15,16]. To match up with the various tapers of Ni-Ti instruments, firms have produced gutta-percha with a large taper (0.04 and 0.06). Gordon [17] found that higher taper gutta-percha points had better adaptation in a study of filling efficacy and reduced the time required for filling the canal compared with the standard tapered cones, using the cold lateral condensation. Nevertheless, some studies found different results [18,19].

A high percentage of endodontic sealer penetration may be an indirect indicator of potential resistance to microbial and fluid filtration between the canalicular system and the periapex, favoring three-dimensional obturations. Several factors may influence sealer penetration, including the effectiveness of the removal of the smear layer, [20] the anatomy of the root canal system, [21,22] the obturation techniques, [23] the physical and chemical properties of the sealer, [24] and the gutta-percha characteristics [17]. Confocal laser scanning microscopy (CLSM) is considered an appropriate technique for evaluating the amount of sealer that has penetrated the dentinal tubules [17,25].

The root filling efficacy of various compaction techniques employing gutta-percha points has yielded inconclusive findings, particularly in the context of hybrid techniques and the influence of different tapered gutta-percha master cones. This study postulates two key hypotheses. Firstly, it is hypothesized that the hybrid compaction technique will yield superior results in terms of root canal sealing when compared to the cold lateral compaction and continuous wave techniques. Secondly, the second hypothesis posits that the utilization of more tapered gutta-percha master cones (0.04) will result in improved sealing proficiency compared to their less tapered counterparts (0.02), leading to greater sealant penetration within the root canal dental tubules.

Accordingly, this study aims to compare the maximum sealer penetration depth and the percentage of sealer penetration into dentinal tubules using three condensation techniques: cold lateral condensation, continuous wave, and a hybrid, while employing two different tapered gutta-percha master cones (0.02 and 0.04).

2. Materials and Methods

The Ethics Committee of the Egas Moniz University Instituteo (CIIEM), Portugal, approved the study protocol (CEPI/0893). The sample size was calculated for the percent of sealer penetration using cold lateral condensation as a reference technique, and information from a confocal study [26], with a mean of 73 and a standard deviation of 8.7; we assumed that the experimental technique (hybrid) had a higher standard deviation (sd 14) than the reference technique. The effect size established was 15 percent points. The type I error alpha was set at 0.05 and the power (1 − β) was 0.80. The sample size obtained was n = 10. The STATA V17 (StataCorp LLC, College Station, TX, USA) program used a sample size calculation.

The root specimens for laboratory tests were obtained from Egas Moniz Instituto Universitrio CIIEM. Sixty extracted fully developed human teeth with single, straight canals were selected and radiographically examined (Kodak 2100; Kodak Dental Systems, Atlanta, GA, USA) with a Trophy RVG Ultimate 6100 digital sensor (Kodak Dental Systems, Atlanta, GA, USA) from facial and proximal views to ensure the presence of a single canal and to evaluate the root canal morphology. The study applied inclusion criteria, which required teeth to be erupted with fully developed apices and straight root canals. Exclusion criteria included teeth with visible root cracks, fractures, calcified root canals, or dental caries affecting the root portion of the tooth. Furthermore, teeth with dental development anomalies were also excluded. The teeth were stored in a 0.2% sodium azide solution.

2.1. Root Canal Preparation and Filling

The root length was standardized as 12 mm from the apex and cut with a 910P diamond disc (Drewdel Zweilinf, Berlin, Germany). The roots were debrided with ultrasonic scalers and washed with distilled water. Subsequently, they were immersed for 15 min at room temperature in a 6% NaOCl solution to remove the remaining organic debris, following Gharib protocol [27].

The working length of each canal was established by measuring the penetration of a 10 K-file (Flexofile; Dentsply Maillefer, Ballaigues, Switzerland) until it reached the apical foramen and then subtracting 0.5 mm. The canal spaces were cleaned and mechanically shaped with Mtwo rotary system files (VDW, Munich, Germany) in conjunction with Slick-Gel ES (SybronEndo Company, Orange, CA, USA) and 1.8 mL 5.25% sodium hypochlorite (NaOCl) between each file size. A handpiece was used with an electric engine (X-Smart; Dentsply Maillefer, Ballaigues, Switzerland) at 280 rpm. The manufacturer's recommendations were followed during the root canal preparation. All the canals were enlarged to an ISO size 35, 0.04 taper, to working length.

A dentist instrumented all the teeth. Apical patency was maintained throughout the instrumentation using a #10 K-file (Flexofile; Dentsply Maillefer, Ballaigues, Switzerland). After preparation, the canals were irrigated for 3 min with 17% ethylenediaminetetraacetic acid (EDTA) to remove the smear layer, followed by 5 mL NaOCl and final irrigation with 10 mL of distilled water to avoid the prolonged effect of the EDTA and NaOCl solutions. The canals were subsequently dried with paper points. AH plus (DeTrey Dentsply, Konstanz, Germany) was used as a sealer in all the cases. This sealer was labelled with rhodamine B (0.1%) (Sigma-Aldrich, St. Louis, MO, USA) to allow analysis under confocal laser scanning microscopy (CLSM). The sealer was applied using a #35 Lentulo Spiral (Zipperer-VDW, Munich, Germany).

2.2. Root Canal Preparation and Filling Technique

Sixty roots were randomly divided into six groups of 10 teeth each. According to the condensation technique and the taper of the gutta-percha master cone, we formed the following groups:

Group 1 (cold lateral condensation 0.02). Ten root canals were filled with 0.02 tapered gutta-percha (VDW, Munich, Germany) using the cold lateral condensation technique. A gutta-percha cone of 0.02 taper was fitted into the root canal at the working length, making firm pressure in an apical direction. A finger spreader (Dentsply Maillefer, Ballaigues, Switzerland) number 20 was introduced at 1 mm short of the working length to laterally compact the gutta-percha to create space and be able to insert auxiliary 0.02 taper gutta-percha cones. This process was repeated until the digital spreader only entered the coronal third of the root canal. A hot metal instrument was used for trimming excess coronary gutta-percha and was subsequently compacted vertically with a Buchanan instrument.

Group 2 (cold lateral condensation 0.04). Ten roots were filled with gutta-percha with a 0.04 taper, using the cold lateral condensation as described in Group 1.

Group 3 (continuous wave 0.02). Ten root canals were sealed with gutta-percha of standardized 0.02 taper using a continuous vertical wave condensation technique with thermoplastic injection.

After inserting a standard gutta-percha point adapted to 1 mm short of the working length, the corresponding tip of the Elements Obturation Unit (EOU) sealing system was heated to 200 °C, and a depth of 3 mm above the canal's length was used. Once the apical third was sealed, the other two-thirds of the root canal was sealed using the thermoplastic gutta-percha injection technique, elements obturation unit EOU system (SybronEndo Company, Glendora, CA, USA) by applying manual vertical condensation, and the corresponding Buchanan Pluggers instrument (Sybron Endodontics, Orange, CA, USA).

Group 4 (continuous wave 0.04). Ten roots were filled with gutta-percha with 0.04 taper, using continuous wave as described in Group 3.

Group 5 (hybrid 0.02). Ten root canals were sealed with a gutta-percha 0.02 taper using a hybrid filling technique. The cold lateral condensation and thermoplastic filling condensation techniques were combined. After filling the root canal using the cold lateral condensation as described for Group I, a hot instrument was used to remove the gutta-percha from the middle and coronal thirds. Subsequently, vertical pressure was applied using the corresponding Buchanan Pluggers (Sybron Endodontics, Orange, CA, USA) within 5 to 7 mm of working lengths to improve the gutta-percha adaptation. The coronal and middle third portions of the root canal were sealed with thermoplastic gutta-percha injected by the corresponding terminal of the elements gutta-percha cartridges (SybronEndo, Glendora, CA, USA) using the elements obturation unit (SybronEndo Company, Glendora, CA, USA). Subsequently, gutta-percha was vertically compacted with a Buchanan Pluggers instrument (Sybron Endodontics, Orange, CA, USA).

Group 6 (hybrid 0.04). Ten roots were filled with gutta-percha with 0.04 taper, using the hybrid technique described in Group 5.

In all the filled root canals, vestibule-lingual and mesiodistal radiographs were taken of each root to verify its correct condensation. Facial and proximal views of digital radiographs of all teeth roots were taken to verify the canal obturations. Figure 1 illustrates radiographic images depicting root canals filled using the three techniques examined in the current study.

The teeth were placed in a Memmert BE 500 heater (Memmert, Heilbronn, Germany) and incubated at 37 °C for three days to set the sealer completely. Each root was embedded in an epofix hardener resin block (Struers, Ballerup, Denmark).

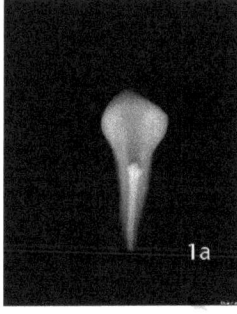 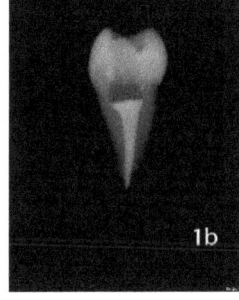

Figure 1. *Cont.*

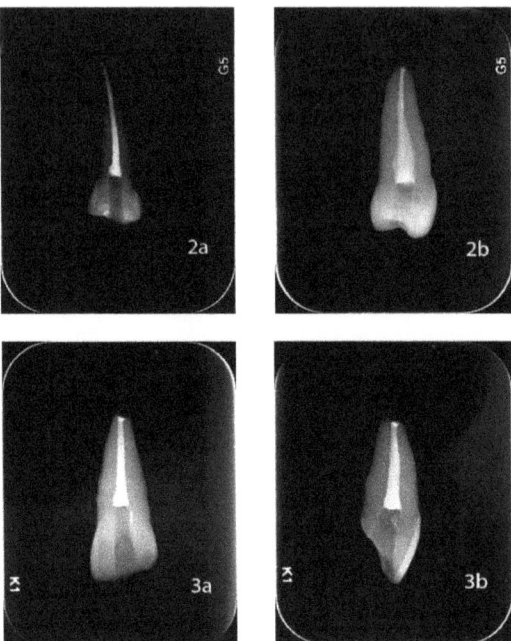

Figure 1. Illustrates radiographic images of teeth filled with each of the three compaction techniques evaluated. Cold lateral condensation ((**1a**) vestibule-lingual and (**1b**) mesiodistal radiograph); continuous wave ((**2a**) vestibule-lingual and (**2b**) mesiodistal radiograph) and hybrid technique ((**3a**) vestibule-lingual and (**3b**) mesiodistal radiograph).

2.3. Sectioning and Image Analysis

One-millimeter transversal sections were made in the 3, 7, and 10 mm levels from the apex of sixty roots using a 0.3 mm Isomet saw (Buehler IsoMet, Lake Bluff, IL, USA) at 200 rpm and continuous water cooling. In this manner, three slices per root were created (coronal, middle, apical), resulting in 180 pieces. The samples were then mounted onto glass slides. Only the apically facing surface of each slice was examined. All the sections were sequentially polished with Sof-Lex discs (3M ESPE, Seefeld, Germany) using running tap water as a lubricant to smooth the surfaces.

Images of the filled areas were acquired using the epifluorescence mode of an inverted Leica TCS-SP2 confocal laser scanning microscopy (CLSM) (Leica, Mannheim, Germany). An argon-mixed gas laser was used (Ar/HeNe) as the light source. Excitation light had a wavelength maximum of 543 nm. The respective absorption and emission wavelengths for rhodamine B were 554 and 649 nm. The images were recorded at 40×, with a 1024 × 1024 pixels resolution. The images were acquired and analyzed using the Leica Confocal software Version 2.1E (Leica Microsystems, Heidelberg, Germany). All the pictures were taken by using 10 sections with a 4 µm step size.

The images were evaluated according to the method used by Gharib et al. [27] for measuring the depth of penetration; each image was imported into the Leica Confocal Software Version 2.1E and, using the distance tool software, the point of deepest penetration was measured from the canal wall to the area of maximum sealer penetration (Figure 2). Each image was imported into the Image J software (Rasband WS, ImageJ, 1.54; US National Institute of Health, Bethesda, MD, USA) to calculate the percentage of sealer penetration, and the root canal's circumference wall was measured. Next, the areas along the canal walls in which the sealer penetrated dentinal tubules (sealer tags) were outlined and measured using the same method. The percentage of the canal walls where the sealer had penetrated was calculated by dividing the canal circumference's outline by the entire circumference (Figure 2).

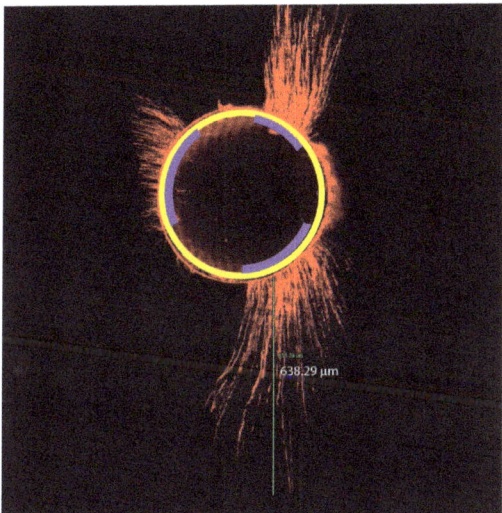

Figure 2. Representative confocal laser microscopic image showing the maximum depth of sealer penetration illustrated by a green line. The root canal wall with sealer penetration is illustrated using a violet curved line, and a yellow line depicts the perimeter.

2.4. Statistical Analysis

The average percentage of penetration and the maximum depth of sealer penetration were calculated in the three root levels analysed: 3, 7, and 10 mm. These indicators were compared among the three condensation techniques used in the levels of the root canal examined using mixed linear regression models, considering that the observations were nested within teeth. Models with and without interaction terms were tested (interactions between the root level and the compaction technique, and between the technique and the gutta-percha taper master cones). Unstandardized β coefficients, and 95% confidence intervals (95% CI) were obtained. Akaike's information criterion was used for the model selection. After fitting the models and obtaining estimates for coefficients ($\beta_0, \beta_1, \ldots, \beta_k$) linear combinations of these estimators were calculated in order to obtain the interaction terms effects as well as their 95% confidence intervals and *p*-values. The statistical significance value was set at $\alpha = 0.05$. Data analysis was performed using Stata V15 (StataCorp LLC., College Station, TX, USA).

3. Results

The results of the percentage sealer penetration using the cold lateral condensation technique presented a mean of 57.49 (±28.9), for continuous wave, 56.8 (±33.1), and, for the hybrid technique, 64.5 (±29.8). Table 1 presents the mean sealer penetration by technique and gutta-percha taper across the root level. In the coronal sections, the lowest percentage of penetration corresponded to the cold lateral condensation technique (74.3%) and values above 80% were observed in the continuous wave and hybrid techniques. In the middle section, a similar pattern was observed, and in the apical third, continuous wave had the lowest percentage of penetration.

None of the groups studied achieved a full adaptation of sealer material on the dentin walls. Figure 3a–c illustrates the root sealer penetration into the coronal (Figure 3a), middle (Figure 3b), and apical (Figure 3c) sections, using the hybrid technique. The higher depth of sealer penetration was observed in the coronal third.

Table 1. Percentage of sealer penetration in μm into dentinal tubules in the coronal (10 mm), the middle (7 mm), and the apical (3 mm) thirds by groups according with technique and gutta-percha point taper size.

Groups Condensation Technique and Gutta-Percha Taper	Root Level
	Coronal (10 mm) Mean (±SD)
Cold Lateral Condensation	74.3 (19.1)
Cold Lateral Condensation 0.02 [1]	75.4 (20.5)
Cold Lateral Condensation 0.04 [2]	73.2 (18.6)
Continuous Wave	82.7 (21.0)
Continuous Wave 0.02 [1]	74.3 (26.1)
Continuous Wave 0.04 [2]	91.3 (9.6)
Hybrid	81.3 (20.9)
Hybrid 0.02 [1]	79.6 (22.3)
Hybrid 0.04 [2]	83.0 (20.4)
	Middle (7 mm) Mean (±SD)
Cold Lateral Condensation	63.9 (25.2)
Cold Lateral Condensation 0.02 [1]	62.9 (24.1)
Cold Lateral Condensation 0.04 [2]	64.8 (27.5)
Continuous Wave	64.8 (19.5)
Continuous Wave 0.02 [1]	63.5 (23.1)
Continuous Wave 0.04 [2]	66.0 (16.4)
Hybrid	69.0 (27.9)
Hybrid 0.02 [1]	75.4 (22.9)
Hybrid 0.04 [2]	62.6 (22.1)
	Apical (3 mm) Mean (±SD)
Cold Lateral Condensation	34.3 (26.4)
Cold Lateral Condensation 0.02 [1]	37.5 (28.8)
Cold Lateral Condensation 0.04 [2]	31.3 (24.9)
Continuous Wave	22.8 (23.9)
Continuous Wave 0.02 [1]	20.1 (31.6)
Continuous Wave 0.04 [2]	25.4 (14.0)
Hybrid	43.1 (31.5)
Hybrid 0.02 [1]	33.5 (28.2)
Hybrid 0.04 [2]	52.8 (33.1)

[1] Gutta-percha master cone taper 0.02, [2] Gutta-percha master cone taper 0.04.

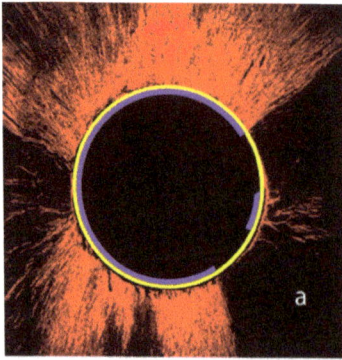

Figure 3. *Cont.*

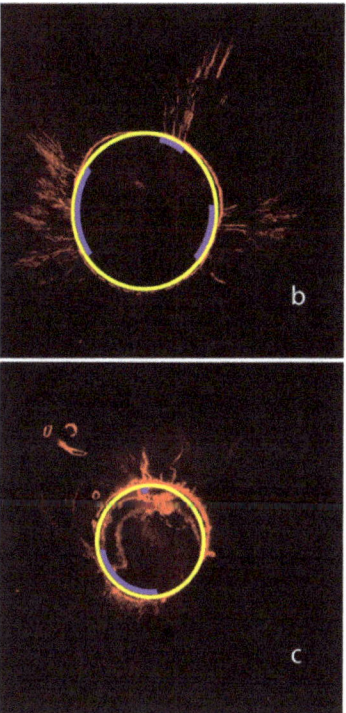

Figure 3. Representative confocal laser microscopic image of root sealer penetration. (**a**) corresponds to the coronal third, (**b**) depicts the sealer penetration in the middle third. And (**c**) depicts sealer penetration in the apical third, using the hybrid technique.

The results of the maximum penetration of sealer using the cold lateral condensation technique showed a mean of 918.2 (±383.2), for continuous wave, 960.1 (±623.4), and for hybrid, 1144.2 (±571.1). Table 2 presents the results of the maximum penetration depth of condensation techniques by root level and taper of the gutta-percha master cones. In the coronal section, the hybrid technique presented a high penetration mean (1401.6 μm), similarly, it was high in the middle section (1423.4 μm). In the coronal and middle root thirds, the lowest penetration depth was observed in the cold lateral condensation groups.

Table 2. Depth of sealer penetration in μm into dentinal tubules in the coronal (10 mm), the middle (7 mm), and the apical (3 mm) thirds, by groups according with condensation technique and gutta-percha taper sizes.

Group by Condensation Technique and Gutta-Percha Taper	Root Level
	Coronal (10 mm) Mean (±SD)
Cold Lateral Condensation	1084.9 (197.9)
Cold Lateral Condensation 0.02 [1]	1294.5 (450.1)
Cold Lateral Condensation 0.04 [2]	875.5 (461.5)
Continuous Wave	1337.1 (291.1)
Continuous Wave 0.02	1271.9 (678.4)
Continuous Wave 0.04	1402.8 (514.0)
Hybrid	1401.6 (477.3)
Hybrid 0.02	1170.7 (796.1)
Hybrid 0.04	1632.9 (585.8)

Table 2. Cont.

Group by Condensation Technique and Gutta-Percha Taper	Root Level
	Middle (7 mm) Mean (±SD)
Cold Lateral Condensation	982.8 (467.4)
Cold Lateral Condensation 0.02 [1]	1187.7 (552.7)
Cold Lateral Condensation 0.04 [2]	778.0 (449.5)
Continuous Wave	1177.3 (694.0)
Continuous Wave 0.02	1152.1 (666.0)
Continuous Wave 0.04	1202.5 (756.1)
Hybrid	1423.4 (442.8)
Hybrid 0.02	1394.7 (506.2)
Hybrid 0.04	1452.0 (394.8)
	Apical (3 mm) Mean (±SD)
Cold Lateral Condensation	686.8 (329.1)
Cold Lateral Condensation 0.02 [1]	711.4 (412.9)
Cold Lateral Condensation 0.04 [2]	662.3 (565.2)
Continuous Wave	366.0 (263.8)
Continuous Wave 0.02	244.7 (280.5)
Continuous Wave 0.04	487.4 (422.5)
Hybrid	607.7 (365.9)
Hybrid 0.02	745.5 (586.9)
Hybrid 0.04	470.0 (501.1)

[1] Gutta-percha master cone taper 0.02, [2] Gutta-percha master cone taper 0.04.

Table 3 presents the results of the mixed linear regression models fitted for percentage of penetration as the outcome variable, using as predictors the root level, technique, and gutta-percha taper size master cone (model 1 without interaction terms). In this model, the taper size was not significant ($p = 0.803$).

Table 3. Regression coefficients of percentage of sealer penetration and root level and type of condensation technique, and gutta-percha cone tapper (model 1), and regression coefficients of maximum penetration depth, technique and interaction between root level and technique (model 2).

Model 1 [1]			
Variable	Coefficient	95% (CI)	p
Root level			
Coronal	ref	-	-
Middle	−13.6	(−20.2, −7.0)	<0.001
Apical	−46.1	(−52.7, −39.5)	<0.001
Technique			
Cold lateral condensation	ref	-	-
Continuous wave	−0.8	(−11.9, 10.4)	0.895
Hybrid	7.0	(−4.2, 18.1)	0.219
Tapper			
0.02	ref	-	-
0.04	−1.2	(−10.3, 7.9)	0.803
Model 2 [1]			
Variable	Coefficient	95% (CI)	p
Root level			
Coronal	ref	-	-
Middle	−10.4	(−21.4, 0.6)	0.063
Apical	−40.0	(−50.9, −29.0)	<0.001
Technique			
Cold lateral condensation	ref	-	-

Table 3. Cont.

Continuous wave	8.5	(−5.8, 22.8)	0.244
Hybrid	7.0	(−7.3, 21.3)	0.336
Root level and technique [2]			
Coronal × Cold lateral condensation	ref	-	-
Middle × Continuous wave	−7.6	(−23.1, 7.9)	0.337
Middle × Hybrid	−1.9	(−17.4, 13.7)	0.812
Apical × Continuous wave	−20.1	(−35.6, −4.5)	0.011
Apical × hybrid	1.8	(−13.8, 17.3)	0.823

[1] Nested model (root level nested in teeth), Likelihood Ratio test vs. linear model: $\chi^2 = 27.32$ $p < 0.001$. [2] Interaction root level and type of technique.

The root level was significant ($p < 0.001$); a higher percentage of sealer penetration was observed in the coronal compared with the middle and apical root thirds (Table 3).

A significant interaction was found between root level and technique. At the apical level, a higher percentage of sealant penetration was observed in the hybrid compared with the continuous wave technique (20.36 (IC95% 6.06, 34.65) $p = 0.005$).

To study the impact of possible interaction between condensation techniques and the root level on the sealer penetration, the corresponding interaction terms were included in the model (Table 3, model 2). A significant difference was observed in the apical third, indicating a higher percentage of sealant penetration in the hybrid compared with the continuous wave technique (−20.1, 95% CI (−35.6, −4.5), $p = 0.011$). Figure 4 depicts the percentage of penetration in each technique across root levels. A lack of parallelism is observed, indicating the interaction between the compaction technique and the root level. The predicted values appear to be close at the coronal and middle root levels; however, in the apical section differences between techniques were observed the continuous wave had the lowest percentage penetration results ($p < 0.05$).

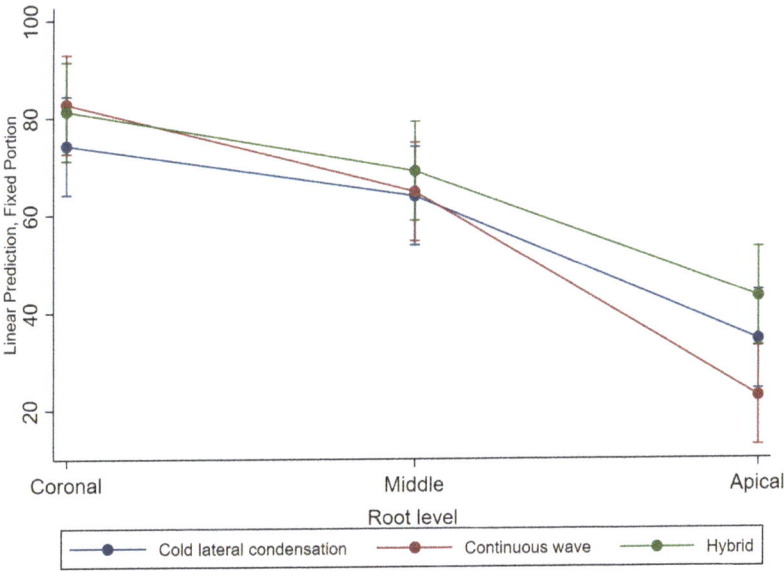

Figure 4. The plot of the adjusted predictors of the percentage of sealer penetration by compaction technique across root levels. Vertical bars represent 95% confidence intervals for the mean estimates.

Table 4, Model 1 presents the results of the mixed linear regression model fitted for maximum penetration depth, including as predictors the root level technique, and gutta-percha taper size master cone ($p = 0.770$), (Model 1). The taper size was not significant in the model, while the root level and technique was significant ($p < 0.001$), similarly to the findings of percentage penetration.

Table 4. Regression coefficients of maximum penetration depth and root level. Type of condensation technique and gutta percha cone tapper (Model 1). Regression coefficients of maximum penetration depth, condensation technique and interaction between root level and technique (Model 2).

Model 1 [1]			
Variable	Coefficient	95% (CI)	p
Root level			
Coronal	ref	-	-
Middle	−102.1	(323.8, 119.6)	0.367
Apical	−398.1	(−619.9, −176.4)	<0.001
Technique			
Cold lateral condensation	ref	-	-
Continuous wave	252.2	(0.739, 503.7)	0.049
Hybrid	316.7	(65.3, 568.2)	0.014
Taper			
0.02	ref	-	-
0.04	−21.2	(−163.6, 121.2)	0.770
Model 2 [2]			
Variable	Coefficient	95% (CI)	p
Root level			
Coronal	ref	-	-
Middle	−102.1	(−323.8, 119.6)	0.367
Apical	−398.1	(−619.9, −176.4)	<0.001
Technique			
Cold lateral condensation	ref	-	-
Continuous wave	252.2	(0.7, 503.7)	0.049
Hybrid	316.8	(65.3, 568.2)	0.014
Root level and technique [3]			
Coronal × Cold lateral condensation	ref	-	-
Middle × Continuous wave	−57.7	(−371.3, 255.9)	0.718
Middle × Hybrid	123.8	(−189.7, 437.4)	0.439
Apical × Continuous wave	−573.0	(−886.6, −259.4)	<0.001
Apical × Hybrid	−395.8	(−709.4, −82.3)	0.013

[1] Nested model (root level nested in teeth). [2] Likelihood Ratio test vs. linear model: $\chi^2 = 8.12$, $p = 0.002$. [3] Interactions terms root level and type of technique.

In Table 4, Model 2 presents the results of the mixed regression model including the interaction terms between the root level and the technique; this interaction was significant. The computation of the effects indicated that in the middle third, the hybrid technique had higher penetration than cold lateral condensation (440.6 95% CI (189.10, 692.06), $p = 0.001$). Additionally, in the apical third continuous wave presented a lower penetration depth than cold lateral condensation (−320.77 95% CI (−572.25, −69.30) $p = 0.012$).

Figure 5 depicts the maximum depth of sealer penetration for each technique across the root level, and an interaction between the technique and the root level is observed. The predicted values of sealer penetration in the coronal third of hybrid and continuous wave are close to each other, and cold lateral condensation shows lower results, while in the apical third this relationship changes and continuous wave has the lowest penetration value.

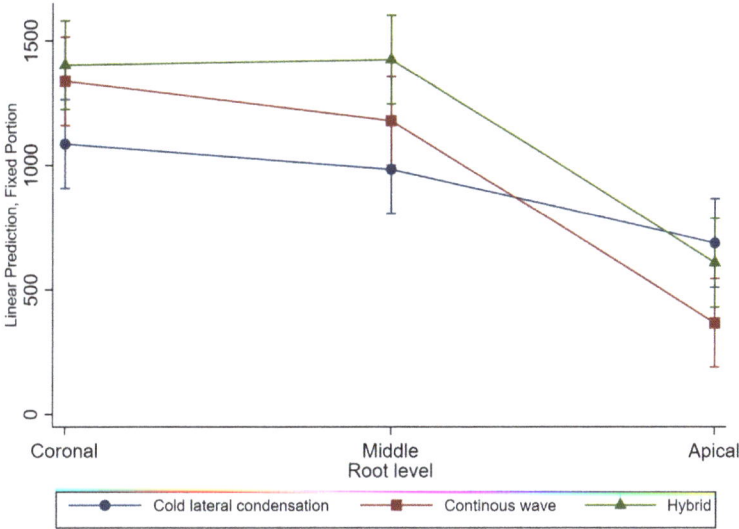

Figure 5. The plot of the adjusted predictors of maximum penetration depth (μm) by compaction technique across root levels. Vertical bars represent 95% confidence intervals for the mean estimates.

4. Discussion

In this study, the penetration of sealer material into dentin tubules using three condensation techniques (cold lateral condensation, continuous-wave and hybrid) were compared. The study alternative hypothesis was that the hybrid technique would provide higher sealer penetration than cold lateral condensation. The results support this hypothesis. The study provided evidence of a significant difference between the cold lateral condensation and the hybrid technic evaluated. The hybrid method presented good results, combining the cold lateral condensation in the apical third and the continuous wave above the middle and coronal thirds.

Similarly, a study of the efficacy of filling techniques in C-1 shaped root canals found fewer voids and a higher percentage of gutta-percha using the cold lateral condensation than using the continuous wave in the apical third [21]. Accordingly, a comparison of the cold lateral condensation and the continuous wave found less sealer and more gutta-percha in the cold lateral condensation sample in the 2 mm sections. Furthermore, the continuous wave technique had more penetration than the cold lateral condensation into the 4, 6 and 8 mm sections [23].

The information obtained in the evaluation of complex root canal anatomies may support using the hybrid technique tested in the present study. Likewise, in a microcomputed tomography-based study comparing Thermafil and the cold lateral condensation, it was identified that using Thermafil voids surrounded by the filling material was mostly in the apical root third [28]. The results of these studies suggest that the middle and coronal thirds of the root canal are better filled with warm gutta-percha techniques compared with the cold lateral condensation; however, the apical third cold lateral condensation appears to have adequate results gutta-percha cones placed against the root wall during cold lateral condensation may facilitate penetration of the sealer, particularly at the apex [29]. Karatekin et al. [23] suggested the need for a modified continuous wave technique in the apical 2 mm section in C1-type canals. The hybrid technique described in the present study may be an adequate option for these cases.

Study findings on the effectiveness of hybrid or "combination" filling techniques are inconsistent. Tagger's hybrid technique applied with the cold lateral condensation and GuttaFlow identified a larger gutta-percha-filled area in the middle and coronal thirds using this hybrid condensation technique, but there was no difference in the apical third regrading the percent of the gutta-percha area, voids and sealer area [13].

Likewise, a longitudinal study examining bacterial penetration into the root canal found no difference in the sealing ability between cold lateral condensation, Thermafill, System B, and ProTaper gutta-percha single cones after two months of observation [30]. A study using nano-computer tomography image found no difference in total obturation and calculated voids between cold lateral condensation and continuous wave [31]. Saberi et al. [32] found that a single cone technique and a hybrid (tapered cone and cold lateral compaction) technique had lower coronal leakages than the cold lateral condensation.

The inconsistencies observed in the results of various studies may be attributed to variations in experimental protocols. These variations encompass factors such as the type of teeth sections utilized, the conditions of the root canal, differences in the preparations of the root canals, the specific type of endodontic sealer selected, the treatment steps, the methodologies employed for assessing sealer penetration, and the overall experimental design, among other variables [33,34]. Clinical variations among teeth may also contribute to disparities, including distinctions in the anatomy of root canals, patient-related factors, and variations in dentin structure across different sections of teeth dentin sclerosis has been found to influence sealer penetration [35].

The apical portion of human teeth exhibits significant structural variations, such as accessory root canals, areas of resorption, pulp stones, irregular secondary dentine, cementum-like lining, and deviations in the apex from the root canal's long axis [36]. As individuals age, dentin undergoes permanent microstructural modifications characterized by the gradual mineral infiltration of tubule lumens. This process, referred to as dental sclerosis, commences at the root apex, progresses towards the crown, and results in a decreased fracture resistance of dentin [37]. This may help elucidate the greater sealer penetration observed in the coronal region compared to the apical region in our current study.

The time elapsed between obturation and the assessment of sealer penetration, as well as environmental factors affecting sealer setting, can exert an impact on the obtained results. It should be recognized that sealer penetration may undergo changes as the sealer sets and interacts with dentin over time [38,39]. Addressing these factors and maintaining standardized methods can help reduce discrepancies in the results of sealer penetration studies conducted using different compaction techniques in endodontics.

The variations in study results can also be influenced by the statistical data analysis methods. In this study, mixed linear models were employed, allowing for the nesting of root sections within the teeth from which they were obtained. This nesting was considered based on a comparison between nested and non-nested models. Furthermore, the analysis of interactions between root level and condensation techniques provided insights into the differences between these techniques. The mixed linear regression model indicated the presence of an interaction between the technique and the root level. Specifically, a higher maximum penetration depth was observed in the apical root level with the hybrid technique compared to lateral condensation.

In the present study, AH Plus endodontic sealer was chosen because it has good penetration, and adequate flow and adaption ability in the root canal system, it has been considered as a gold standard [40–42]. The teeth were evaluated using confocal laser scanning microscopy with the incorporation of a fluorescent dye (rhodamine B). This technique displays the sealing material's adaptation through the dentinal tubules in the specimen cross-sections [27]. In the present study, using overexposure images by the confocal laser scanning microscopy program, it was possible to obtain the offset of the dentinal tubules' undulating path. This process provides detailed information and reduces the risk of cracking artefacts since the sample does not require drying.

The rhodamine B concentration (0.1%) was considered adequate for identifying the sealer in dentinal tubules. This fluorophore does not harm the sealer and behaves satisfactorily when it is used in combination with an epoxy resin-based material, such as the

AH-plus used in the present study [13,15]. Nevertheless, the results of a study conducted by Donnermeyer et al. [43] indicated that Rhodamine B may leach into dentine beyond the sealant penetration and may be inadequate to assess sealing capacity.

However, a study by Eğemen and Belli [44] found adequate results utilizing this fluorescent dye. They investigated the effect on dentin tubules penetration of resin-based (AH-plus) and calcium silicate-based sealers. The authors conducted a pilot study to select the dyes to be used for the evaluation of sealant penetration, rhodamine (Rhod-2) and Fluo-3 were tested. The results indicated that these two dyes were appropriated to identify the sealant tubules' penetration for the original obturation and for root canal retreatment [44].

In the present study, there were no substantial variations observed in terms of depth of penetration or the percentage of sealer penetration when comparing 0.02 tapered master cones to their 0.04 tapered counterparts. Consequently, the study did not corroborate the hypothesis proposing enhanced results with less tapered cones. Hembrough et al. [45] consistently did not detect a significant difference when measuring the percentage surface of the root canal taken up by gutta-percha, comparing 0.02 and 0.06 taper cones.

Other studies had similar results using the cold lateral condensation [17,18]. Moreover, in a study applying area-metric analysis comparing 0.02 and 0.04 taper guttapercha, no statistically significant difference was found in the sealer-filling canal area with the cold lateral condensation or single cone techniques [19]. When assessing curved root canals, a study found no significant difference in apical leakage between 0.06 and 0.02 gutta-percha taper cones. However, canals filled with a 0.02 master cone had a lower average leakage [46]. In a study by Schäfer et al. [47], it was observed that matching the preparation with single cones in the apical section led to a higher percentage of gutta-percha-filled areas when using constant taper gutta-percha compared to variable tapered single-cone gutta-percha. The inconsistency in the results of studies with larger taper compared with standard taper gutta-percha cones may be primarily due to the instruments selected for the root canals preparation, the microleakage assessment method and the evaluation of the sealer penetration technique.

The study found that none of the compaction techniques that were evaluated achieved complete adaptation to dentinal walls, a result in line with earlier research [48]. Even though root canal treatment has a high success rate, the search for the ideal compaction technique is an ongoing endeavor.

Irrespective of the technique applied and the gutta-percha taper selected, higher penetration depth and percentage of sealer penetration were observed in the coronal third followed by the middle third and, last, the apical third. Similar results have been reported by Akcay et al. [25] when comparing different types of sealers. Moreover, these results are consistent with several studies' findings using the confocal laser scanning microscopy technique [26,27]. In an evaluation of bonding to the root canal, significantly greater coronal dentin permeability was observed than the apical third and was influential in root bonding [49]. Higher sealer penetration in the coronal third may be explained by the reduced accumulation of the smear layer or its easier removal in this third than the middle and the apical thirds. Furthermore, the dentinal tubules' setup in the apical region is irregular and more prone to obliteration, presenting dentin sclerosis, which hinders the penetration of the sealer cement [50]. The consistency of these results suggests that the most influential factor of this observation is the root canal anatomy. This aspect makes us reflect on the importance of performing several observations along the root canal when studying root canal compaction techniques, including the middle and coronary root levels, avoiding the omission of important information.

A limitation of the current study pertains to the exclusive inclusion of single-rooted teeth with straight canals. Root canals exhibiting diverse anatomical variations may yield distinct outcomes. Another limitation was the absence of a control group. However, all the technique steps were carefully followed and samples without root canal compaction were tested before-hand, including the experimental groups, to confirm the fluorescent dye's penetration. Those samples covered with nail polish exhibited no dye penetration. In future studies, it is essential to explore the use of fluorescent dyes specifically designed for dentin tubule penetration. Additionally, a limitation of the fluorescent confocal laser scanning microscopy method is that the number of measurements performed in each root canal could impact the percentage and the depth of penetration the percentage and depth of penetration results. To address this limitation, the ImageJ program was utilized to measure the area and collect pixel value statistics, enabling the evaluation of both depth and the percent sealer penetration, as previously demonstrated in other studies [27].

In the realm of future research, innovative imaging methods, notably microcomputed tomography (Micro-CT), may be integrated to unlock valuable insights into the dynamic interactions between sealers and dentin. Micro-CT's three-dimensional capabilities empower a comprehensive assessment of sealer penetration, revealing its volumetric characteristics and spatial distribution within dentin. This technique can effectively complement the information offered by confocal laser scanning microscopy (CLSM), a potent imaging tool recognized for its high-magnification examination of dentin surfaces and sealer distribution patterns [51]. In addition, the integration of Micro-CT or 2D printed replicas presents an opportunity to enhance the precision of tooth comparison in endodontic procedures, effectively mitigating potential anatomical discrepancies. Furthermore, the necessity for long-term scrutiny of sealer penetration becomes apparent, as the longevity of felling materials may become a significant factor [51].

In a systematic review and meta-analysis conducted by Mekhdieva et al. [52] the objective was to evaluate the effectiveness of bioceramic endodontic sealers in reducing postoperative pain when compared to traditional filling techniques. Their analysis revealed that patients who received treatment with bioceramic sealers, whether in a single visit or across multiple visits, reported experiencing lower levels of postoperative pain [52]. Future research can investigate the effects of innovative biocompatible sealing materials, such as bioceramic sealers, on hybrid compaction techniques like the one introduced in our present study.

This study adds to the knowledge on sealer penetration in favor of using hybrid techniques. The combination of cold lateral condensation and continuous wave has the advantage of using a classic technic, which has a relative low cost and is taught in most of dental schools, with continuous wave that requires lower obturation time and allows good adaption to the root canal complexities [6].

This study significantly contributes to the existing body of knowledge pertaining to sealer penetration, underscoring the merits of employing hybrid techniques in endodontic treatment. The combination of traditional cold lateral condensation alongside the modern continuous wave method offers a distinctive advantage. It combines a well-established, cost-effective classic technique that is widely integrated into dental education curricula with the efficiency of the continuous wave approach, resulting in reduced obturation time and enhanced adaptability to the intricate configurations of the root canal system.

5. Conclusions

In conclusion, the depth of the penetration of root canal sealers into the dentinal tubules and the percentage of sealer penetration into the root canal walls were significantly influenced by the root canal level, with a lower penetration into the root canal apical third. Teeth filled with gutta-percha master point taper 0.04 had a similar maximum sealer penetration and percentage sealant penetration to conventional 0.02 taper points. The ability to obtain good sealer penetration was different between the techniques across root levels. The hybrid technique evaluated, combining the cold lateral condensation in the apical root third and continuous wave above the apical third, presented a higher maximum sealer penetration into the apical third than the continuous wave technique, and higher penetration than the cold lateral condensation was observed into the middle and coronal thirds. The evaluated hybrid technique may be a good alternative in root canal treatment.

Author Contributions: Conceptualization, I.B.-N. and D.V.-G.; methodology, I.B.-N.; software, P.M.; validation, I.B.-N. and P.M.; formal analysis, M.A.Z.-Z.; investigation, I.B.-N. and D.V.-G.; data curation, M.E.I.-C. and M.A.Z.-Z.; writing—original draft preparation, I.B.-N.; writing—review and editing, M.E.I.-C., M.A.Z.-Z. and D.R.-P.; supervision, A.C.-S. All authors have read and agreed to the published version of the manuscript.

Funding: This research received no external funding.

Institutional Review Board Statement: The study was conducted in accordance with the Declaration of Helsinki, and aproved by The Ethics Committee of the Egas Moniz University Institute (CIIEM), Portugal, with the register number CEPI/0893.

Informed Consent Statement: Informed consent was obtained from all subjects involved in the study.

Data Availability Statement: Data will be available from corresponding authors.

Conflicts of Interest: The authors declare no conflict of interest.

References

1. Suguro, H.; Takeichi, O.; Hayashi, M.; Okamura, T.; Hira, A.; Hirano, Y.; Ogiso, B. Microcomputed tomographic evaluation of techniques for warm gutta-percha obturation. *J. Oral Sci.* **2018**, *60*, 165–169. [CrossRef] [PubMed]
2. Campello, A.F.; Marceliano-Alves, M.F.; Siqueira, J.F.; Fonseca, S.C.; Lopes, R.T.; Alves, F.R.F. Unprepared surface areas, accumulated hard tissue debris, and dentinal crack formation after preparation using reciprocating or rotary instruments: A study in human cadavers. *Clin. Oral Investig.* **2021**, *25*, 6239–6248. [CrossRef] [PubMed]
3. Qualtrough, A.J.E.; Whitworth, J.M.; Dummer, P.M.H. Preclinical endodontology: An international comparison. *Int. Endod. J.* **1999**, *32*, 406–414. [CrossRef] [PubMed]
4. Bhandi, S.; Mashyakhy, M.; Abumelha, A.S.; Alkahtany, M.F.; Jamal, M.; Chohan, H.; Raj, A.T.; Testarelli, L.; Reda, R.; Patil, S. Complete Obturation—Cold Lateral Condensation vs. Thermoplastic Techniques: A Systematic Review of Micro-CT Studies. *Materials* **2021**, *14*, 4013. [CrossRef]
5. Dummer, P.M.H. Comparison of undergraduate endodontic teaching programmes in the United Kingdom and in some dental schools in Europe and the United States. *Int. Endod. J.* **1991**, *24*, 169–177. [CrossRef]
6. Bhagat, K.; Jasrotia, A.; Bhagat, R.K. A comparison of cold lateral compaction and warm vertical compaction using continuous wave of compaction technique. *Int. J. Appl. Dent. Sci.* **2021**, *7*, 244–246. [CrossRef]
7. Llena-Puy, M.C.; Forner-Navarro, L.; Barbero-Navarro, I. Vertical root fracture in endodontically treated teeth: A review of 25 cases. *Oral Surg. Oral Med. Oral Pathol. Oral Radiol. Endodontol.* **2001**, *92*, 553–555. [CrossRef]
8. Lertchirakarn, V.; Palamara, J.E.; Messer, H.H. Load and strain during lateral condensation and vertical root fracture. *J. Endod.* **1999**, *25*, 99–104. [CrossRef]
9. Schilder, H. Filling root canals in three dimensions. *Dent. Clin. N. Am.* **1967**, *11*, 723–744. [CrossRef]
10. Buchanan, L. The continuous wave of obturation technique: 'centered' condensation of warm gutta percha in 12 seconds. *Dent. Today* **1996**, *15*, 60–67.
11. Yee, F.S.; Marlin, J.; Krakow, A.A.; Gron, P. Three-dimensional obturation of the root canal using injection-molded, thermoplasticized dental gutta-percha. *J. Endod.* **1977**, *3*, 168–174. [CrossRef]
12. Tagger, M. Use of thermo-mechanical compactors as an adjunct to lateral condensation. *Quintessence Int. Dent. Dig.* **1984**, *15*, 27–30.
13. Marciano, M.A.; Bramante, C.M.; Duarte, M.A.H.; Delgado, R.J.R.; Ordinola-Zapata, R.; Garcia, R.B. Evaluation of single root canals filled using the lateral compaction, tagger's hybrid, microseal and guttaflow techniques. *Braz. Dent. J.* **2010**, *21*, 411–415. [CrossRef] [PubMed]
14. Robberecht, L.; Colard, T.; Claisse-Crinquette, A. Qualitative evaluation of two endodontic obturation techniques: Tapered single-cone method versus warm vertical condensation and injection system An in vitro study. *J. Oral Sci.* **2012**, *54*, 99–104. [CrossRef] [PubMed]
15. Haupt, F.; Pult, J.R.W.; Hülsmann, M. Micro–computed Tomographic Evaluation of the Shaping Ability of 3 Reciprocating Single-File Nickel-Titanium Systems on Single- and Double-Curved Root Canals. *J. Endod.* **2020**, *46*, 1130–1135. [CrossRef] [PubMed]
16. Schafer, E.; Schulzbongert, U.; Tulus, G. Comparison of Hand Stainless Steel and Nickel Titanium Rotary Instrumentation: A Clinical Study. *J. Endod.* **2004**, *30*, 432–435. [CrossRef] [PubMed]
17. Gordon, M.P.J.; Love, R.M.; Chandler, N.P. An evaluation of 0.06 tapered gutta-percha cones for filling of 0.06 taper prepared curved root canals. *Int. Endod. J.* **2005**, *38*, 87–96. [CrossRef] [PubMed]
18. Motamedi, M.R.K.; Mortaheb, A.; Jahromi, M.Z.; Gilbert, B.E. Micro-CT Evaluation of Four Root Canal Obturation Techniques. *Scanning* **2021**, *2021*, 1–7. [CrossRef]

19. Romania, C.; Beltes, P.; Boutsioukis, C.; Dandakis, C. Ex-vivo area-metric analysis of root canal obturation using gutta-percha cones of different taper. *Int. Endod. J.* **2009**, *42*, 491–498. [CrossRef]
20. Haupt, F.; Meinel, M.; Gunawardana, A.; Hülsmann, M. Effectiveness of different activated irrigation techniques on debris and smear layer removal from curved root canals: A SEM evaluation. *Aust. Endod. J.* **2020**, *46*, 40–46. [CrossRef]
21. Gok, T.; Capar, I.D.; Akcay, I.; Keles, A. Evaluation of Different Techniques for Filling Simulated C-shaped Canals of 3-dimensional Printed Resin Teeth. *J. Endod.* **2017**, *43*, 1559–1564. [CrossRef] [PubMed]
22. Du, Y.; Soo, I.; Zhang, C.F. A case report of six canals in a maxillary first molar. *Chin. J. Dent. Res.* **2011**, *14*, 151–153. Available online: http://www.ncbi.nlm.nih.gov/pubmed/22319758 (accessed on 2 February 2022). [PubMed]
23. Karatekin, A.O.; Keleş, A.; Gençoğlu, N. Comparison of continuous wave and cold lateral condensation filling techniques in 3D printed simulated C-shape canals instrumented with Reciproc Blue or Hyflex EDM. *PLoS ONE* **2019**, *14*, e0224793. [CrossRef] [PubMed]
24. Komabayashi, T.; Colmenar, D.; Cvach, N.; Bhat, A.; Primus, C.; Imai, Y. Comprehensive review of current endodontic sealers. *Dent. Mater. J.* **2020**, *39*, 703–720. [CrossRef] [PubMed]
25. Akcay, M.; Arslan, H.; Durmus, N.; Mese, M.; Capar, I.D. Dentinal tubule penetration of AH Plus, iRoot SP, MTA fillapex, and guttaflow bioseal root canal sealers after different final irrigation procedures: A confocal microscopic study. *Lasers Surg. Med.* **2016**, *48*, 70–76. [CrossRef] [PubMed]
26. Furtado, T.C.; de Bem, I.A.; Machado, L.S.; Pereira, J.R.; Só, M.V.R.; da Rosa, R.A. Intratubular penetration of endodontic sealers depends on the fluorophore used for CLSM assessment. *Microsc. Res. Tech.* **2020**, *84*, 305–312. [CrossRef]
27. Gharib, S.R.; Tordik, P.A.; Imamura, G.M.; Baginski, T.A.; Goodell, G.G. A Confocal Laser Scanning Microscope Investigation of the Epiphany Obturation System. *J. Endod.* **2007**, *33*, 957–961. [CrossRef]
28. Kierklo, A.; Tabor, Z.; Pawińska, M.; Jaworska, M. A microcomputed tomography-based comparison of root canal filling quality following different instrumentation and obturation techniques. *Med. Princ. Pract.* **2015**, *24*, 84–91. [CrossRef]
29. De Macedo, L.M.D.; Silva-Sousa, Y.; Da Silva, S.R.C.; Baratto, S.S.P.; Baratto-Filho, F.; Rached-Júnior, F.J.A. Influence of Root Canal Filling Techniques on Sealer Penetration and Bond Strength to Dentin. *Braz. Dent. J.* **2017**, *28*, 380–384. [CrossRef]
30. Yücel, A.Ç.; Çiftçi, A. Effects of different root canal obturation techniques on bacterial penetration. *Oral Surg. Oral Med. Oral Pathol. Oral Radiol. Endodontol.* **2006**, *102*, e88–e92. [CrossRef]
31. Holmes, S.; Gibson, R.; Butler, J.; Pacheco, R.; Askar, M.; Paurazas, S. Volumetric Evaluation of 5 Root Canal Obturation Methods in TrueTooth 3-dimensional–Printed Tooth Replicas Using Nano–computed Tomography. *J. Endod.* **2021**, *47*, 485–491.e4. [CrossRef] [PubMed]
32. Saberi, E.; Akbari, N.; Ebrahimipour, S.; Jalilpour, H. In-vitro evaluation of coronal microbial leakage after post space tooth preparation. *Minerva Stomatol.* **2016**, *65*, 127–133. Available online: http://www.ncbi.nlm.nih.gov/pubmed/27075369 (accessed on 2 March 2022). [PubMed]
33. Peters, O.A.; Paqué, F. Root Canal Preparation of Maxillary Molars With the Self-adjusting File: A Micro-computed Tomography Study. *J. Endod.* **2011**, *37*, 53–57. [CrossRef] [PubMed]
34. Haji, T.H.; Selivany, B.J.; Suliman, A.A. Sealing ability in vitro study and biocompatibility in vivo animal study of different bioceramic based sealers. *Clin. Exp. Dent. Res.* **2022**, *8*, 1582–1590. [CrossRef]
35. Ordinola-Zapata, R.; Bramante, C.M.; Graeff, M.S.; Perochena, A.d.C.; Vivan, R.R.; Camargo, E.J.; Garcia, R.B.; Bernardineli, N.; Gutmann, J.L.; de Moraes, I.G. Depth and percentage of penetration of endodontic sealers into dentinal tubules after root canal obturation using a lateral compaction technique: A confocal laser scanning microscopy study. *Oral Surg. Oral Med. Oral Pathol. Oral Radiol. Endodontol.* **2009**, *108*, 450–457. [CrossRef]
36. Mjör, I.A.; Smith, M.R.; Ferrari, M.; Mannocci, F. The structure of dentine in the apical region of human teeth. *Int. Endod. J.* **2001**, *34*, 346–353. [CrossRef]
37. Yan, W.; Chen, H.; Fernandez-Arteaga, J.; Paranjpe, A.; Zhang, H.; Arola, D. Root fractures in seniors: Consequences of acute embrittlement of dentin. *Dent. Mater.* **2020**, *36*, 1464–1473. [CrossRef]
38. Allan, N.A.; Walton, R.E.; Schaffer, M. Setting Times for Endodontic Sealers Under Clinical Usage and In Vitro Conditions. *J. Endod.* **2001**, *27*, 421–423. [CrossRef]
39. Donfrancesco, O.; Del Giudice, A.; Zanza, A.; Relucenti, M.; Petracchiola, S.; Gambarini, G.; Testarelli, L.; Seracchiani, M. SEM Evaluation of Endosequence BC Sealer Hiflow in Different Environmental Conditions. *J. Compos. Sci.* **2021**, *5*, 99. [CrossRef]
40. Balguerie, E.; van der Sluis, L.; Vallaeys, K.; Gurgel-Georgelin, M.; Diemer, F. Sealer penetration and adaptation in the dentinal tubules: A scanning electron microscopic study. *J. Endod.* **2011**, *37*, 1576–1579. [CrossRef]
41. Vo, K.; Daniel, J.; Ahn, C.; Primus, C.; Komabayashi, T. Coronal and apical leakage among five endodontic sealers. *J. Oral Sci.* **2022**, *64*, 95–98. [CrossRef] [PubMed]
42. Piai, G.G.; Duarte, M.A.H.; Nascimento, A.L.D.; da Rosa, R.A.; Só, M.V.R.; Vivan, R.R. Penetrability of a new endodontic sealer: A confocal laser scanning microscopy evaluation. *Microsc. Res. Tech.* **2018**, *81*, 1246–1249. [CrossRef] [PubMed]
43. Donnermeyer, D.; Schmidt, S.; Rohrbach, A.; Berlandi, J.; Bürklein, S.; Schäfer, E. Debunking the concept of dentinal tubule penetration of endodontic sealers: Sealer staining with rhodamine B fluorescent dye is an inadequate method. *Materials* **2021**, *14*, 3211. [CrossRef] [PubMed]
44. Eğemen, A.; Belli, S. The Effect of Primary Root Canal Treatment on Dentinal Tubule Penetration of Calcium Silicate–based Sealers during Endodontic Retreatment. *J. Endod.* **2022**, *48*, 1169–1177. [CrossRef] [PubMed]

45. Hembrough, M.; Robertsteiman, H.; Belanger, K. Lateral condensation in canals prepared with nickel-titanium rotary instruments: An evaluation of the use of three different master cones. *J. Endod.* **2002**, *28*, 516–519. [CrossRef]
46. Pérez Heredia, M.; Clavero González, J.; Ferrer Luque, C.M.; González Rodríguez, M.P. Apical seal comparison of low-temperature thermoplasticized gutta-percha technique and lateral condensation with two different master cones. *Med. Oral Patol. Oral Cirugía Bucal.* **2007**, *12*, E175–E179. Available online: http://www.ncbi.nlm.nih.gov/pubmed/17322810 (accessed on 3 March 2022).
47. Schäfer, E.; Köster, M.; Bürklein, S. Percentage of Gutta-percha–filled Areas in Canals Instrumented with Nickel-Titanium Systems and Obturated with Matching Single Cones. *J. Endod.* **2013**, *39*, 924–928. [CrossRef]
48. Lea, C.; Apicella, M.; Mines, P.; Yancich, P.; Parker, M. Comparison of the obturation density of cold lateral compaction versus warm vertical compaction using the continuous wave of condensation technique. *J. Endod.* **2005**, *31*, 37–39. [CrossRef]
49. Ferrari, M.; Mannocci, F.; Vichi, A.; Cagidiaco, M.C.; Mjör, I.A. Bonding to root canal: Structural characteristics of the substrate. *Am. J. Dent.* **2000**, *13*, 255–260. Available online: http://www.ncbi.nlm.nih.gov/pubmed/11764112 (accessed on 3 March 2022).
50. Paqué, F.; Luder, H.U.; Sener, B.; Zehnder, M. Tubular sclerosis rather than the smear layer impedes dye penetration into the dentine of endodontically instrumented root canals. *Int. Endod. J.* **2006**, *39*, 18–25. [CrossRef]
51. De-Deus, G.; Souza, E.M.; Silva, E.J.N.L.; Belladonna, F.G.; Simões-Carvalho, M.; Cavalcante, D.M.; Versiani, M.A. A critical analysis of research methods and experimental models to study root canal fillings. *Int. Endod. J.* **2022**, *55* (Suppl. S2), 384–445. [CrossRef] [PubMed]
52. Mekhdieva, E.; Del Fabbro, M.; Alovisi, M.; Comba, A.; Scotti, N.; Tumedei, M.; Carossa, M.; Berutti, E.; Pasqualini, D. Postoperative Pain following Root Canal Filling with Bioceramic vs. Traditional Filling Techniques: A Systematic Review and Meta-Analysis of Randomized Controlled Trials. *J. Clin. Med.* **2021**, *10*, 4509. [CrossRef] [PubMed]

Disclaimer/Publisher's Note: The statements, opinions and data contained in all publications are solely those of the individual author(s) and contributor(s) and not of MDPI and/or the editor(s). MDPI and/or the editor(s) disclaim responsibility for any injury to people or property resulting from any ideas, methods, instructions or products referred to in the content.

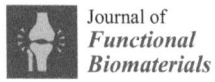

Review

The Use of Graphene Oxide in Orthodontics—A Systematic Review

Joanna Rygas [1], Jacek Matys [2,3,*], Magdalena Wawrzyńska [4], Maria Szymonowicz [4] and Maciej Dobrzyński [5]

1. Dental Practice, Wojciecha z Brudzewa 10, 51-601 Wroclaw, Poland; joanna.rygas@gmail.com
2. Oral Surgery Department, Wroclaw Medical University, Krakowska 26, 50-425 Wroclaw, Poland
3. Department of Orthodontics, Technische Universitat Dresden, 01307 Dresden, Germany
4. Pre-Clinical Research Centre, Wroclaw Medical University, Bujwida 44, 50-345 Wroclaw, Poland; magdalena.wawrzynska@umw.edu.pl (M.W.); maria.szymonowicz@umw.edu.pl (M.S.)
5. Department of Pediatric Dentistry and Preclinical Dentistry, Wroclaw Medical University, Krakowska 26, 50-425 Wroclaw, Poland; maciej.dobrzynski@umw.edu.pl
* Correspondence: jacek.matys@umw.edu.pl

Abstract: Background: Graphene-based materials have great prospects for application in dentistry and medicine due to their unique properties and biocompatibility with tissues. The literature on the use of graphene oxide in orthodontic treatment was reviewed. Methods: This systematic review followed the PRISMA protocol and was conducted by searching the following databases: PubMed, Scopus, Web of Science, and Cochrane. The following search criteria were used to review the data on the topic under study: (Graphene oxide) AND (orthodontic) ALL FIELDS. For the Scopus database, results were narrowed to titles, authors, and keywords. A basic search structure was adopted for each database. Initially, a total of 74 articles were found in the considered databases. Twelve articles met the inclusion criteria and were included in the review. Results: Nine studies demonstrated the antibacterial properties of graphene oxide, which can reduce the demineralization of enamel during orthodontic treatment. Seven studies showed that it is biocompatible with oral tissues. Three studies presented that graphene oxide can reduce friction in the arch-bracket system. Two studies showed that it can improve the mechanical properties of orthodontic adhesives by reducing ARI (Adhesive Remnant Index). Three studies demonstrated that the use of graphene oxide in the appropriate concentration can also increase the SBS (shear bond strength) parameter. One research study showed that it can increase corrosion resistance. One research study suggested that it can be used to accelerate orthodontic tooth movement. Conclusion: The studies included in the systematic review showed that graphene oxide has numerous applications in orthodontic treatment due to its properties.

Keywords: adhesive remnant index; antibacterial effect; corrosion resistance; demineralization; shear bond strength; white spots

1. Introduction

Discovered in 2004, graphene oxide (GO) is considered one of the most promising nanomaterials. This two-dimensional carbon material acts as the fundamental graphite unit and is composed of a single layer of hexagonally arranged sp2 carbon atoms [1,2]. Furthermore, graphene possesses extraordinary characteristics, including a significant surface area and exceptional mechanical, electrical, and thermal properties [3–5]. These attributes enable graphene to be utilized in diverse applications [1,6]. Nevertheless, the application of graphene may encounter restrictions due to issues such as agglomeration and challenges in processing. To overcome these limitations, chemical modification becomes necessary in order to generate derivatives of graphene, like graphene oxide (GO) and reduced graphene oxide (rGO). These modified forms prove to be more versatile and find applications across various fields [1,6–11]. The provided illustration depicts the structures of graphene, graphene oxide (GO), and reduced graphene oxide (rGO). GO is derived from the oxidation process applied to graphene, whereas rGO is obtained through the chemical or thermal reduction of GO [1] (Figure 1).

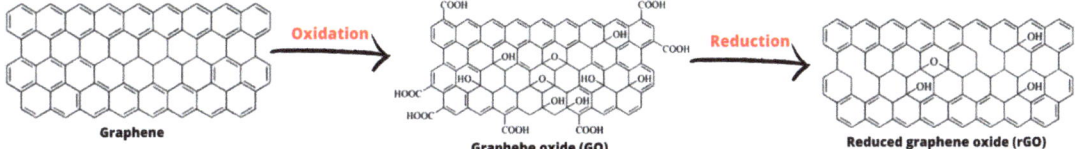

Figure 1. The figure illustrates the structural composition of graphene, graphene oxide (GO), and reduced graphene oxide (rGO) (created with Canva.com (accessed on 1 September 2023)).

The majority of research conducted on the antimicrobial properties of graphene-based nanomaterials (GBNs) has proposed three potential mechanisms to explain their antimicrobial activity against various microorganisms [1,12,13]. The first is the induction of oxidative stress in bacterial cells through the formation of reactive oxygen species, which damage bacterial cell membranes and thereby disrupt their metabolic activity [1,7,14–16]. The second involves killing pathogens with the sharp edges of graphene oxide particles—the so-called "nano-sharpening effect" [1,3,14]. It causes leakage of the bacterial cytoplasmic fluid and consequently, cell death. The third is the isolation of the bacterial cell from the external environment—the so-called "wrapping effect" [1,7,14]. Graphene oxide nanoparticles wrap around bacterial cells and isolate them from the environment, thus preventing bacterial proliferation and cell membrane activity [1,14]. The mechanical disruption caused by electrostatic forces can result in the disturbance of bacterial cells, leading to alterations in membrane potential, depolarization, and compromised integrity of the bacterial cell membrane. This process eventually leads to osmotic imbalance, disruption of cellular respiration, cell lysis, and ultimately, the demise of the bacterial cell [1] (Figure 2).

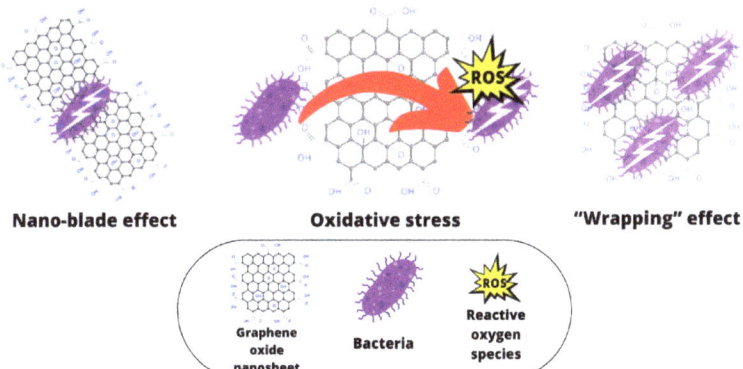

Figure 2. The diagram illustrates three distinct antibacterial mechanisms of graphene oxide (created with Canva.com (accessed on 1 September 2023)).

The bactericidal effect of graphene oxide is influenced not only by intrinsic and extrinsic factors but also by the composition, structure, and maturity stage of microbial cells [1,7]. Researchers have acknowledged the impact of bacterial structure on antimicrobial activity. Understanding the underlying mechanisms of graphene-based nanomaterials can contribute to the development of dental materials resistant to microbial infections [1,8]. Nano-scale nanoparticles possess a higher surface area to volume ratio compared to non-nano particles, allowing for closer interaction with microbial membranes and enhanced antimicrobial activity [17,18]. To enhance antimicrobial properties, dental materials often incorporate antimicrobial agents such as chlorhexidine and quaternary ammonium compounds [1]. However, these additions often result in a compromise between antimicrobial effectiveness and mechanical properties [1,7]. In contrast, graphene oxide has the unique ability to associate with other biomaterials like polymers, ceramics, and metals, facilitating the design of biomaterials with desired properties. For instance, graphene and its derivatives can be incorporated into dental materials through methods such as colloidal dispersion, direct synthesis, sintering, and conjugation [1].

Recently, the use of graphene-oxide-based materials has become very beneficial in the field of dental research [7,8,19]. This is due to its favourable biological properties, high specific surface area, biocompatibility, physico-chemical stability, mechanical strength, electronic properties, and easy synthesis process, while also being low-cost [1,7,20]. Moreover, thanks to the mechanisms of antibacterial effect, graphene oxide can reduce the total amount of *S. mutans* (*Streptococcus mutans*) in the oral cavity and reduce the formation of white spot lesions [4,14,16,21]. This not only reduces the risk of carious cavities, but also improves the aesthetic effect at the end of orthodontic treatment [14,16]. It is also essential for orthodontists to assess the impact of graphene on the bonding of brackets to the tooth surface. Due to these properties, graphene oxide may not only have a wide range of uses in dentistry, but also in medicine. In recent studies [14,16], GO has been identified as a potential carrier in nanomedicine, especially for cancer treatment and controlled drug delivery systems. It can be an alternative to fight against bacterial infection [22,23]. Furthermore, recent research in the field of dental materials suggests the potential of graphene oxide usage as a sealer component in endodontic treatment [24]. The failure of endodontic treatment is directly associated with microbial infection in the root canal or periapical areas. An endodontic sealer that is both bactericidal and biocompatible is essential for the success of a root canal. The study [16] showed that graphene-oxide-based composites show promise as endodontic sealers for protection against reinfection in root canal treatment and enhance success in endodontic treatment overall treatments.

The main objective of this systematic review was to explore the impact of graphene oxide properties on its use in orthodontic treatment. Based on the analysed articles on the use of graphene oxide in orthodontic treatment, it was concluded that, due to its unique properties and biocompatibility, it is worth writing a systematic review on this topic. Furthermore, a systematic review on this topic has not yet been published. Such a review of the literature may encourage researchers to carry out further studies, which could be of great benefit to both orthodontists and patients in the future.

2. Materials and Methods

2.1. Focused Question

The systematic review followed the PICO framework as follows.

PICO question: in the case of orthodontic materials (population), will the addition of graphene oxide (investigated condition) cause a change in their properties (outcome) compared to orthodontic materials without the addition of graphene (comparison condition)?

2.2. Protocol

The selection process for articles in the systematic review was carefully outlined following the PRISMA flow diagram (Figure 3) [25].

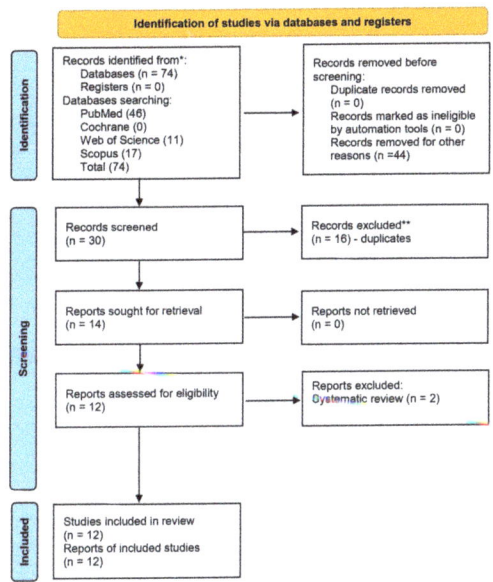

Figure 3. The PRISMA 2020 flow diagram [25].

2.3. Eligibility Criteria

The review included studies that adhered to the following criteria: studies investigating the use of graphene materials in orthodontics, both in vitro and in vivo studies, studies published in English, and studies with a control group. The reviewers collectively decided to exclude studies that met the following criteria: non-English studies, opinion pieces, review articles and meta-analyses, letters to the editor, editorial papers, clinical reports, studies without full-text accessibility, and duplicated publications. No restrictions were imposed on the year of publication.

2.4. Information Sources, Search Strategy, and Study Selection

On 1 February 2023, electronic searches were conducted in the following databases: Pubmed, Cochrane, Web of Science, and Scopus. For the Scopus database, results were narrowed to titles, authors and keywords. Searches were limited to individuals and studies that met the eligibility criteria. The study was then supplemented with a literature search of the articles considered not found during the database search. Only articles with full-text versions available were considered.

2.5. Data Collection Process and Data Items

Two reviewers autonomously gathered data from articles that fulfilled the inclusion criteria. The extracted information was then entered into a standardized Excel file.

2.6. Assessing Risk of Bias in Individual Studies

At the initial stage of study selection, the titles and abstracts of each study were independently checked by the authors to minimise potential reviewer bias. The level of agreement among reviewers was determined using Cohen's κ test [26]. Any differences of opinion on the inclusion or exclusion of a study were resolved through discussion between authors.

2.7. Quality Assessment

Two independent reviewers (J.M., M.D.) evaluated the procedural quality of each study included in the article. The assessment criteria were based on the presence of key information related to the association of graphene oxide use in orthodontic treatment. To evaluate the study design, implementation, and analysis, the following criteria were used: a minimum group size of 10 subjects, the presence of a control group, a clear description of the performed procedure technique, the specific orthodontic adhesive used in the research, a biocompatibility test for graphene oxide, consideration of the type of orthodontic arch in the study, and analysis of the effect of graphene oxide on friction in the bracket–arch system, including parameters such as shear bond strength (SBS) and adhesive remnant index (ARI). The studies were scored on a scale of 0 to 9 points, with a higher score indicating higher study quality. The risk of bias was assessed as follows: 0–3 points denoted a high risk, 4–6 points denoted a moderate risk, and 7–9 points indicated a low risk. Any discrepancies in scoring were resolved through discussion until a consensus was reached.

3. Results

3.1. Study Selection

An initial search of the database identified 74 articles that were potentially eligible for the literature review. A first selection of article titles and abstracts allowed the exclusion of 44 articles as unrelated to the reviewed topic. Among the remaining 30 articles, there were 16 duplicates. Two non-research articles were rejected. Finally, 12 articles were qualified for the systematic review. All of the included studies were in vitro studies.

3.2. General Characteristics of the Included Studies

Twelve studies were included in this review. The general characteristics of each study (purpose of the study, control and study group, results, and conclusions) are presented in Table 1.

Shear bond strength (SBS) and adhesive remnant index (ARI) coefficients are essential parameters for describing the mechanical properties of orthodontic adhesives [27]. In the research conducted by Maryam Pourhajibagher et al. [19], Roghayeh Ghorbanzadeh et al. [8], and Nozha M. Sawana et al. [6], no significant difference in ARI value was observed between the control samples and the modified experimental groups. However, in another study by Nozha M. Sawana et al. [28], orthodontic adhesive samples treated with 0.35 wt% Ag-GS (graphene sheets decorated with silver nanoparticles) showed the lowest ARI score among all the experimental groups after thermocycling. Additionally, in the study conducted by Mohammad Alnatheera et al. [16], the samples treated with 0.25 wt% SGO-modified adhesive (silanized graphene oxide) exhibited the lowest ARI scores.

According to the investigation by Roghayeh Ghorbanzadeh et al. [8] and Maryam Pourhajibagher et al. [19], Transbond XT with 5% wt. nGO (nanographene oxide) exhibited the highest shear bond strength (SBS) value. In the study conducted by Seung-Min Lee et al. [14], the SBS of the control group showed no significant difference compared to the BAG@GO (graphene oxide with a bioactive glass mixture) group, whereas adhesives with 1 wt% BAG@GO showed a small gain in SBS. In the Nozha M. Sawana et al. [28] study, there was no significant difference in SBS between 0.35 wt% Ag-GS and the commercial adhesive after 2 h of storage in distilled water. However, a notable difference in SBS was observed when the nanoparticle concentration was improved (0.55 wt% Ag-GS) compared to the commercial adhesive, indicating that higher nanoparticle concentrations reduced SBS. In the study conducted by Mohammad Alnatheera et al. [16], the samples treated with 0.25 wt% SGO-modified adhesive showed the highest mean SBS. Lastly, in the study by Nozha M. et al. [6], the effect of GNP-Ag (graphene nanoplatelets with silver nanoparticles) concentration on SBS was explored over a 24 h period of storage in distilled water. The findings revealed a gradual decline in SBS with an increase in GNP-Ag concentration in the experimental adhesive. This temporal insight highlights the importance of considering the long-term performance and stability of nanoparticle-infused adhesives in orthodontic treatment.

The research conducted by Maryam Pourhajibagher et al. [12,19] and Roghayeh Ghorbanzadeh et al. [8] demonstrated that the addition of nGO to Transbond XT led to a significant reduction in *S. mutans* colony counts, indicating antimicrobial properties. However, Maryam Pourhajibagher et al. [12] specifically noted that only the concentration of 10 wt% nGO showed a statistically significant decrease in the colony-forming units of test microorganisms after 60 days. The anti-microbial activity of the eluted components from the modified orthodontic adhesive discs against *S. mutans* was directly related to the concentration of nGO. Moreover, the study by Maryam Pourhajibagher et al. [19] revealed a gradual increase in biofilm inhibition with increasing nGO concentrations, without a concurrent increase in the failure rates of brackets. On the other hand, it was observed that concentrations higher than 5 wt% nGO significantly inhibited the growth of *S. mutans*, but this was accompanied by a decrease in the average bond strength of the adhesive to the enamel as the nGO concentration exceeded 5%. The ideal orthodontic adhesive (composite) should possess antimicrobial properties and be capable of inducing enamel remineralization without adversely affecting the bond strength of the brackets to the enamel.

The studies conducted by Maryam Pourhajibagher et al. [12,19] and Roghayeh Ghorbanzadeh et al. [8] revealed that adding nGO to Transbond XT resulted in a significant reduction in *S. mutans* colony counts, indicating its antimicrobial properties. Notably, Maryam Pourhajibagher et al. [12] specifically emphasized that only the concentration of 10 wt% nGO demonstrated a statistically significant decrease in the colony-forming units of test microorganisms after 60 days. The antimicrobial activity of the eluted components from the modified orthodontic adhesive discs against *S. mutans* was directly correlated with the concentration of nGO. Additionally, Maryam Pourhajibagher et al. [19] observed a gradual increase in biofilm inhibition with increasing nGO concentrations without a concurrent increase in the failure rates of brackets. However, it was also observed that concentrations higher than 5 wt% nGO led to significant inhibition of *S. mutans* growth, but this was accompanied by a decrease in the average bond strength of the adhesive to the enamel as the nGO concentration exceeded 5%. This highlights the importance of balancing antimicrobial properties with maintaining strong bonding to the enamel for an ideal orthodontic adhesive (composite), which should possess both antimicrobial capabilities and the ability to induce enamel remineralization without compromising the bond strength of the brackets to the enamel.

Nozha M. et al. [6] conducted a study with the objective of formulating and characterizing functionalized graphene nanoplatelets (GNPs) combined with silver nanoparticles (AgNPs) to evaluate the antimicrobial and mechanical properties of GNP-Ag-modified adhesives used in bonding orthodontic brackets. The research yielded noteworthy results regarding the viability of human gingival fibroblast (HGF) cells when exposed to the modified experimental adhesive (Transbond XT) [6]. The experimental adhesive containing 0.25 wt% and 0.5 wt% of GNP-Ag (graphene nanoplatelets with silver nanoparticles) showed low cytotoxicity, with cell survival rates exceeding 80%. However, after 48 h, the adhesive with 0.5 wt% of GNPAg exhibited considerable cytotoxic behaviour. On the other hand, the adhesive with 0.25 wt% of GNP-Ag demonstrated a substantial increase in antibacterial properties, making it suitable for bonding orthodontic brackets to the enamel surface without compromising bond strength.

In a separate study conducted by Nozha M. et al. [28], their primary objective was to modify orthodontic adhesive by skilfully incorporating graphene sheets adorned with silver nanoparticles (Ag-GS). After bonding the orthodontic brackets, they aimed to evaluate the ensuing mechanical and antibacterial properties. The investigation demonstrated a clear trend of decreasing relative microbiological viability with a proportional increase in the weight percentage (wt%) of nanoparticles in the adhesives. However, it was observed that the orthodontic adhesive containing 0.55 wt% of Ag-GS exhibited considerable cytotoxic behaviour after 48 h. These findings underscore the crucial significance of meticulously optimizing the nanoparticle concentration in orthodontic adhesives to ensure both biocompatibility and effective antimicrobial properties. In the study conducted by Mohammad Alnatheera et al. [16], their research focus was on modifying the Transbond XT (control adhesive) by skilfully incorporating 0.25 wt% and 0.5 wt% of SGO-modified adhesive (silanized graphene oxide). The 0.25 wt% SGO-modified adhesive group showed the most effective bactericidal properties and exhibited the least cytotoxicity when compared to the 0.5 wt% SGO-modified adhesive and Transbond XT. Furthermore, Jung-Hwan Lee et al. [29] investigated the antimicrobial-adhesive effects of PMMA with and without nGO incorporation. Specimens with higher amounts of nGO exhibited more robust anti-adhesion effects against all microbial species, and no significant cytotoxicity was observed when compared to the control group. While this innate nGO did not significantly enhance mechanical properties compared to the control, it did not exhibit any systemic toxic effects in humans from fully polymerized PMMA products, as reported in previous studies.

Pengfei Wang et al. [15] and Zonglin Pan et al. [30] conducted a comprehensive study exploring the fretting friction and wear behaviours of stainless steel archwires coated with a carbon film that contained embedded graphene sheets (GSEC). They specifically investigated how these GSEC-coated orthodontic stainless steel archwires performed in contact with untextured and microgroove textured stainless steel brackets within an artificial saliva environment. The research findings strongly suggested that the combined effect of the GSEC film on the archwire surface and the micro-groove textures on the brackets had a remarkable positive influence on the overall friction and wear characteristics of the stainless steel archwire–bracket sliding contacts. As a result, the study demonstrated great promise for utilizing GSEC-coated archwires in various clinical orthodontic treatment applications (Figure 4).

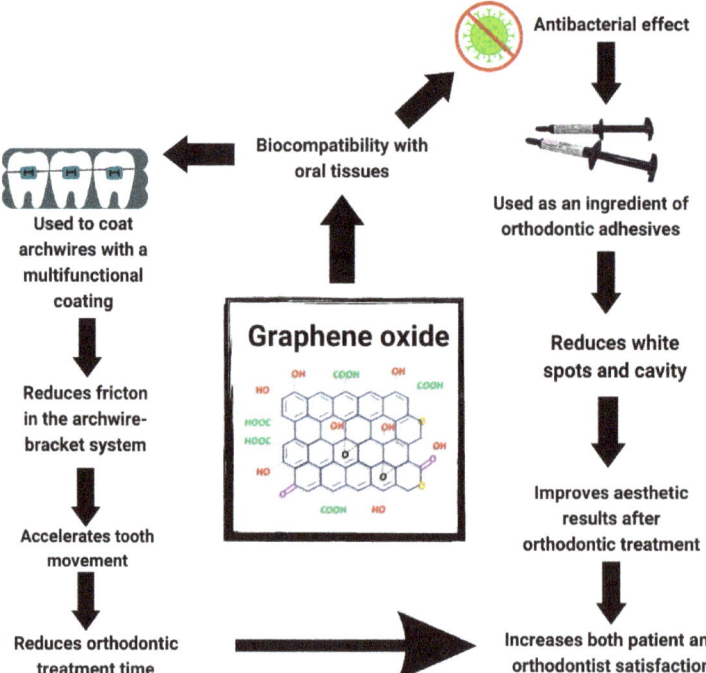

Figure 4. Figure illustrates the use of graphene oxide in orthodontic treatment (created with Canva.com (accessed on 1 September 2023)).

Zonglin Pan et al. [30] conducted a study with comparable outcomes. Their research demonstrated that GSEC film-coated archwires exhibited low friction coefficients and exceptional wear resistance when interacting with stainless steel brackets in artificial saliva environments. The authors concluded that applying the surface coating technique with GSEC film could lead to more effective and efficient orthodontic treatment. On the other hand, Danni Daia et al. [7] focused on graphene oxide (GO) coatings on NiTi (nickel titanium) alloys. Their study revealed that the coating did not sufficiently cover the substrate at low GO concentrations, providing only minor enhancements to NiTi alloy's tribological and anti-corrosion properties. However, as the GO concentration increased, the GO coating exhibited significantly improved antibacterial activity. It was cautioned that higher GO concentrations might compromise the biocompatibility of GO-coated NiTi alloys. The authors suggested their study offered a controllable and straightforward process to enhance NiTi alloy surface properties, including corrosion resistance, friction resistance, and antimicrobial properties, while ensuring biocompatibility. Additionally, Delong Jiao et al. [6] conducted a series of experiments in vitro and in vivo (on mice), demonstrating that the application of GOG (gelatine reduced graphene oxide) can accelerate orthodontic tooth movement. The results indicated accelerated bone remodelling in the GOG-treated group, with enhanced osteoblasto-/osteoclasto-genesis and angiogenesis.

3.3. Main Study Outcomes

Nine studies [6–9,12,14,16,18,20] demonstrated the antibacterial properties of graphene oxide, which can reduce the demineralisation of enamel during orthodontic treatment. Seven studies [6,8,12,14,16,18,20] showed that it is biocompatible with oral tissues. Three studies [4,7,15] showed that graphene oxide can reduce friction in the arch-bracket system. Two studies [16,20] showed that it can improve the mechanical properties of orthodontic adhesives by reducing ARI (Adhesive Remnant Index). Three studies [8,16,19] demonstrated that graphene oxide used in the appropriate concentration can also increase the SBS (shear bond strength) parameter. One research study [7] showed that it can increase the corrosion resistance. One research study [18] suggested that it can be used to accelerate orthodontic tooth movement. It can be used to coat the surface of orthodontic arches [4,6,15] and as an additive to orthodontic adhesives [6,8,12,14,16,19,20].

3.4. Quality Assessment

Out of the articles included in the review, four [6,8,16,20] were deemed high-quality, with a score of 7/9 points. Two studies [9,18] were classified as low-quality. Additionally, six studies [4,7,12,14,15,19] were considered to have a moderate risk of bias, scoring between 4 and 6 points (Table 2). Distribution of bias risk of eligible studies is presented in Figure 5.

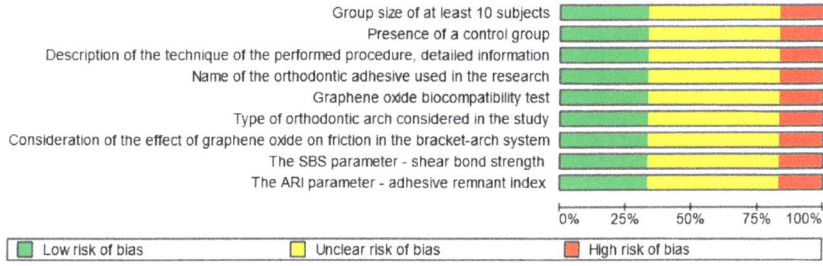

Figure 5. Distribution of bias risk of eligible studies (created with RevMan Web, Cochrane, UK).

Table 1. General characteristics of the included studies.

Studies	Purpose of the Study	Control and Study Group	Results	Conclusions
Maryam Pourhajibagher et al. [19]	SBS and ARI scores of orthodontic adhesive were incorporated with nGO. The antimicrobial activities of the modified orthodontic adhesive were compared against *S. mutans*.	Transbond XT (3M Unitek, Monrovia, CA, USA) with 0 (as the control), 1, 2, 5, and 10 wt% nGO.	- The orthodontic adhesive containing 5 wt% nGO exhibited the highest concentration of nGO and shear bond strength (SBS) value. - It also showed no significant differences in adhesive remnant index compared to the control group. - SBS in the 1%, 2%, and 5% nGO groups was significantly higher than that in the 10% nGO group.	- Addition of 5 wt% nGO to the orthodontic adhesive can be deemed effective in reducing microbial count and biofilm formation without negatively impacting shear bond strength (SBS) and adhesive remnant index (ARI).
Delong Jiao et al. [18]	The aim of the study was to find out if gelatine reduced graphene oxide (GOG) accelerated orthodontic tooth movement.	In the experimental group, GOG solution was administered via buccal submucous local injection around the maxillary left first molar, while the control group received phosphate buffer saline (PBS) solution injection.	- The administration of GOG led to accelerated bone remodelling, promoting the generation of osteoblasts and osteoclasts as well as stimulating angiogenesis.	- Serial experiments in vitro and in vivo showed that application of GOG can accelerate orthodontic tooth movement.
Roghayeh Ghorbanzadeh et al. [8]	Physiomechanical and antimicrobial effectiveness of a novel orthodontic composite (OC-nGO) containing nGO following photodynamic therapy (PDT) and photothermal therapy (PTT) was compared against Streptococcus mutans.	Transbond XT (3M Unitek, Monrovia, CA, USA) with 0 (as the control), 1, 2, 5, and 10 wt% nGO.	- *S. mutans* metabolic activity and biofilm susceptibility were most affected by diode laser light when 5% wt. nGO was present for up to 150 days of rinsing. - Transbond XT with 5% wt. nGO exhibited the highest shear bond strength (SBS) value, along with potent antimicrobial and anti-biofilm activities. - All test concentrations of nGO in OC-nGO demonstrated adhesive remnant index (ARI) scores similar to the control group.	- Photo-activated 5% wt. OC-nGO can be used as an additive in orthodontic composites/adhesives to effectively control cariogenic bacterial biofilms.

Table 1. *Cont.*

Studies	Purpose of the Study	Control and Study Group	Results	Conclusions
Maryam Pourhajibagher et al. [12]	Antimicrobial and cytotoxic effects of a conventional orthodontic adhesive infused with varying concentrations of nanographene oxide (nGO).	Transbond XT (3M Unitek, Monrovia, CA, USA) with 0 (as the control), 1, 2, 5, and 10 wt% nGO.	- The modified orthodontic adhesive did not exhibit any cytotoxic effects on HGF cells. - The Transbond XT adhesive infused with 5% and 10% nGO significantly reduced the mean total viable counts of *S. mutans* for up to 30 days. - However, after 60 days, only the adhesive containing 10% nGO showed a statistically significant decrease in the colony-forming units of the test microorganisms.	- The antimicrobial activity against *S. mutans* in cariogenic biofilms is notably significant when using a modified orthodontic adhesive containing nGO at concentrations of 5% and 10%.
Seung-Min Lee et al. [14]	Mechanical and biological properties of orthodontic bonding adhesive enriched with graphene oxide and bioactive glass.	Transbond™ Supreme Low-Viscosity Light Cure Adhesive, 3M, Monrovia, CA, USA) with 0 (as the control), 1, 3, and 5 wt% of BAG@GO.	- There was no statistically significant difference in shear bond strength (SBS) between the control group and the BAG@GO group. - The adhesives with 1 wt% BAG@GO exhibited a slight increase in SBS. - However, the adhesive group with 5 wt% BAG@GO showed lower SBS, although this difference was not statistically significant.	- The mechanical properties of the orthodontic bonding adhesive enriched with graphene oxide and bioactive glass were suitable for clinical use. - The biological properties were found to be safe for application to patients.
Pengfei Wang et al. [15]	Fretting friction and wear behaviour of the graphene sheets embedded carbon (GSEC) stainless steel archwire in the archwire–bracket contact.	Graphene sheets embedded carbon (GSEC) films were produced with a high substrate bias voltage. The control group consisted of uncoated stainless steel archwire sliding against a conventional stainless steel bracket.	- The combined influence of the GSEC films on the archwires and the micro-groove textures on the brackets led to outstanding friction and wear performance in the archwire–bracket sliding contacts.	- The study suggested great potential of the GSEC films for clinical orthodontic treatment applications.

Table 1. *Cont.*

Studies	Purpose of the Study	Control and Study Group	Results	Conclusions
Jung-Hwan Lee et al. [29]	Antimicrobial-adhesive effects of PMMA with and without nGO incorporation.	In nGO and nGO-incorporated PMMA (up to 2 wt%), the 3-point flexural strength and hardness were assessed. To examine the anti-adhesive effects, the experimental specimens were tested against four different microbial species. The control group involved bacteria only.	- Specimens containing higher levels of nGO exhibited more potent anti-adhesion effects against all microbial species. - None of the specimens showed any signs of cytotoxicity when compared to the control group, and there have been no reports of systemic toxic effects in humans from fully polymerized PMMA products. - However, the innate nGO did not significantly enhance the mechanical properties compared to the control.	The data indicate that nGO-incorporated PMMA holds promise for various applications, including removable or provisional prosthodontics, as well as implantable biomaterials, thanks to its documented antimicrobial and anti-adhesive properties.
Nozha M. et al. [28]	Incorporating graphene sheets decorated with silver nanoparticles (Ag-GS) and investigating how these modifications impact the mechanical and antibacterial properties after bonding with orthodontic brackets.	Ag-GS was added to the orthodontic adhesive (Transbond XT orthodontic adhesive (3 M, Unitek, USA)) in two distinct concentrations (0.35 and 0.55 wt%). As a control adhesive, a Transbond XT adhesive was utilized.	- After 2 h of storage in distilled water, there was no significant difference in shear bond strength (SBS) between the 0.35 wt% Ag-GS modified adhesive and the commercial adhesive. - However, as the nanoparticle concentration increased (0.55 wt% Ag-GS), a noticeable decrease in SBS was observed compared to the commercial adhesive, indicating that higher nanoparticle concentrations negatively affected SBS. - The orthodontic adhesive with 0.55 wt% Ag-GS demonstrated significant cytotoxic behaviour after 48 h.	Incorporating 0.35 wt% of nanoparticles significantly enhances the antibacterial capabilities of the orthodontic adhesives. This concentration demonstrated promising outcomes for bonding orthodontic brackets to enamel without compromising the adhesive strength.

Table 1. Cont.

Studies	Purpose of the Study	Control and Study Group	Results	Conclusions
Mohammad Alnatheera et al. [16]	Creating and analysing silanized graphene oxide (SGO) nanoparticles and evaluating their spectral, microbiological, and mechanical properties when incorporated into orthodontic adhesive for bonding to orthodontic brackets.	Transbond XT (control adhesive) was modified by incorporating 0.25 wt% and 0.5 wt% SGO-modified adhesive.	The samples treated with 0.25 wt% SGO-modified adhesive exhibited the highest mean SBS and the lowest ARI scores. The 0.25 wt% SGO-modified adhesive group demonstrated the most potent bactericidal effect and the least cytotoxicity compared to the 0.5 wt% SGO-modified adhesive and Transbond XT groups.	Incorporating 0.25 wt% of SGO into Transbond XT resulted in improved antimicrobial and mechanical properties, making it a promising option for bonding orthodontic brackets.
Zonglin Pan et al. [30]	Influence of coating stainless steel archwires with graphene sheets embedded carbon (GSEC) film on friction on archwire–bracket contact.	Carbon films were produced using an electron cyclotron resonance plasma sputtering system at substrate bias voltages ranging from +5 to +50 V. Uncoated stainless steel archwires were used as the control.	When sliding against stainless steel brackets in artificial saliva environments, the GSEC film-coated archwires demonstrated low friction coefficients and high wear resistance.	The application of the GSEC film surface coating technique is anticipated to enhance the effectiveness and efficiency of orthodontic treatments.
Nozha M. et al. [6]	Creating and analysing graphene nanoplatelets (GNPs) functionalised with silver nanoparticles (AgNPs) and assessing the antimicrobial and mechanical properties of the resulting GNP-Ag-modified adhesives when used to bond orthodontic brackets.	Graphene conjugated with Ag nanoparticles were incorporated into the Transbond XT orthodontic adhesive (3 M, Unitek, USA) at 0.25 wt% and 0.5 wt%. Unmodified Transbond XT was kept as a control group.	The ARI values showed no significant difference between the control samples and the modified experimental groups. After 24 h of storage in distilled water, the SBS decreased with an increase in GNP-Ag concentration in the experimental adhesive. The study revealed a notable difference in the viability of HGF cells between the modified and unmodified experimental adhesive. The experimental adhesive containing 0.25 and 0.5 wt% of GNP-Ag demonstrated low cytotoxicity, with the cell survival rate being above 80%. However, after 48 h, the experimental adhesive with 0.5 wt% GNP-Ag exhibited significant cytotoxic behaviour.	Incorporating silver nanoparticle-doped graphene nanoplatelets could serve as a potential antimicrobial modification for orthodontic adhesives. Addition of 0.25 wt% of this composite resulted in a significant increase in antibacterial properties, making it a suitable choice for bonding orthodontic brackets to the enamel surface without compromising bond strength.

Table 1. *Cont.*

Studies	Purpose of the Study	Control and Study Group	Results	Conclusions
Danni Daia et al. [7]	Exploration of the impact of different concentrations of graphene oxide (GO) coatings for NiTi alloy on corrosion resistance, friction performance, and antibacterial properties.	Specially prepared samples were coated with 0 (as the control), 0.5, 2, or 5 mg/mL GO concentrations.	- At low GO concentrations, the coating on the substrate was insufficient, leading to limited improvements in the tribological and anti-corrosion properties of the NiTi alloy. - As the GO concentration increased, the antibacterial activity of the coating improved continuously. - However, higher GO concentrations may compromise the biocompatibility of the GO-coated NiTi.	By applying a multifunctional GO nanocoating, the surface of NiTi can be enhanced to improve its corrosion resistance, friction resistance, and antimicrobial properties while ensuring biocompatibility.

SBS—shear bond strength; ARI—adhesive remnant index; GOG—gelatine reduced graphene oxide; HGF—human gingival fibroblast; BAG@GO—Graphene oxide (GO) with a bioactive glass (BAG) mixture; Ag-GS—graphene sheets decorated with silver nanoparticles; SGO—silanized graphene oxide; GNP-Ag—graphene nanoplatelets (GNPs) with silver nanoparticles (AgNPs).

Table 2. Assessing risk of bias, presence (1) or its absence (0).

Criteria/Authors	Maryam Pourhajibagher [19]	Delong [18]	Roghayeh Ghorbanzadeh [8]	Maryam Pourhajibagher [12]	Seung-Min [14]	Pengfei Wang [15]	Jung-Hwan [29]	Nozha M. [28]	Alnatheera [16]	Zonglin [30]	Nozha M. [6]	Danni [7]
Group size of at least 10 subjects	1	0	1	1	0	0	0	1	1	0	1	0
Control group	1	1	1	1	1	1	1	1	1	1	1	1
Description of the technique of the performed procedure, detailed information, e.g., additional instruments supporting the procedure, duration of the procedure	1	1	1	1	1	1	1	1	1	1	1	1
Name of the orthodontic adhesive used in the research	1	0	1	1	1	0	0	1	1	0	1	0
Graphene oxide biocompatibility test	0	1	1	1	1	0	1	1	1	0	1	1
Type of orthodontic arch considered in the study	0	0	0	0	0	1	0	0	0	1	0	1
Consideration of the effect of graphene oxide on friction in the bracket-arch system	0	0	0	0	0	1	0	0	0	1	0	1
The SBS parameter—shear bond strength	1	0	1	0	1	0	0	1	1	0	1	0
The ARI parameter—adhesive remnant index	1	0	1	0	1	0	0	1	1	0	1	0
Total points	6	3	7	5	6	4	3	7	7	4	7	5
Risk of bias	Moderate	High	Low	Moderate	Moderate	Moderate	High	Low	Low	Moderate	Low	Moderate

4. Discussion

In modern dentistry, tremendous efforts have been made to prevent oral diseases and promote oral hygiene [2]. Restorative materials with excellent biological properties, improved mechanical properties, and longer service life have always been sought [5]. Graphene oxide has been shown to possess antibacterial properties and biocompatibility, making it a safe and beneficial material for use in oral cavity biomaterials [21]. Several studies meeting the inclusion criteria in this review have demonstrated various potential applications of graphene oxide in orthodontic treatment. Some of these studies [6,8,19] found no significant difference in the adhesive remnant index (ARI) between the control and modified experimental groups. Conversely, other studies [16,20] reported that orthodontic adhesive samples modified with graphene oxide exhibited the lowest ARI scores among all the groups studied. Regarding shear bond strength (SBS), some authors [14,19,20] did not find a statistically significant difference between the study and control groups. However, other studies [5,8,16] suggested that Transbond XT modified with nGO showed the highest SBS value. In contrast, the study by Maryam Pourhajibagher et al. [19] indicated that SBS in the 10% nGO group was statistically lower than in the control group. Furthermore, the SBS value for the 1%, 2%, and 5% nGO groups was significantly higher than that in the 10% nGO group. Similarly, a significant reduction in SBS was observed with increasing nanoparticle concentration (0.55 wt% Ag-GS) [8]. Overall, graphene oxide has the potential to enhance the mechanical properties of orthodontic adhesives, provided that it is added at the appropriate concentration.

Numerous studies [6–9,12,14,16,18,20] have highlighted the antibacterial properties of graphene oxide, which can effectively reduce enamel demineralization during orthodontic treatment. Authors [14] have even suggested that the anti-demineralization effect increases as the concentration of BAG@GO (graphene oxide coated with bioactive glass) rises. Similar findings were reported by Maryam Pourhajibagher et al. [19], demonstrating a gradual increase in biofilm inhibition (decrease in *S. mutans* growth) with higher nGO concentrations, without compromising the bond strength of the brackets (SBS). On the other hand, studies conducted by Nozha M. et al. [6] and Nozha M. et al. [28] revealed significant cytotoxic behaviour for 0.5 wt% of GNPAg experimental adhesive and 0.55 wt% of Ag-GS orthodontic adhesive, respectively, after 48 h. These results underscore the importance of using graphene oxide in appropriate concentrations to avoid potential cytotoxicity and impairment of bonding strength in orthodontic adhesives.

Several studies [4,7,15] have demonstrated that graphene oxide (GO) can effectively reduce friction in the archwire–bracket system. For instance, GO can be used to coat stainless steel archwires with a graphene sheet embedded carbon (GSEC) film, leading to reduced friction in the archwire–bracket contact [4,15]. In another study by Danni Daia et al. [7], a multifunctional GO nanocoating was applied to the surface of NiTi to enhance its corrosion resistance, friction resistance, and antimicrobial properties. The authors suggested that the GO nanocoating could also improve the mechanical properties of orthodontic arches, such as corrosion resistance [7] and high wear resistance [6,15]. However, Danni Daia et al. [7] also pointed out that when the GO concentration was low, the GO coating inadequately covered the substrate, resulting in only slight improvements in the tribological and anti-corrosion properties of NiTi alloy. As the GO concentration increased, the GO coating exhibited enhanced antibacterial activity, but a higher concentration could compromise the biocompatibility of GO-coated NiTi. Therefore, the application of surface coating techniques using the GSEC film or GO nanocoating holds promise for making orthodontic treatment more effective and efficient. However, it is crucial to carefully control the concentration of graphene oxide coating to achieve a balance of desired surface properties. By optimizing the GO concentration, clinicians and patients can benefit from the improved performance of orthodontic materials.

Finally, it is worth noting that a study [18] presented compelling evidence for the potential of graphene oxide (GOG) to accelerate orthodontic tooth movement due to its unique properties. The authors demonstrated that the GOG-treated group exhibited accelerated bone remodelling with increased osteoblastic and osteoclastic activity, as well as enhanced angiogenesis [18]. The results consistently indicated the biocompatibility of GOG and its ability to stimulate bone marrow stromal cells (BMSCs) to promote bone remodelling and tooth movement [18].

These findings open up promising avenues for further research in this area. However, the limitations of the present systematic review need to be highlighted. Given the diverse array of articles, conducting a meta-analysis proved unfeasible. To enhance the assessment of this subject matter, further research is warranted, ideally with a larger sample size and encompassing both clinical and in vivo studies.

5. Conclusions

Thanks to its properties, graphene oxide may have prospects for use in orthodontic treatment. First of all, due to its biocompatibility, it can be used safely in the oral cavity. It has an antibacterial effect and can be added as an ingredient in orthodontic adhesives. It can reduce carious white spots and, consequently, cavities. Fewer white spots will also lead to improved aesthetic results after orthodontic treatment. Graphene oxide can be used to coat arches with a multifunctional coating. Reduction of friction in the archwire–bracket system improves the mechanical properties of orthodontic arches and increases corrosion resistance. Also, reduced friction contributes to faster tooth movement. Research also indicates graphene oxide's ability to accelerate orthodontic tooth movement, which could speed up orthodontic treatment.

The development of technology gives better opportunities to both the patient and the orthodontist due to the new physicochemical, mechanical, and antibacterial properties of nanosized materials that can be used in coating orthodontic wires and producing orthodontic bonding materials. Not only can we control biofilm formation, reduce bacterial activity, and facilitate anticariogenic action, but also, through the desired tooth movement, shorten the treatment time. This offers great prospects for the further development of research using graphene oxide in orthodontic treatment, especially in vivo.

Author Contributions: Conceptualization, J.R., J.M. and M.D.; methodology, J.R., J.M. and M.D.; formal analysis, M.S. and M.W., data curation, J.R., J.M. and M.S.; writing—original draft preparation, J.R. and J.M.; writing—review and editing, M.D., J.M. and M.S.; project administration, M.D. and M.W.; supervision and funding acquisition, M.D. and M.W. All authors have read and agreed to the published version of the manuscript.

Funding: This work was financed by a subsidy from Wroclaw Medical University, number SUBZ. B180.23.054.

Data Availability Statement: Availability of supporting data—the datasets used and/or analysed during the current study are available from the corresponding author on reasonable request.

Conflicts of Interest: The authors declare no conflict of interest.

References

1. Radhi, A.; Mohamad, D.; Rahman, F.S.A.; Abdullah, A.M.; Hasan, H. Mechanism and factors influence of graphene-based nanomaterials antimicrobial activities and application in dentistry. *J. Mater. Res. Technol.* **2021**, *11*, 1290–1307. [CrossRef]
2. Zare, P.; Aleemardani, M.; Seifalian, A.; Bagher, Z.; Seifalian, A.M. Graphene Oxide: Opportunities and Challenges in Biomedicine. *Nanomaterials* **2021**, *11*, 1083. [CrossRef]
3. Powell, C.; Beall, G.W. Graphene oxide and graphene from low grade coal: Synthesis, characterization and applications. *Curr. Opin. Colloid Interface Sci.* **2015**, *20*, 362–366. [CrossRef]
4. Ge, Z.; Yang, L.; Xiao, F.; Wu, Y.; Yu, T.; Chen, J.; Lin, J.; Zhang, Y. Graphene Family Nanomaterials: Properties and Potential Applications in Dentistry. *Int. J. Biomater.* **2018**, *2018*, 1539678. [CrossRef] [PubMed]
5. Qi, X.; Jiang, F.; Zhou, M.; Zhang, W.; Jiang, X. Graphene oxide as a promising material in dentistry and tissue regeneration: A review. *Smart Mater. Med.* **2021**, *2*, 280–291. [CrossRef]
6. Sawan, N.M.; AlSagob, E.I.; Ben Gassem, A.A.; Alshami, A.A. Graphene functionalized with nanosilver particle-modified methacrylate-based bonding agent improves antimicrobial capacity and mechanical strength at tooth orthodontic bracket interface. *Polym. Compos.* **2021**, *42*, 5850–5858. [CrossRef]

7. Dai, D.; Zhou, D.; He, L.; Wang, C.; Zhang, C. Graphene oxide nanocoating for enhanced corrosion resistance, wear resistance and antibacterial activity of nickel-titanium shape memory alloy. *Surf. Coat. Technol.* **2022**, *431*, 128012. [CrossRef]
8. Ghorbanzadeh, R.; Nader, A.H.; Salehi-Vaziri, A. The effects of bimodal action of photodynamic and photothermal therapy on antimicrobial and shear bond strength properties of orthodontic composite containing nano-graphene oxide. *Photodiagn. Photodyn. Ther.* **2021**, *36*, 102589. [CrossRef]
9. Nizami, M.Z.I.; Takashiba, S.; Nishina, Y. Graphene oxide: A new direction in dentistry. *Appl. Mater. Today* **2020**, *19*, 100576. [CrossRef]
10. Silveira, S.R.; Sahm, B.D.; Kreve, S.; dos Reis, A.C. Osseointegration, antimicrobial capacity and cytotoxicity of implant materials coated with graphene compounds: A systematic review. *Jpn. Dent. Sci. Rev.* **2023**, *59*, 303–311. [CrossRef]
11. Nizami, M.Z.I.; Yin, I.X.; Lung, C.Y.K.; Niu, J.Y.; Mei, M.L.; Chu, C.H. In Vitro Studies of Graphene for Management of Dental Caries and Periodontal Disease: A Concise Review. *Pharmaceutics* **2022**, *14*, 1997. [CrossRef] [PubMed]
12. Pourhajibagher, M.; Ghorbanzadeh, R.; Salehi-Vaziri, A.; Bahador, A. In Vitro assessments of antimicrobial potential and cytotoxicity activity of an orthodontic adhesive doped with nano-graphene oxide. *Folia Medica* **2022**, *64*, 110–116. [CrossRef]
13. Kuropka, P.; Dobrzynski, M.; Bazanow, B.; Stygar, D.; Gebarowski, T.; Leskow, A.; Tarnowska, M.; Szyszka, K.; Malecka, M.; Nowak, N.; et al. A Study of the Impact of Graphene Oxide on Viral Infection Related to A549 and TC28a2 Human Cell Lines. *Materials* **2021**, *14*, 7788. [CrossRef] [PubMed]
14. Lee, S.-M.; Yoo, K.-H.; Yoon, S.-Y.; Kim, I.-R.; Park, B.-S.; Son, W.-S.; Ko, C.-C.; Son, S.-A.; Kim, Y.-I. Enamel Anti-Demineralization Effect of Orthodontic Adhesive Containing Bioactive Glass and Graphene Oxide: An In-Vitro Study. *Materials* **2018**, *11*, 1728. [CrossRef]
15. Wang, P.; Luo, X.; Qin, J.; Pan, Z.; Zhou, K. Effect of Graphene Sheets Embedded Carbon Films on the Fretting Wear Behaviors of Orthodontic Archwire–Bracket Contacts. *Nanomaterials* **2022**, *12*, 3430. [CrossRef]
16. Alnatheer, M.; Alqerban, A.; Alhazmi, H. Graphene oxide-modified dental adhesive for bonding orthodontic brackets. *Int. J. Adhes. Adhes.* **2021**, *110*, 102928. [CrossRef]
17. Zakrzewski, W.; Dobrzynski, M.; Dobrzynski, W.; Zawadzka-Knefel, A.; Janecki, M.; Kurek, K.; Lubojanski, A.; Szymonowicz, M.; Rybak, Z.; Wiglusz, R.J. Nanomaterials Application in Orthodontics. *Nanomaterials* **2021**, *11*, 337. [CrossRef]
18. Jiao, D.; Wang, J.; Yu, W.; Zhang, K.; Zhang, N.; Cao, L.; Jiang, X.; Bai, Y. Biocompatible reduced graphene oxide stimulated BMSCs induce acceleration of bone remodeling and orthodontic tooth movement through promotion on osteoclastogenesis and angiogenesis. *Bioact. Mater.* **2022**, *15*, 409–425. [CrossRef]
19. Pourhajibagher, M.; Bahador, A. Orthodontic adhesive doped with nano-graphene oxide: Physico-mechanical and antimicrobial properties. *Folia Medica* **2021**, *63*, 413–421. [CrossRef]
20. Tahriri, M.; Del Monico, M.; Moghanian, A.; Yaraki, M.T.; Torres, R.; Yadegari, A.; Tayebi, L. Graphene and its derivatives: Opportunities and challenges in dentistry. *Mater. Sci. Eng. C* **2019**, *102*, 171–185. [CrossRef] [PubMed]
21. Zhao, M.; Shan, T.; Wu, Q.; Gu, L. The Antibacterial Effect of Graphene Oxide on *Streptococcus mutans*. *J. Nanosci. Nanotechnol.* **2020**, *20*, 2095–2103. [CrossRef] [PubMed]
22. Itoo, A.M.; Vemula, S.L.; Gupta, M.T.; Giram, M.V.; Kumar, S.A.; Ghosh, B.; Biswas, S. Multifunctional Graphene Oxide Nanoparticles for Drug Deliver in Cancer. *J. Control. Release* **2022**, *350*, 26–59. [CrossRef]
23. Geng, Z.; Cao, Z.; Liu, J. Recent advances in targeted antibacterial therapy basing on nanomaterials. *Exploration* **2023**, *3*, 20210117. [CrossRef] [PubMed]
24. Nizami MZ, I.; Gorduysus, M.; Shinoda-Ito, Y.; Yamamoto, T.; Nishina, Y.; Takashiba, S.; Arias, Z. Graphene Oxide-based Endodontic Sealer: An in Vitro Study. *Acta Medica Okayama* **2022**, *76*, 715–721. [PubMed]
25. Page, M.J.; McKenzie, J.E.; Bossuyt, P.M.; Boutron, I.; Hoffmann, T.C.; Mulrow, C.D.; Shamseer, L.; Tetzlaff, J.M.; Akl, E.A.; Brennan, S.E.; et al. The PRISMA 2020 statement: An updated guideline for reporting systematic reviews. *BMJ* **2021**, *372*, n71. [CrossRef]
26. Watson, P.; Petrie, A. Method agreement analysis: A review of correct methodology. *Theriogenology* **2010**, *73*, 1167–1179. [CrossRef]
27. Cehreli, S.B.; Polat-Ozsoy, O.; Sar, C.; Cubukcu, H.E.; Cehreli, Z.C. A comparative study of qualitative and quantitative methods for the assessment of adhesive remnant after bracket debonding. *Eur. J. Orthod.* **2011**, *34*, 188–192. [CrossRef]
28. Sawan, N.M.; Alshami, A.A.; Aldegheishem, A.; Alsagob, E.I. Graphene sheets decorated with silver in orthodontic bonding. *Int. J. Adhes. Adhes.* **2022**, *117*, 103113. [CrossRef]
29. Lee, J.-H.; Jo, J.-K.; Kim, D.-A.; Patel, K.D.; Kim, H.-W.; Lee, H.-H. Nano-graphene oxide incorporated into PMMA resin to prevent microbial adhesion. *Dent. Mater.* **2018**, *34*, e63–e72. [CrossRef]
30. Pan, Z.; Zhou, Q.; Wang, P.; Diao, D. Robust low friction performance of graphene sheets embedded carbon films coated orthodontic stainless steel archwires. *Friction* **2021**, *10*, 142–158. [CrossRef]

Disclaimer/Publisher's Note: The statements, opinions and data contained in all publications are solely those of the individual author(s) and contributor(s) and not of MDPI and/or the editor(s). MDPI and/or the editor(s) disclaim responsibility for any injury to people or property resulting from any ideas, methods, instructions or products referred to in the content.

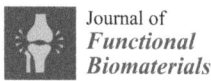

Article

Synthesis and Characterization of Dental Nanocomposite Resins Reinforced with Dual Organomodified Silica/Clay Nanofiller Systems

Maria Saridou [1,†], Alexandros K. Nikolaidis [2,*,†], Elisabeth A. Koulaouzidou [2] and Dimitris S. Achilias [1]

[1] Laboratory of Polymer and Color Chemistry and Technology, Department of Chemistry, Aristotle University Thessaloniki, 541 24 Thessaloniki, Greece; axilias@chem.auth.gr (D.S.A.)
[2] Division of Dental Tissues' Pathology and Therapeutics (Basic Dental Sciences, Endodontology and Operative Dentistry), School of Dentistry, Aristotle University Thessaloniki, 541 24 Thessaloniki, Greece; koulaouz@dent.auth.gr
* Correspondence: nikolchem@dent.auth.gr; Tel.: +30-2310-99616
† These authors contributed equally to this work.

Abstract: Quaternary ammonium (QA) compounds have been widely studied as potential disinfectants in dental restorative materials. The present work investigates whether the gradual displacement of nanosilica by QA-clay nanoparticles may have an impact on the physicochemical and mechanical properties of dental nanocomposite resins. For this purpose, Bis-GMA/TEGDMA-based composite resins were initially synthesized by incorporating 3-(trimethoxysilyl)propyl methacrylate (γ-MPS)-modified nanosilica/QA-clay nanoparticles at 60/0, 55/5, 50/10, 40/20, and 30/30 wt% filler loadings. Their structural characterization was performed by means of scanning electron microscopy (SEM) and X-ray diffraction analysis (XRD). The degree of double bond conversion (DC) over time and the polymerization shrinkage were determined with Fourier transform infrared spectroscopy (FTIR) and a linear variable displacement transducer (LVDT), respectively. Mechanical properties as well as water sorption and solubility parameters were also evaluated after storage of nanocomposites in water for 7 days at 37 °C. Spectral data revealed intercalated clay configurations along with areas characterized by silica-clay clusters for clay loadings up to 30 wt%. Furthermore, the insertion of 10 wt% QA-clay enhanced the auto-acceleration effect also sustaining the ultimate (DC), reduced the setting contraction and solubility, and, finally, yielded flexural modulus and strength very close to those of the control nanocomposite resin. The acquired results could herald the advanced design of dental restorative materials appropriate for contemporary clinical applications.

Keywords: dental nanocomposite resins; quaternary ammonium compounds; organomodified nanosilica; clay nanoparticles; nanotechnology

Citation: Saridou, M.; Nikolaidis, A.K.; Koulaouzidou, E.A.; Achilias, D.S. Synthesis and Characterization of Dental Nanocomposite Resins Reinforced with Dual Organomodified Silica/Clay Nanofiller Systems. *J. Funct. Biomater.* 2023, *14*, 405. https://doi.org/10.3390/jfb14080405

Academic Editors: Lavinia Cosmina Ardelean, Laura-Cristina Rusu and Nikolaos Silikas

Received: 30 June 2023
Revised: 18 July 2023
Accepted: 30 July 2023
Published: 1 August 2023

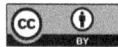

Copyright: © 2023 by the authors. Licensee MDPI, Basel, Switzerland. This article is an open access article distributed under the terms and conditions of the Creative Commons Attribution (CC BY) license (https://creativecommons.org/licenses/by/4.0/).

1. Introduction

Over the last decades, dental composite resins have been widely applied in both anterior and posterior tooth restorations. Aesthetic characteristics and toxicity reasons associated with amalgam fillings have strongly motivated the dental industry to promote composite resins to direct restorations [1]. Nevertheless, the oral cavity constitutes a dynamic regime governed by high masticatory stresses in combination with several biological and chemical threats that can affect the longevity of dental composites [2,3]. To overcome these limiting factors, composites' formulations are usually manipulated by the utilization of dimethacrylate monomers such as Bis-GMA, UDMA, and TEGDMA reinforced with diverse inorganic fillers that are conjugated with the polymer matrix through silane coupling agents. Nowadays, contemporary trends involve dental composite resins reinforced with zirconia [4,5], silica nanoparticles [6], halloysite nanotubes [7], and even composites derived from biomass rice husk silica that demonstrate excellent performance [8]. Although fillers with specific size distribution can contribute to the achievement of good mechanical and physicochemical performance, dental composites are still a challenge with secondary caries originating from the metabolic activity of pathogenic bacteria [9].

Several approaches have been adopted in order to enhance the microbial resistance of dental restorative materials. Although the direct incorporation of leachable disinfectants [10] such as fluoride [11], chlorhexidine (CHX) [12], benzalkonium chloride [13], essential oils [14], and a wide range of nanoparticles [15] into dental composites can induce antimicrobial ability in the composite, there are still some ambiguities related to loss activity, weakening of the remaining restoration, and discoloration over time [16]. Furthermore, mesoporous silica nanoparticles loaded with CHX might reinforce the dental composite against plaque formation, but these may also affect its mechanical performance due to the release and recharge mechanism of the biocide agent [17]. Considering the exploitation of biocide agents through such nanoscale vehicles, their unstable position is attributed to the physical absorption of nanoparticles within the polymer network. Other well-established approaches involve the incorporation of non-leachable quaternary ammonium monomers (QA) [18,19], or QA combined with a nanofiller such as silica (QASi) [20,21], clay (QA-clay) [22], or in the form of polymeric QA polyethyleneimine particles (QPEI) [23]. In this manner, it is believed that functional groups of QA are chemically bound to the organic matrix, and the antimicrobial component remains entrapped in the polymer network of the dental composite, thus ensuring an optimum antibacterial action over time [24].

To the best of our knowledge, there is no literature data describing dental composite resins reinforced with both potentially antimicrobial QA-clay nanofillers [25,26] and silica nanoparticles sustaining the overall physicomechanical performance [27,28]. The aim of this study was to investigate the effect of the displacement of nanosilica by QA-clay nanoparticles on the physicochemical and mechanical properties of the obtained dental nanocomposite resins. For this purpose, experimental dental nanocomposites based on a BisGMA/TEGDMA matrix and filled with 3-(trimethoxysilyl)propyl methacrylate (γ-MPS) modified nanosilica were initially synthesized as control samples (golden standards). Silica nanoparticles were then replaced by different types of QA-clays at different filler loadings to produce pure nano-filled resin composites. The null hypothesis was that the type and amount of nanoclay might influence the structural configurations and final properties of the developed nanocomposites. The obtained results are supposed to be conducive to the design of contemporary dental nanocomposite resins, meeting the requirements of modern clinical applications.

2. Materials and Methods

2.1. Materials

The monomers triethylene glycol dimethacrylate (TEGDMA), 95%, and 2,2-Bis[p-(2'-hydroxy-3'-methacryloxypropoxy)phenylene]propane (Bis-GMA) were both provided by SIGMA-ALDRICH CHEMIE GmbH (Steinheim, Germany). The co-initiator 2-(dimethylamino) ethylmethacrylate (DMAEMA), 99%, and initiator camphorquinone, 98%, were purchased from J&K Scientific GmbH (Pforzheim, Germany). Organically modified silica nanopowder (S.MPS) with 3-(trimethoxysilyl)propyl methacrylate (γ-MPS) was synthesized and subsequently characterized in our previous work [29]. The commercially available organomodified montmorillonite Nanomer® I.34MN, i.e., an –onium ion modified clay containing 25 to 30 wt% methyl dixydroxyethyl hydrogenated tallow ammonium ion (QA-clay), was produced by Nanocor Company (Hoffman Estates, IL, USA) and supplied by Aldrich (Taufkirchen, Germany). Two experimental QA-clays, namely, a clay type intercalated with cetyltrimethylammonium chloride (MMT-CTAC), as well as its surface-modified analog with 3-(trimethoxysilyl)propyl methacrylate (S.MMT-CTAC), were both prepared and characterized in our previous works [22,30]. The particular structures of the above QA-clays are presented in Scheme 1. All other chemicals used were of reagent grade.

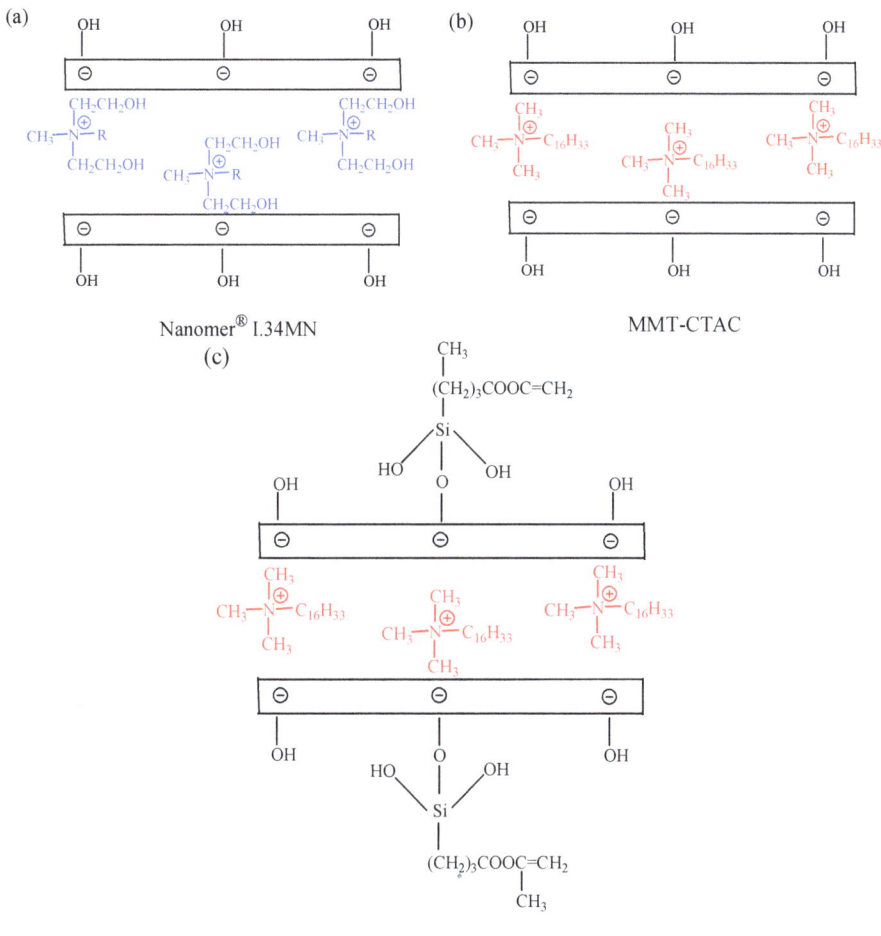

Scheme 1. Structural configurations of: (**a**) Nanomer® I.34MN; (**b**) MMT-CTAC; (**c**) S.MMT-CTAC clay used for the synthesis of dental nanocomposite resins (R stands for hydrogenated tallow).

2.2. Preparation of the Uncured Dental Composite Pastes

Seven groups of experimental composites were prepared by initially mixing a Bis-GMA/TEGDMA base (50:50 wt/wt) that contained camphorquinone (0.2 wt%) and DMAEMA (0.8 wt%) as a photo-initiating system. Afterward, neat S.MPS and nanoparticle combinations of S.MPS/Nanomer® I.34MN, S.MPS/MMT-CTAC, and S.MPS/S.MMT-CTAC were individually inserted in the resin by manual mixing until the powder was completely wetted with organic matrix, and the obtained mixture was ultrasonicated for 10 min. Environmental conditions were kept constant (22 °C, 40% relative humidity, 1 atm) during the mixing process. The specific composition of each prepared nanocomposite is described in Table 1. The overall nanofiller loading was kept at 60 wt% to ensure paste handling properties almost similar to a commercial dental composite resin.

Table 1. Abbreviated names of the studied materials based on their particular composition.

Dental Nanocomposite Resin	S.MPS (wt%)	Nanomer® I.34MN (wt%)	MMT-CTAC (wt%)	S.MMT-CTAC (wt%)
S.MPS 60	60	-	-	-
S.MPS/Nanomer 55/5	55	5	-	-
S.MPS/Nanomer 50/10	50	10	-	-
S.MPS/Nanomer 40/20	40	20	-	-
S.MPS/Nanomer 30/30	30	30	-	-
S.MPS/CTAC 50/10	50	-	10	-
S.MPS/S.CTAC 50/10	50	-	-	10

2.3. Measurements

2.3.1. Structural Characterization of the Experimental Dental Resins

A JEOL JSM-6390LV (JEOL USA, Inc., Peabody, MA, USA) scanning electron microscope system (SEM) operated within 0.5–30 kV (3 nm resolution) was utilized in order to examine the surface of the prepared materials. A protective carbon black coating against charging was applied on the sample surfaces prior to the scanning process. Microphotos were taken by focusing electron beams on the studied surfaces and using Smile Shot™ software. Elemental analysis of the samples was performed by means of the INCAPentaFETx3 (Oxford Instruments, Abingdon, UK) energy-dispersive X-ray (EDX) microanalytical system, and the percentage of the targeted elements was determined by averaging different areas acquisitions.

A Miniflex II X-ray diffractometer (XRD) supplied by RigakuCo. (Tokyo, Japan) was used to record the spectral patterns of the obtained nanocomposites within the scanning range (2 theta) of 2–12°. The following operation conditions were selected: Cu Kα radiation with wavelength 0.154 nm, angle steps of 0.05°, 5 s/angle step.

2.3.2. Setting Contraction Kinetics

The "bonded-disk" technique established by Watts et al. [31–33] was applied in order to calculate the real-time contraction due to polymerization process. Particularly, an unpolymerized sample in the form of a disk (1.0 × 8.0 mm) was placed on the surface of a glass plate (3 mm thickness) within a mounted metal ring (internal diameter ~15 mm). A flexible membrane was used to adhere the upper surface of the sample. A uniaxial transducer (LVDT) was placed on the center of the membrane, in order to measure the linear variable displacement of the specimen over time. A dual system combining a transducer indicator (E 309, RDP Electronics Ltd., Wolverhampton, UK) and a high-resolution analog-to-digital converter (ADAM-4016) was utilized to transmit the signal from the LVDT module to the computer. The data were acquired by means of AdvantechAdam/Apax.NET Utility software (version 2.05.11). An LED light-curing device (Bluephase® Style M8, Ivoclar Vivadent AG, FL-9494, Schaan, Liechtenstein) with an intensity of 800 mW·cm^{-2} ± 10% was positioned above the glass plate to continuously irradiate the unset samples for 5 min. A radiometer (Hilux, Benlioglu Dental Inc., Ankara, Turkey) was utilized to check the output intensity of the photo-curing unit. Environmental conditions were kept constant (22 °C, 40% relative humidity, 1 atm) during the photo-curing process. Each dental nanocomposite was measured five times (n = 5). The calculation of the strain (%) was based on the following formula:

$$\varepsilon(\%) = 100 \times \frac{\Delta L}{L_0} \quad (1)$$

where ε (%) represents the strain (%), and DL (mm) and L_0 (mm) are the deformation due to setting and the initial thickness of the nanocomposite, respectively.

2.3.3. Degree of Conversion

Polymerization kinetics were performed by placing a small amount of each composite between two translucent Mylar strips, which were pressed to produce a very thin film. The upper surface of the films of unpolymerized composites was exposed to visible light of the above LED unit and directly measured by a FTIR spectrometer (Spectrum One, PerkinElmer Inc., Waltham, MA, USA) at diverse setting moments (0, 5, 10, 15, 20, 25, 30, 40, 60, 80, 120, 180 s). Spectral acquisition of the nanocomposite films (n = 5) was conducted in the wavenumber region of 4000–600 cm^{-1}, performing 32 scans per sample at 4 cm^{-1} resolution. Environmental conditions were kept constant (22 °C, 40% relative humidity, 1 atm) during the photo-curing process. The obtained records were manipulated with specific software (Spectrum v5.0.1, Perkin-Elmer LLC 1500F2429). The degree of conversion (DC%) over time was calculated based on the area of the absorption band at 1637 cm^{-1} (aliphatic C=C bonds) and the band at 1580 cm^{-1} (aromatic C=C bonds) as well as on the best fit baseline method according to the Beer–Lambert law [34]. For this purpose, the following equation was used:

$$\text{DC}(\%) = \left[1 - \frac{\left(\frac{A_{1637}}{A_{1580}}\right)_{\text{polymer}}}{\left(\frac{A_{1637}}{A_{1580}}\right)_{\text{monomer}}}\right] \times 100 \quad (2)$$

2.3.4. Mechanical Properties

A Teflon mold (2 × 2 × 25 mm) was filled with the unset material, in order to prepare bar-shaped specimens for three-point bending tests according to the ISO 4049. Each side of the mold was irradiated for 40 s with the aforementioned LED lamp, by overlapping the unset areas. Environmental conditions were kept constant (22 °C, 40% relative humidity, 1 atm) during the photo-curing process. Ten specimens (n = 10) per dental resin were formed and subsequently immersed in deionized water for 1 week at 37 ± 1 °C. Then, they were placed on a three-point bending module between two supports of 20 mm distance. The bend tests were conducted in a universal testing machine (Testometric AX, M350-10 kN, Testometric Co., Ltd., Rochdale, UK at a cross-head speed of 0.5 mm·min^{-1}). The exerted load (N) versus deformation were recorded, and the acquired data were manipulated with the WinTestAnalysis CX software (Version 3.5.30.10). The flexural modulus (E, GPa) and strength (σ, GPa) were calculated based on the following formulae:

$$E = \frac{F_1 l^3}{4bd_1 h^3} 10^{-3} \quad \text{and} \quad \sigma = \frac{3F_{\max} l}{2bh^2} \quad (3)$$

where F_1 is the measured load (N), $F_{\max}$ is the highest load measured prior to mechanical failure (N), l is the distance between the supports (20 mm), b is the width of the sample (mm), h is the height of the sample (mm), and d_1 is the deformation (mm) related to the load F_1.

2.3.5. Water Sorption and Solubility

The determination of the water sorption and solubility parameters was performed in accordance with the requirements of ISO 4049. A Teflon mold was filled with each unset dental nanocomposite, in order to produce disc-shaped specimens (15 mm × 1 mm). The specimens (n = 5) were set with the aforementioned LED curing unit by irradiating for 40 s each side and targeting to nine preselected overlapping irradiation areas. Environmental conditions were kept constant (22 °C, 40% relative humidity, 1 atm) during the photo-curing process. The discs were stored in a desiccator, and then they were pre-conditioned at 37 ± 1 °C for 24 h. Afterwards, the specimens were transferred into another desiccator (23 ± 1 °C) to remain for 2 h. Then, they were weighed (±0.1 mg accuracy) by means of an analytical balance (Sartorius TE 124S, Sartorius AG, Goetingen, Germany). The above procedure was repeated until the materials reach a constant mass (m_1). Their volume (V) was calculated upon their mean thickness and diameter, which were previously measured with a digital micrometer (±0.02 mm accuracy). Subsequently, the specimens were stored in water at 37 ± 1 °C. After 1 week, they were isolated, left to dry and weighed (m_2). The discs were then placed in desiccator until a constant mass (m_3) was achieved.

The water sorption parameter, W_{sp} (µg/mm^3), was calculated from the formula:

$$W_{sp} = \frac{m_2 - m_3}{V} \quad (4)$$

where m_2 is the mass of the disc (µg) after storage in water for 1 week, m_3 is the mass of the reconditioned disc (µg), and V is the volume of the disc (mm^3).

The solubility parameter, W_{sl} (µg/mm^3), was calculated according to the following equation:

$$W_{sl} = \frac{m_1 - m_3}{V} \quad (5)$$

where m_1 is the conditioned mass (µg) of the disc before the storage in water.

2.3.6. Statistical Analysis

The assumption of normal distribution was investigated for the variables using the Shapiro–Wilk test. One-way analysis of variance (ANOVA) was used to compare the flexural modulus, sorption, solubility, and strain between the seven groups. The Kruskal–Wallis test was used to compare flexural strength between the seven groups. Bonferroni corrections were made to adjust for multiple tests. Statistical analysis was performed using IBM SPSS Statistics 28. The statistical significance level was set at p-value ≤ 0.05.

3. Results and Discussion

3.1. Limitations of Research

In the framework of the evaluation of the developed dental nanocomposite resins, certain possible restrictions affecting the research outputs could be considered. The common hand spatulation mixing method was applied to prepare the starting nanocomposite paste. The above technique may have an effect on the extent of fillers' dispersion and on the overall performance of the obtained composite. Moreover, the prevention of bias could not be supported by randomization methods, and the determined sample size for the majority of the conducted tests was mainly dictated by ISO 4049 "Dentistry-Polymer Based Restorative Materials". The above limitations mainly originate from the limited availability of the experimentally synthesized silica and clay nanoparticles used in composites' formulations. As the current research targeted the basic requirements of ISO 4049, which are always necessary for the dental industry, antimicrobial and cytotoxicity tests were not conducted in parallel. Future experimental cycles would provide particular data in order to estimate the potential antimicrobial effect of the proposed dental nanocomposite resins due to the presence of the QA-clays utilized here.

3.2. Morphological Characterization of the Prepared Materials

SEM images captured for the produced dental nanocomposite resins are presented in Figure 1. Regarding the composite loaded with 60 wt% S.MPS nanoparticles (Figure 1a), it is apparent that an adequate dispersion of silica was accomplished (white spots) into the formed polymer network (dark regions), even if some small aggregates can be discriminated. Similar clustering tendencies have also been observed by other researchers and ascribed to the widely applied hand spatulation mixing technique of monomers with inorganic fillers [35–39]. The desirable distribution of the total filler content seems to be retained when the amount of Nanomer® I.34MN clay was elevated up to 30 wt% (Figure 1e). A stepwise size increment of the created agglomerates is also observed in the range of 10–30 wt% clay (Figure 1c–e). The aforementioned behavior could be attributed to the intermolecular hydrogen bonding between the intercalating agents of the hydrophylic Nanomer® I.34MN particles. On the other hand, more bulky agglomerates occurred for the

S.MPS/Nanomer 55/5 (Figure 1b), denoting not only the equivalent clay–clay interactions but also the possible formation of silica-clay clusters due to the hydrogen bonding interactions between the free unreacted hydroxy groups originating from the organomodified silica and the hydroxy groups of the Nanomer® I.34MN quaternary ammonium intercalant (Scheme 1). Furthermore, the insertion of 10 wt% MMT-CTAC (Figure 1f) and S.MMT-CTAC clay (Figure 1g) in the dimethacrylated organic matrix can also lead to sufficient dispersion of the used nanoparticles similar to that of S.MPS/Nanomer 50/10. In particular, the filler agglomeration detected for the S.MPS/S.CTAC 50/10 nanocomposite maybe due to the side reactions of the double bonds attached on the S.MMT-CTAC and/or the double bond reactions between both the silane modified silica and clay nanofillers (Scheme 1).

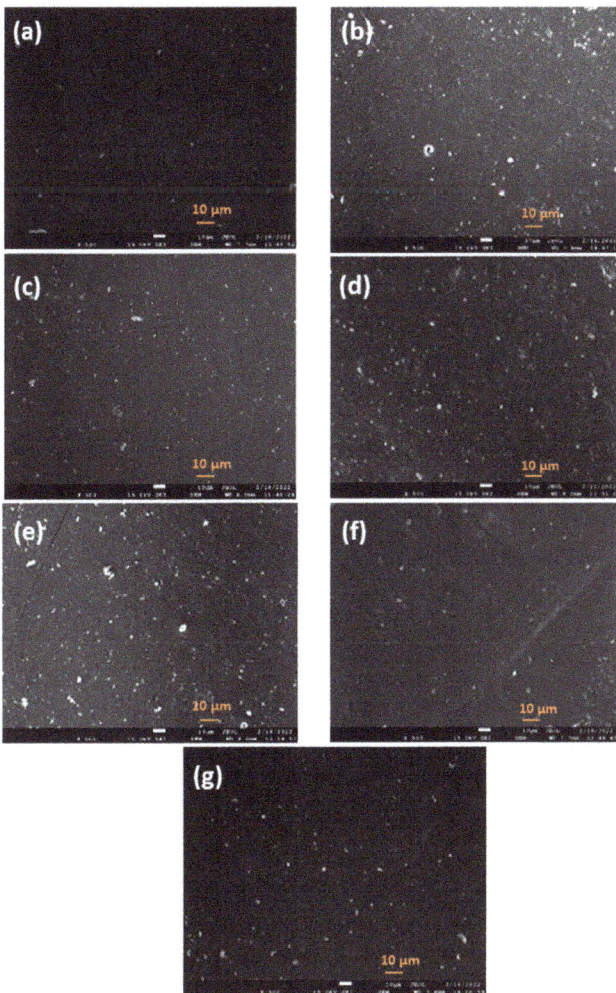

Figure 1. SEM microphotos taken for dental nanocomposites reinforced with: (**a**) pure nanosilica (S.MPS); (**b–e**) Nanomer® I.34MN clay particles (5–30 wt%) in the presence of nanosilica; (**f**) MMT-CTAC clay; (**g**) S.MMT-CTAC clay nanoparticles (10 wt%) in the presence of nanosilica.

Table 2 encompasses the data derived from the EDX spectra of the studied dental nanocomposites. A constant enrichment of nanocomposites with Al is observed by increasing the content of Nanomer clay from 5 to 30 wt%, thus ensuring the good dispersion of clay particles into the formed polymer network over the tested filler concentration range. The Al content also remained for composites with 10 wt% MMT-CTAC and S.MMT-CTAC at higher levels than Nanomer, probably due to the occurrence of larger agglomerates revealed by SEM images. Under this regime, the accumulation of Al species could be favored, resulting in their high abundance over the scanned surfaces.

Table 2. Content of clay elements (%) in dental nanocomposite resins measured by means of EDX.

Dental Nanocomposite Resin	Si (%) Mean (SD)	Al (%) Mean (SD)	O (%) Mean (SD)
S.MPS 60	46.74 (0.00)	-	53.26 (0.00)
S.MPS/Nanomer 55/5	46.33 (0.08)	0.47 (0.09)	53.20 (0.01)
S.MPS/Nanomer 50/10	46.05 (0.13)	0.78 (0.15)	53.16 (0.02)
S.MPS/Nanomer 40/20	44.55 (0.41)	2.48 (0.46)	52.97 (0.05)
S.MPS/Nanomer 30/30	43.30 (0.17)	3.90 (0.19)	52.80 (0.02)
S.MPS/CTAC 50/10	45.37 (0.28)	1.56 (0.31)	53.07 (0.04)
S.MPS/S.CTAC 50/10	45.62 (0.21)	1.27 (0.24)	53.11 (0.03)

The XRD spectra recorded for the synthesized dental nanocomposite resins are illustrated in Figure 2. It is observed that even though clay nanoparticles exhibit diffraction peaks at 2θ = 5.14° (Nanomer® I.34MN clay, Figure 2a), 4.42°, and 4.31° (MMT-CTAC and S.MMT-CTAC, Figure 2b), their corresponding S.MPS nanocomposites always display X-ray diffractions at higher angles. Provided that amorphous nanosilica develops diffuse scattering at the angular region of 20–25° [40], possible cluster formation through amorphous silica–Nanomer® I.34MN interactions could be responsible for the shifts in clay reflections (001) to higher 2θ values. These interactions seem to be even stronger when the clay loading remains at 5–10 wt%, as the dominant silica nanoparticles (55–50 wt%) clearly impede the diffraction pattern of clay, regardless of the chemical structure of the intercalating agent (Figure 2a,b). Further incorporation of clay nanoparticles up to 30 wt% gradually enhances the peak intensities of dental composites, thus implying the amplified presence of intercalated clay configurations (Figure 2a). Although the intercalation of macromolecular chains within clay galleries governs the morphological characteristics of the synthesized dental nanocomposites, there might still be some areas characterized by silica-clay clusters over the nanocomposite structures. These findings could be also supported by the SEM observations, as previously described.

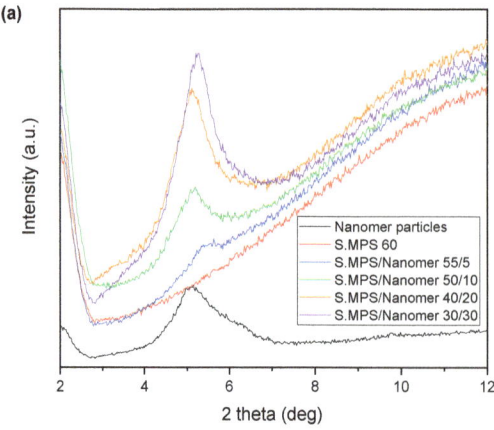

Figure 2. *Cont.*

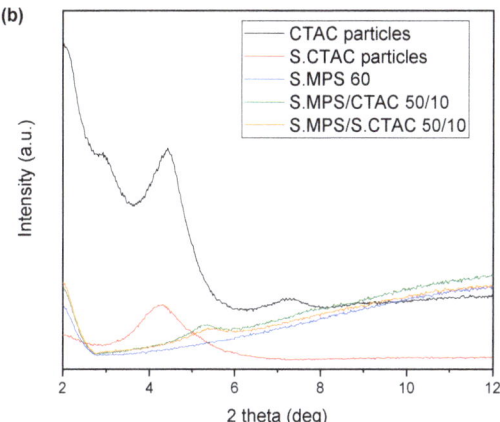

Figure 2. Comparative XRD spectra of the investigated dental nanocomposite resins filled with nanosilica and. (**a**) Nanomer ® I.34MN clay (5–30 wt%); (**b**) MMT-CTAC and S.MMT-CTAC clay nanoparticles at 10 wt% filler loading.

3.3. Polymerization Reaction Kinetics

Figure 3 illustrates the degree of conversion versus time curves recorded for dental nanocomposites filled with silica-clay nanoparticles. The DC (%) values calculated after 180 min curing are listed in Table 3. Concerning the different clay mass fraction, the plots of the free radical polymerization kinetics revealed the occurrence of the auto-acceleration or gel effect phenomenon as it was mainly expressed by a steep increase in the slope mostly in the range of 20–25 min of the setting procedure (Figure 3a). In general, the gel effect is controlled by diffusion phenomena [41], where the free volume inside the developed polymer network can be limited due to the presence of inorganic fillers along with the developed macromolecular chains. Under such circumstances, the mobility of macroradicals is restricted, leading to further difficulty in their finding each other and terminating the polymerization reaction. Hence, their local concentration is increased, resulting in the augmentation of the reaction rate. The auto-acceleration phenomenon was found to be stronger for the S.MPS 60 and S.MPS/Nanomer 50/10 nanocomposites, approaching DC values of (17.31–31.8%) and (19.01–33.54%), respectively. This attitude was attenuated almost sequentially for S.MPS/Nanomer 40/20 (19.66–26.18%), S.MPS/Nanomer 30/30 (18.67–25.30%), and S.MPS/Nanomer 55/5 (19.46–24.39%) composites. The most comprehensive distribution of nanoclay into the organic matrix that was proved by SEM for S.MPS/Nanomer 50/10 nanocomposite could better constrain the macroradical movement due to the decrease in the total free volume of the polymer network, and it could extensively sustain the auto-acceleration phenomenon. The DC value found for S.MPS 60 nanocomposite (48.41%, Table 3) was comparable to 46.84% reported by Liu et al. for Bis-GMA/TEGDMA-based composites containing 30 wt% silica nanoparticles [42]. Wang et al. also described dental resin composites filled with 60 wt% silica nanoclusters exhibiting 49.8% [43]. Moreover, it is obvious that the step-by-step enrichment of dental composites with 10 to 30 wt% Nanomer clay leads to the descending of double bond conversion from 44.89 to 37.86% (Table 3). The relatively low determined degree of conversion could be attributed to the glass effect phenomenon occurring when the extensive network has been developed, thus provoking the high viscosity of the reaction mixture. The phenomenon is controlled by the limited diffusion of both the monomers and the initial initiator radicals and finally affects the rate constant of chain propagation [41,44–46]. In addition, the DC value for S.MPS/Nanomer 55/5 was further lowered to 30.34%. Regarding the S.MPS/Nanomer 40/20, S.MPS/Nanomer 30/30, and S.MPS/Nanomer 55/5 composites, the SEM findings denoted larger silica-clay aggregates that might act as microfillers, affecting the light absorption and scattering, and thus weakening the light photo-initiation process [47]. The gel effect phenomenon was also observed for S.MPS/S.CTAC 50/10 and S.MPS/CTAC 50/10 nanocomposites during the period of time from 20–25 min (Figure 3b). Particularly, the S.MPS/S.CTAC 50/10 yielded almost similar conversions (17.89–32.59%) as the S.MPS/Nanomer 50/10 composite during auto-acceleration phenomenon, whereas lower DC values (17.96–24.96%) were calculated for S.MPS/CTAC 50/10. The vinyl functionalities attached on the surface of S.MMT-CTAC nanoparticles (Scheme 1) could account for the comparatively enhanced DC throughout the gel effect, as methacrylate groups of clay might react with those originated from Bis-GMA and TEGDMA monomers. The ultimate DC measured for S.MPS/S.CTAC 50/10 (43.61%) was close to that of S.MPS/Nanomer 50/10, and for S.MPS/CTAC, the DC was found to be 32.28% (Table 3). The absence of any functional groups in the structure of MMT-CTAC clay (Scheme 1) in combination with some nanofiller agglomeration (Figure 1f) may be responsible for the weaker glass effect phenomenon during the photo-polymerization of the S.MPS/CTAC composite.

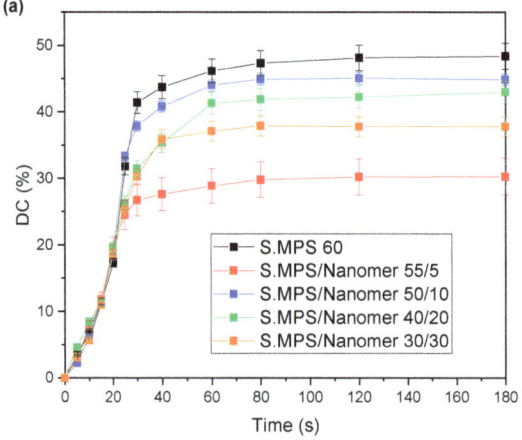

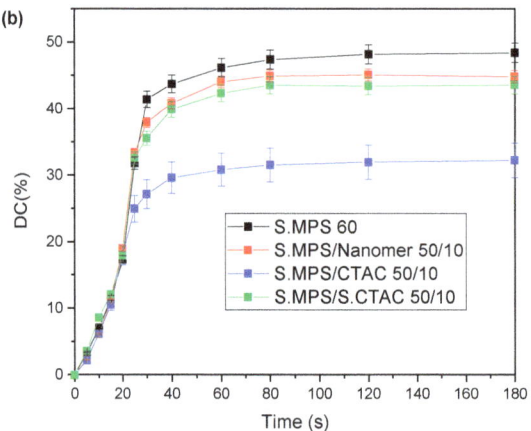

Figure 3. Plots of degree of conversion (DC%) versus time for dental nanocomposites containing: (**a**) different silica/clay nanoparticle ratios (up to 30/30 wt%); (**b**) diverse types of nanoclay at silica/clay nanoparticle ratio 50/10 wt%.

Table 3. Curing kinetics data and polymerization shrinkage, solubility, and sorption values calculated for the synthesized dental nanocomposite resins. Different superscript indicates statistically significant difference ($p < 0.05$).

Dental Nanocomposite Resin	DC (%) Mean (SD)	Strain (%) Mean (Min, Max)	Sorption, Wsp (µg/mm^3) Mean (Min, Max)	Solubility, Wsl (µg/mm^3) Mean (Min, Max)
S.MPS 60	48.41 (1.94)	3.51 (3.31, 3.75) [a]	27.54 (24.82, 30.37) [a,b,g]	6.21 (4.77, 7.18) [a,b]
S.MPS/Nanomer 55/5	30.34 (2.73)	2.76 (2.52, 2.93) [a]	28.48 (26.84, 30.38) [b,c]	6.61 (6.12, 7.20) [a,b]
S.MPS/Nanomer 50/10	44.89 (0.90)	2.93 (2.43, 3.19) [a]	33.77 (31.16, 38.47) [c,d,g]	4.79 (4.59, 4.97) [a,b]
S.MPS/Nanomer 40/20	43.00 (1.72)	5.22 (4.20, 6.00) [b]	37.07 (30.38, 40.13) [d,f]	5.67 (2.55, 9.35) [a,b]
S.MPS/Nanomer 30/30	37.86 (1.51)	6.14 (5.09, 7.39) [b]	44.97 (41.83, 46.13) [e,f]	7.27 (5.48, 10.00) [a]
S.MPS/CTAC 50/10	32.28 (2.58)	3.68 (3.40, 3.92) [a]	41.12 (40.12, 41.81) [f]	5.72 (4.79, 7.05) [a,b]
S.MPS/S.CTAC 50/10	43.61 (1.31)	2.63 (2.50, 2.79) [a]	31.59 (30.41, 33.39) [g]	3.02 (1.62, 4.39) [b]

3.4. Water Sorption and Solubility

Water sorption of the composite resin materials constitutes a physicochemical process of clinical importance due to its significant impact on strength and wear performance [48]. The weight values per volume unit of the obtained nanocomposites after aging in water for 7 days are listed in Table 3. Statistically significant differences ($p < 0.05$) between the seven studied groups are also included. Regarding the increasing nanoclay content in dental nanocomposite resins, it is shown that the sorption characteristics are influenced by the gradual addition of Nanomer® I.34MN clay, reaching experimental values in the range of 28.48–44.97 µg/mm^3. The composite reinforcement with clay nanofiller up to 20 wt% yields W_{sl} results that conform with the sorption requirements of ISO 4049 (<40 µg/mm^3) [49]. Janda et al. highlighted the correlation between the filler loading of resin-based filling materials and water sorption [50]. It seems that the hydrophilic nature of Nanomer® I.34MN clay promotes the attraction of water molecules via hydrogen bonding as the clay amount becomes larger. Consequently, the penetration of water proceeds intensively and, hence, affects the sorption resistance of the highly reinforced nanocomposites. Moreover, the S.MPS/S.CTAC 50/10 nanocomposite exhibited a remarkable resistance against water sorption (31.59 µg/mm^3) in comparison to the S.MPS/Nanomer (33.37 µg/mm^3) and S.MPS/CTAC (41.12 µg/mm^3) counterparts. In that case, the surface silanized S.MMT-CTAC clay could serve as a supplementary crosslinking agent that further enhances the polymer network against the entry of water molecules.

The solubility of dental composite resins is closely related to the release of unreacted monomers from the polymer matrix to the aqueous environment during the aging process conducted at 37 °C, which somehow simulates the oral conditions. All the solubility data presented in Table 3 are in accordance with the solubility criteria of ISO 4049 (<7.5 µg/mm^3) [49]. Statistically significant differences ($p < 0.05$) are also included in Table 3. Indeed, the incorporation of 5 wt% Nanomer® I.34MN clay does not vitally affect the ability of the material to withstand the elution of the entrapped monomers from the crosslinked polymer structure to the outer aqueous environment. It is worth pointing out that the S.MPS/Nanomer 50/10 presented better resistance (4.79 µg/mm^3) when compared to the control sample S.MPS 60 (6.21 µg/mm^3). Al-Shekhli et al. reported solubility results for the commercial dental composite resins Premise, Herculite, and Supreme XT (4.36, 4.02 and 4.02 µg/mm^3) that are relatively close to that of S.MPS/Nanomer 50/10 [51]. The relatively high DC value found for the S.MPS/Nanomer 50/10 (44.89%) and the well-dispersed intercalated clay platelets (Figures 1c and 2a) capable of acting as barriers against the diffusion of the remaining monomers may account for the observed low solubility level. Although the additional clay loading can render the nanocomposite more susceptible to monomer release, the determined solubility values did not exceed the corresponding values of the control dental nanocomposite. S.MPS/CTAC 50/10 and S.MPS/S.CTAC 50/10 composites also mitigated the monomer migration to the aqueous medium, as revealed by their measured solubilities (5.72 and 3.02 µg/mm^3). In particular, both the DC found for the S.MPS/S.CTAC dental nanocomposite resin (43.61%) and the sufficient dispersion of the silicate layers into the polymer network (Figure 1g) may account for the performance mentioned above.

3.5. Polymerization Shrinkage Kinetics

Figure 4 depicts the kinetics of polymerization shrinkage for the total of the synthesized dental nanocomposite resins. In addition, Table 3 summarizes the strain values (%) calculated for the studied materials, also involving statistically significant differences ($p < 0.05$) between the seven studied groups. It is well accepted that light-cured composite resins are challenged with dimensional alterations caused by polymerization reactions of the organic monomers [52]. The process involves the conversion of van der Waals interactions into covalent bonds, resulting in a decrease in free volume, internal stresses, and, finally, in the formation of microleakage at the tooth restoration interface [33]. The variations in the filler type may have a strong effect on the polymerization shrinkage–stress kinetics of resin composites [53]. According to Figure 4, an abrupt increase in the strain curves at the early stages of the setting procedure (<10 min curing) was recorded for all studied materials, and this trend was more intense for S.MPS/Nanomer 30/30 (Figure 4a) and S.MPS/CTAC 50/10 (Figure 4b). Regarding the Nanomer® I.34MN clay incorporation, the lowest setting contraction was determined for the S.MPS/Nanomer 55/5 composite (2.76%), followed by S.MPS/Nanomer 50/10 (2.93%), which are limited in comparison to S.MPS 60 (3.51%). Organomodified clay nanoparticles are known to swell through the insertion of the developed macromolecular chains between silicate lamellae, leading to the increment in the internal free volume of the clay and eventually to the decrease in the total strain of the nanocomposite [54,55]. However, the higher mass fractions of clay at 20 and 30 wt% resulted in the ultimate strains of 5.22% and 6.14%, respectively. The possible formation of inorganic agglomerates into the intercalated nanocomposite structures, as previously supported by SEM and XRD results, might decrease the expansion and free volume of Nanomer® I.34MN clay and subsequently the polymerization shrinkage of the cured nanocomposite. Regarding the different type of clay at 10 wt% content, the S.MPS/CTAC nanocomposite experienced larger setting contraction (3.68%) than S.MPS/Nanomer, possibly due to the different degree of clay swelling effect. On the contrary, the S.MPS/S.CTAC 50/10 composite displayed the highest dimensional stability (2.63%), perhaps owing to the higher extension of clay platelet disorientation, as proved by the lowest-intensity peak in the XRD diffractogram (Figure 2b). This configuration could contribute to the increase in the free volume of S.MMT-CTAC clay and maintain the nanocomposite's polymerization shrinkage at a relatively low level.

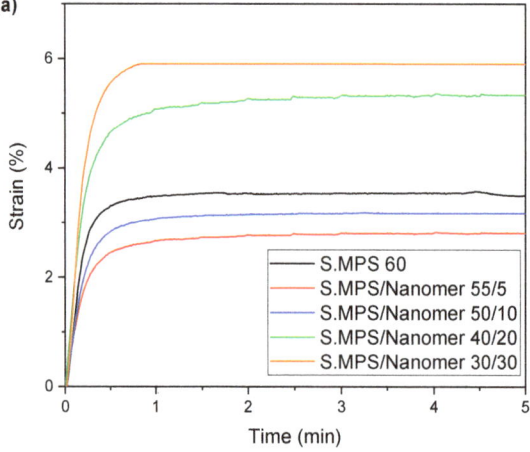

Figure 4. *Cont.*

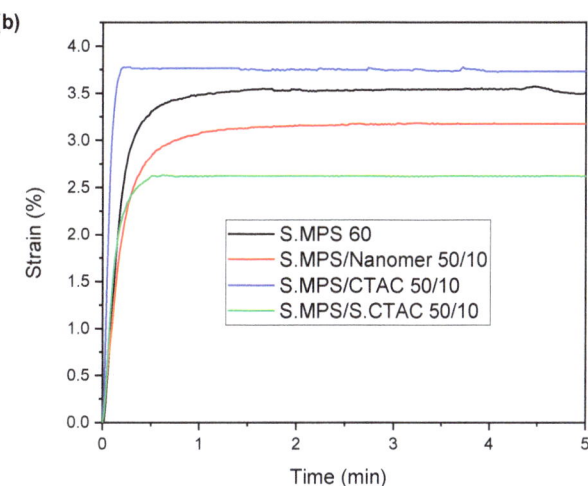

Figure 4. Time dependence of polymerization shrinkage of the studied dental nanocomposites reinforced with: (**a**) specific silica/clay nanoparticle ratios (up to 30/30 wt%); (**b**) several types of nanoclays at silica/clay nanoparticle ratio 50/10 wt%.

3.6. Flexural Properties

The flexural modulus tendencies determined for dental nanocomposites containing silica along with clay nanoparticles are presented in Figure 5, and the corresponding values involving statistically significant differences ($p < 0.05$) are listed in Table 4. Regarding the variation in clay loading (Figure 5a), it is clear that the displacement of the total content of silica nanoparticles by 10 wt% nanoclay in the dental composite formulation can retain the stiffness of the ultimate nanocomposite (2.61 GPa) at a similar level as the control S.MPS 60 (2.69 GPa). These findings are very close to the elastic modulus assessed by Atali et al. for the universal resin composites Omnichroma (2.87 GPa) and Admira Fusion x-tra (2.33 GPa) [56]. Further incorporation of clay nanoparticles may lead to a stepwise decrease in modulus up to 22%, corresponding to the elasticity attitude of S.MPS/Nanomer 30/30 (2.03 MPa), and the largest part of this descent (19%) is due to the transition from the S.MPS/Nanomer 40/20 (2.50 GPa) to the S.MPS/Nanomer 30/30 nanocomposite. Though there is information in the literature correlating the elastic modulus with the DC [57], the aforementioned trend could be attributed to the decrease in DC values (Table 3) by clay loading elevation from 10 to 30 wt%. In addition, the increase in sorption values implies a possible plasticizing effect of water molecules during the aging of specimens, which expands the macromolecular chains of the network, resulting in the observed flexural modulus results. Figure 5b shows that at 10 wt% amount of nanoclay, the rigidity of dental nanocomposite resin with Nanomer® I.34MN particles is at least 20–29% higher than the corresponding resins with MMT-S.CTAC (2.10 GPa) and MMT-CTAC nanofillers (1.85 MPa). The highest DC value determined for S.MPS/Nanomer 50/10 (44.89%) could justify the improvement in the flexural modulus versus S.MPS/S.CTAC 50/10 and S.MPS/CTAC 50/10 composites. Despite the above differences, it was also found that the presence of MMT-S.CTAC (10 wt%) can sustain the final stiffness of the nanocomposite between the values achieved when the Nanomer® I.34MN was used at 20 and 30 wt% mass fractions.

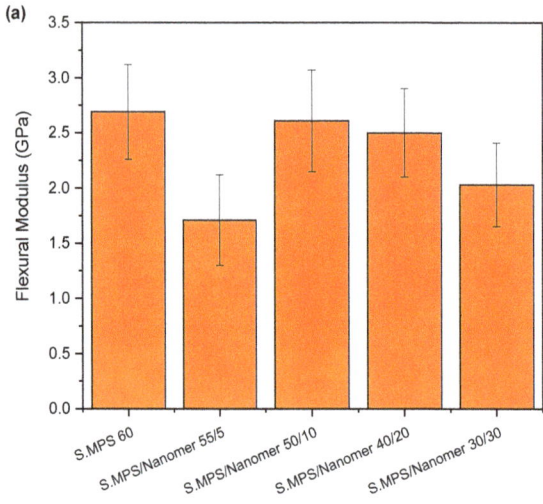

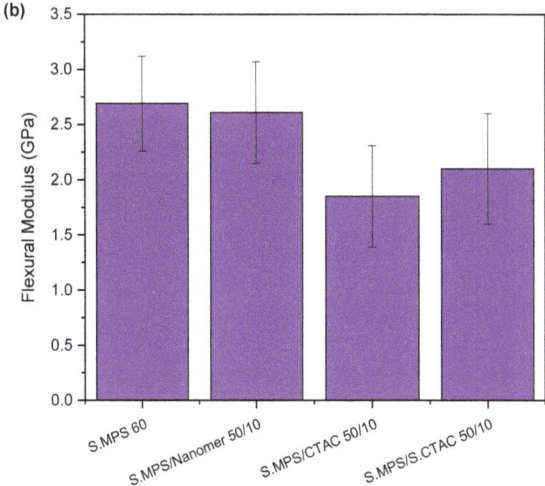

Figure 5. Flexural modulus of the synthesized dental nanocomposite resins nanofilled with silica and: (**a**) Nanomer® I.34MN clay at different nanoclay loadings (5–30 wt%); (**b**) different organoclay types at 10 wt% concentration.

Table 4. Mean values (SD) of flexural modulus and median values (interquartile range, IQR) of strength as measured for the synthesized dental nanocomposite resins. Different superscript indicates statistically significant difference ($p < 0.05$).

Dental Nanocomposite Resin	Flexural Modulus (GPa) Mean (SD)	Flexural Strength (MPa) Median (IQR)
S.MPS 60	2.69 (0.43) [a,c,d]	39.75 (34.59, 56.09) [a]
S.MPS/Nanomer 55/5	1.71 (0.41) [b,d]	32.66 (32.17, 35.39) [a,b]
S.MPS/Nanomer 50/10	2.61 (0.46) [c,d]	41.04 (32.85, 46.37) [a]
S.MPS/Nanomer 40/20	2.50 (0.40) [d]	37.88 (33.91, 39.39) [a]
S.MPS/Nanomer 30/30	2.03 (0.38) [b,c,d]	32.57 (30.86, 36.10) [a,b]
S.MPS/CTAC 50/10	1.85 (0.46) [b]	33.22 (22.80, 37.97) [a,b]
S.MPS/S.CTAC 50/10	2.10 (0.50) [a,b,c,d]	22.46 (15.12, 28.85) [b]

Figure 6 shows that the flexural strength is also vitally influenced by the incorporation of the different amount and type of organoclay nanoparticles. The determined values for each nanocomposite along with statistically significant differences ($p < 0.05$) are presented in Table 4. The majority of the assessed strength values were found to be superior to that of 25 MPa for dental resin composites filled with 60 wt% S.MPS nanoparticles, as mentioned by Rodriguez et al. [49]. Herein, the experimental procedure for the estimation of the nanocomposites' mechanical behavior involved 7 days of aging in aqueous medium, so as to better simulate the oral conditions and intensify the penetration effectiveness of water molecules within the polymer network. On the contrary, other studies applied shorter aging time periods, thus presenting higher flexural strength values [28,58]. In particular, dental nanocomposites filled with 10 wt% Nanomer® I.34MN clay (Figure 6a) exhibited almost the same resistance against flexural stresses (41.04 MPa) when compared with the conventional nanocomposite S.MPS 60 (39.75 MPa), followed by the slightly weaker S.MPS/Nanomer 40/20 (37.88 MPa), and, finally, the S.MPS/Nanomer 30/30 dental composite (32.57 MPa). Moreover, the descending strength of S.MPS/Nanomer 55/5 (32.66 MPa) is similar to that of S.MPS/Nanomer 30/30. The combination of SEM and XRD data could support the latter mechanical position, as the presence of clay-clay agglomerates and silica-clay clusters can result in irregular distribution of flexural stresses, thus accumulating them in limited sites, which contributes to crack propagation (Figures 1 and 2). In terms of the different types of nanoclay (Figure 6b), it seems that at relatively low clay loading levels (10 wt%), the flexural strength level is better sustained for the S.MPS/CTAC 50/10 (33.32 MPa) in comparison to the composite resin containing MMT-S.CTAC (22.46 MPa). Furthermore, the S.MPS/Nanomer 50/10 dental nanocomposite resin exhibits a 23% and 82% improvement in ultimate strength in relation to S.MPS/CTAC 50/10 and S.MPS/S.CTAC 50/10 nanocomposites. The extremely weaker resistance of the latter nanocomposite resin can be explained by the filler aggregated units detected by the SEM technique (Figure 1).

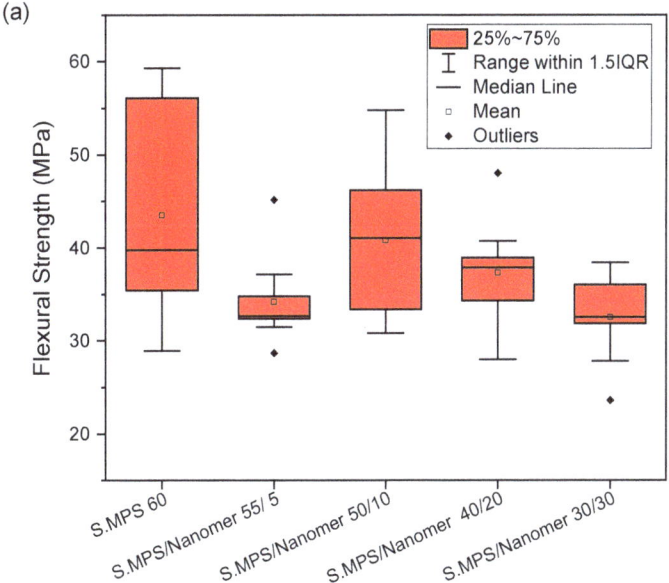

Figure 6. *Cont.*

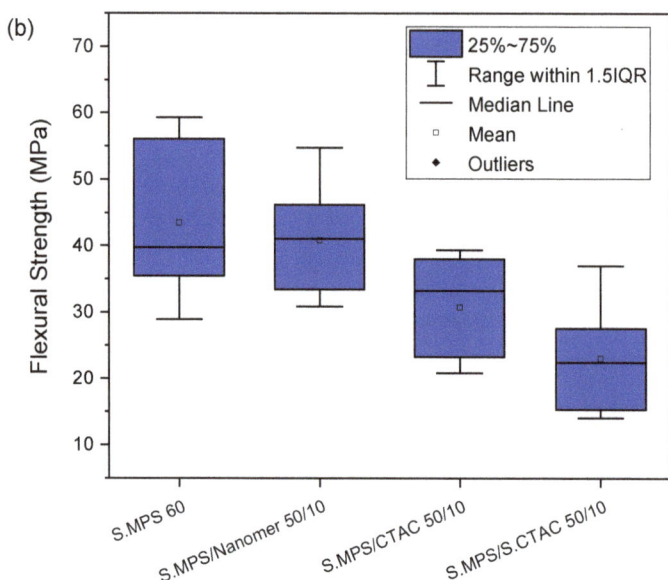

Figure 6. Flexural resistance of the synthesized dental nanocomposite resins nanofilled with silica and: (**a**) Nanomer clay at different nanoclay loadings (up to 30 wt%); (**b**) different organoclay types at 10 wt% concentration.

4. Conclusions

Herein, novel dental nanocomposite resins were synthesized by incorporating organically modified silica along with QA-clay nanoparticles at different clay loadings. It was proved that both the different type and the amount of nanoclay might influence not only the structural characteristics but also the physicochemical and mechanical properties of the obtained nanocomposites, thus confirming the null hypothesis. More particularly, SEM and XRD results showed the intercalation of macromolecular chains within clay galleries, along with some areas characterized by silica-clay clusters over the nanocomposite structures, when the amount of clay reached up to 30 wt%. The degree of conversion, setting contraction, and sorption parameters of the obtained nanocomposite resins were found to decrease by elevating the nanoclay concentration. In particular, the utilization of 10 wt% Nanomer® I.34MN amplified the auto-acceleration effect within the 20–25 min of setting reaction, also keeping the obtained final DC value at almost 45%. The aforementioned mass fraction of clay also decreased the shrinkage strain (2.93%) and solubility (4.79 $\mu g/mm^3$), without affecting the flexural modulus (2.61 GPa) and ultimate strength (41.04 MPa) of the dental nanocomposite resin. These findings are expected to provide scientific information to the dental industry in terms of the correlations between the structural configurations and the ultimate properties of modern dental nanocomposite resins based on novel nanofiller systems. The awareness of the aforementioned results in combination with a comprehensive future study evaluating dental nanocomposites' antibacterial activity could contribute to the integrated design of multifunctional dental restorative materials for modern clinical applications.

Author Contributions: Conceptualization, M.S., A.K.N., E.A.K. and D.S.A.; methodology, M.S. and A.K.N.; validation, E.A.K. and D.S.A.; formal analysis, A.K.N.; investigation, M.S. and A.K.N.; resources, E.A.K.; data curation, A.K.N.; writing—original draft preparation, A.K.N.; writing—review and editing, E.A.K. and D.S.A.; supervision, E.A.K. and D.S.A.; project administration, E.A.K. and D.S.A. All authors have read and agreed to the published version of the manuscript.

Funding: This research received no external funding.

Data Availability Statement: The data presented in this study are available from the corresponding author upon request.

Acknowledgments: The experimental procedures were performed at the Department of Basic Dental Sciences, Division of Dental Tissues' Pathology and Therapeutics, School of Dentistry, Faculty of Health Sciences, Aristotle University of Thessaloniki, Greece, and at the Laboratory of Polymer and Color Chemistry and Technology, Department of Chemistry, Aristotle University of Thessaloniki, Greece. The authors would also like to thank the EVONIK GmbH (Hanau-Wolfgang, Germany) company for the donation of silica nanoparticles. The authors would like to thank the native English speaker Eleni Vlachta, Linguistics MSc, for her valuable contribution to the English revision of the manuscript.

Conflicts of Interest: The authors declare no conflict of interest.

References

1. Smith, L.; Ali, M.; Agrissais, M.; Mulligan, S.; Koh, L.; Martin, N. A Comparative Life Cycle Assessment of Dental Restorative Materials. *Dent. Mater.* **2023**, *39*, 13–24. [CrossRef] [PubMed]
2. Fugolin, A.P.; Pfeifer, C.S. Engineering a New Generation of Thermoset Self-Healing Polymers Based on Intrinsic Approaches. *JADA Found. Sci.* **2022**, *1*, 100014. [CrossRef] [PubMed]
3. Yang, B.; Aregawi, W.; Chen, R.; Zhang, L.; Wang, Y.; Fok, A.S.L. Accelerated Fatigue Model for Predicting Composite Restoration Failure. *J. Dent. Res.* **2022**, *101*, 1606–1612. [CrossRef] [PubMed]
4. Yan, Y.; Chen, C.; Chen, B.; Shen, J.; Zhang, H.; Xie, H. Effects of Hydrothermal Aging, Thermal Cycling, and Water Storage on the Mechanical Properties of a Machinable Resin-Based Composite Containing Nano-zirconia Fillers. *J. Mech. Behav. Biomed. Mater.* **2020**, *102*, 103522. [CrossRef]
5. Yang, J.; Shen, J.; Wu, X.; He, F.; Xie, H.; Chen, C. Effects of Nano-zirconia Fillers Conditioned with Phosphate Ester Monomers on the Conversion and Mechanical Properties of Bis-GMA-and UDMA-based Resin Composites. *J. Dent.* **2020**, *94*, 103306. [CrossRef]
6. Yang, D.L.; Sun, Q.; Niu, H.; Wang, R.L.; Wang, D.; Wang, J.X. The Properties of Dental Resin Composites Reinforced with Silica Colloidal Nanoparticle Clusters: Effects of Heat Treatment and Filler Composition. *Compos. Part B* **2020**, *186*, 107791. [CrossRef]
7. Cho, K.; Rajan, G.; Farrar, P.; Prentice, L.; Prusty, B.G. Dental Resin Composites: A Review on Materials to Product Realizations. *Compos. Part B* **2022**, *230*, 109495. [CrossRef]
8. Lin, G.S.S.; Cher, C.Y.; Cheah, K.K.; Noorani, T.Y.; Ismail, N.H.; Ghani, N.R.N.A. Novel Dental Composite Resin Derived from Rice Husk Natural Biowaste: A Systematic Review and Recommendation for Future Advancement. *J. Esthet. Restor. Dent.* **2022**, *34*, 503–511. [CrossRef]
9. Moro, B.L.P.; Michou, S.; Cenci, M.S.; Mendes, F.M.; Ekstrand, K.R. Secondary Caries Detection and Treatment Decision According to Two Criteria and the Impact of Three-Dimensional Intraoral Scanner on Gap Evaluation. *Caries Res.* **2023**, *57*, 141–151. [CrossRef]
10. Chen, L.; Suh, B.I.; Yang, J. Antibacterial Dental Restorative Materials: A Review. *Am. J. Dent.* **2018**, *31*, 6B–12B.
11. Łukomska-Szymańska, M.; Zarzycka, B.; Grzegorczyk, J.; Sokołowski, K.; Półtorak, K.; Sokołowski, J.; Łapińska, B. Antibacterial Properties of Calcium Fluoride-Based Composite Materials: In Vitro Study. *Biomed Res. Int.* **2016**, *2016*, 1048320. [CrossRef] [PubMed]
12. Boaro, L.C.C.; Campos, L.M.; Varca, G.H.C.; dos Santos, T.M.R.; Marques, P.A.; Sugii, M.M.; Saldanha, N.R.; Cogo-Müller, K.; Brandt, W.C.; Braga, R.R.; et al. Antibacterial Resin-Based Composite Containing Chlorhexidine for Dental Applications. *Dent. Mater.* **2019**, *35*, 909–918. [CrossRef] [PubMed]
13. Chan, D.C.; Hu, W.; Chung, K.-H.; Larsen, R.; Jensen, S.; Cao, D.; Gaviria, L.; Ong, J.L.; Whang, K.; Eiampongpaiboon, T. Reactions: Antibacterial and Bioactive Dental Restorative Materials: Do They Really Work? *Am. J. Dent.* **2018**, *31*, 32B–36B. [PubMed]
14. Lapinska, B.; Szram, A.; Zarzycka, B.; Grzegorczyk, J.; Hardan, L.; Sokolowski, J.; Lukomska-Szymanska, M. An In Vitro Study on the Antimicrobial Properties of Essential Oil Modified Resin Composite against Oral Pathogens. *Materials* **2020**, *13*, 4383. [CrossRef]
15. Butler, J.; Handy, R.D.; Upton, M.; Besinis, A. Review of Antimicrobial Nanocoatings in Medicine and Dentistry: Mechanisms of Action, Biocompatibility Performance, Safety, and Benefits Compared to Antibiotics. *ACS Nano* **2023**, *17*, 7064–7092. [CrossRef]
16. Featherstone, J.D.B. Dental Restorative Materials Containing Quaternary Ammonium Compounds Have Sustained Antibacterial Action. *J. Am. Dent. Assoc.* **2022**, *153*, 1114–1120. [CrossRef]
17. Zhang, J.F.; Wu, R.; Fan, Y.; Liao, S.; Wang, Y.; Wen, Z.T.; Xu, X. Antibacterial Dental Composites with Chlorhexidine and Mesoporous Silica. *J. Dent. Res.* **2014**, *93*, 1283–1289. [CrossRef]
18. Melo, M.; Weir, M.; Passos, V.; Rolim, J.; Lynch, C.; Rodrigues, L.; Xu, H. Human In Situ Study of the Effect of Bis(2-Methacryloyloxyethyl) Dimethylammonium Bromide Immobilized in Dental Composite on Controlling Mature Cariogenic Biofilm. *Int. J. Mol. Sci.* **2018**, *19*, 3443. [CrossRef]
19. Wang, W.; Wu, F.; Zhang, G.; Zhu, S.; Ban, J.; Wang, L. Preparation of a Highly Crosslinked Biosafe Dental Nanocomposite Resin with a Tetrafunctional Methacrylate Quaternary Ammonium Salt Monomer. *RSC Adv.* **2019**, *9*, 41616–41627. [CrossRef]

20. Rechmann, P.; Le, C.Q.; Chaffee, B.W.; Rechmann, B.M.T. Demineralization Prevention with a New Antibacterial Restorative Composite Containing QASi Nanoparticles: An in Situ Study. *Clin. Oral Investig.* **2021**, *25*, 5293–5305. [CrossRef]
21. Dekel-Steinkeller, M.; Weiss, E.I.; Samovici, T.L.-D.; Abramovitz, I. Antibacterial Performance of Composite Containing Quaternary Ammonium Silica (QASi) Filler–A Preliminary Study. *J. Dent.* **2022**, *123*, 104209. [CrossRef] [PubMed]
22. Nikolaidis, A.K.; Koulaouzidou, E.A.; Gogos, C.; Achilias, D.S. Synthesis and Characterization of Dental Nanocomposite Resins Filled with Different Clay Nanoparticles. *Polymers* **2019**, *11*, 730. [CrossRef] [PubMed]
23. Zaltsman, N.; Weiss, E.I. Compositions and Medical Devices Comprising Anti-Microbial Particles. EP3675802A4, 27 February 2019.
24. Zhang, Y.; Chen, Y.; Hu, Y.; Huang, F.; Xiao, Y. Quaternary Ammonium Compounds in Dental Restorative Materials. *Dent. Mater. J.* **2018**, *37*, 183–191. [CrossRef]
25. Matsuo, K.; Yoshihara, K.; Nagaoka, N.; Makita, Y.; Obika, H.; Okihara, T.; Matsukawa, A.; Yoshida, Y.; Van Meerbeek, B. Rechargeable Anti-Microbial Adhesive Formulation Containing Cetylpyridinium Chloride Montmorillonite. *Acta Biomater.* **2019**, *100*, 388–397. [CrossRef]
26. Lee, M.; Kim, D.; Kim, J.; Oh, J.K.; Castaneda, H.; Kim, J.H. Antimicrobial Activities of Thermoplastic Polyurethane/Clay Nanocomposites against Pathogenic Bacteria. *ACS Appl. Bio. Mater.* **2020**, *3*, 6672–6679. [CrossRef]
27. Niu, H.; Yang, D.-L.; Fu, J.-W.; Gao, T.; Wang, J.-X. Mechanical Behavior and Reinforcement Mechanism of Nanoparticle Cluster Fillers in Dental Resin Composites: Simulation and Experimental Study. *Dent. Mater.* **2022**, *38*, 1801–1811. [CrossRef] [PubMed]
28. Rodríguez, H.A.; Kriven, W.M.; Casanova, H. Development of Mechanical Properties in Dental Resin Composite: Effect of Filler Size and Filler Aggregation State. *Mater. Sci. Eng. C* **2019**, *101*, 274–282. [CrossRef]
29. Karkanis, S.; Nikolaidis, A.K.; Koulaouzidou, E.A.; Achilias, D.S. Effect of Silica Nanoparticles Silanized by Functional/Functional or Functional/Non-Functional Silanes on the Physicochemical and Mechanical Properties of Dental Nanocomposite Resins. *Appl. Sci.* **2021**, *12*, 159. [CrossRef]
30. Nikolaidis, A.K.; Achilias, D.S.; Karayannidis, G.P. Effect of the Type of Organic Modifier on the Polymerization Kinetics and the Properties of Poly(Methyl Methacrylate)/Organomodified Montmorillonite Nanocomposites. *Eur. Polym. J.* **2012**, *48*, 240–251. [CrossRef]
31. Watts, D.; Marouf, A. Optimal Specimen Geometry in Bonded-Disk Shrinkage-Strain Measurements on Light-Cured Biomaterials. *Dent. Mater.* **2000**, *16*, 447–451. [CrossRef]
32. Watts, D. Photo-Polymerization Shrinkage-Stress Kinetics in Resin-Composites: Methods Development. *Dent. Mater.* **2003**, *19*, 1–11. [CrossRef] [PubMed]
33. Al Sunbul, H.; Silikas, N.; Watts, D.C. Polymerization Shrinkage Kinetics and Shrinkage-Stress in Dental Resin-Composites. *Dent. Mater.* **2016**, *32*, 998–1006. [CrossRef] [PubMed]
34. Rueggeberg, F.A.; Hashinger, D.T.; Fairhurst, C.W. Calibration of FTIR Conversion Analysis of Contemporary Dental Resin Composites. *Dent. Mater.* **1990**, *6*, 241–249. [CrossRef]
35. Wilson, K.S.; Zhang, K.; Antonucci, J.M. Systematic Variation of Interfacial Phase Reactivity in Dental Nanocomposites. *Biomaterials* **2005**, *26*, 5095–5103. [CrossRef] [PubMed]
36. Wilson, K.S.; Antonucci, J.M. Interphase Structure–Property Relationships in Thermoset Dimethacrylate Nanocomposites. *Dent. Mater.* **2006**, *22*, 995–1001. [CrossRef] [PubMed]
37. Halvorson, R.H.; Erickson, R.L.; Davidson, C.L. The Effect of Filler and Silane Content on Conversion of Resin-Based Composite. *Dent. Mater.* **2003**, *19*, 327–333. [CrossRef]
38. Sideridou, I.D.; Karabela, M.M. Effect of the Structure of Silane-Coupling Agent on Dynamic Mechanical Properties of Dental Resin-Nanocomposites. *J. Appl. Polym. Sci.* **2008**, *110*, 507–516. [CrossRef]
39. Gonçalves, F.; Kawano, Y.; Pfeifer, C.; Stansbury, J.W.; Braga, R.R. Influence of BisGMA, TEGDMA, and BisEMA Contents on Viscosity, Conversion, and Flexural Strength of Experimental Resins and Composites. *Eur. J. Oral Sci.* **2009**, *117*, 442–446. [CrossRef] [PubMed]
40. Maddalena, R.; Hall, C.; Hamilton, A. Effect of Silica Particle Size on the Formation of Calcium Silicate Hydrate [C-S-H] Using Thermal Analysis. *Thermochim. Acta* **2019**, *672*, 142–149. [CrossRef]
41. Achilias, D.S. A Review of Modeling of Diffusion Controlled Polymerization Reactions. *Macromol. Theory Simul.* **2007**, *16*, 319–347. [CrossRef]
42. Liu, X.; Wang, Z.; Zhao, C.; Bu, W.; Na, H. Preparation and Characterization of Silane-Modified SiO_2 Particles Reinforced Resin Composites with Fluorinated Acrylate Polymer. *J. Mech. Behav. Biomed. Mater.* **2018**, *80*, 11–19. [CrossRef] [PubMed]
43. Wang, R.; Zhang, M.; Liu, F.; Bao, S.; Wu, T.; Jiang, X.; Zhang, Q.; Zhu, M. Investigation on the Physical–Mechanical Properties of Dental Resin Composites Reinforced with Novel Bimodal Silica Nanostructures. *Mater. Sci. Eng. C* **2015**, *50*, 266–273. [CrossRef] [PubMed]
44. Achilias, D.S.; Verros, G.D. Modeling of Diffusion-Controlled Reactions in Free Radical Solution and Bulk Polymerization: Model Validation by DSC Experiments. *J. Appl. Polym. Sci.* **2010**, *116*, 1842–1856. [CrossRef]
45. Verros, G.D.; Achilias, D.S. Modeling Gel Effect in Branched Polymer Systems: Free-Radical Solution Homopolymerization of Vinyl Acetate. *J. Appl. Polym. Sci.* **2009**, *111*, 2171–2185. [CrossRef]
46. Verros, G.D.; Latsos, T.; Achilias, D.S. Development of a Unified Framework for Calculating Molecular Weight Distribution in Diffusion Controlled Free Radical Bulk Homo-Polymerization. *Polymer* **2005**, *46*, 539–552. [CrossRef]

47. De Menezes, L.R.; da Silva, E.O. The Use of Montmorillonite Clays as Reinforcing Fillers for Dental Adhesives. *Mater. Res.* **2016**, *19*, 236–242. [CrossRef]
48. Göhring, T.; Besek, M.; Schmidlin, P. Attritional Wear and Abrasive Surface Alterations of Composite Resin Materials in Vitro. *J. Dent.* **2002**, *30*, 119–127. [CrossRef]
49. ISO 4049:2019; Dentistry-Polymer Based Restorative Materials. ISO: Geneva, Switzerland, 2019; p. 29.
50. Janda, R.; Roulet, J.-F.; Latta, M.; Rüttermann, S. Water Sorption and Solubility of Contemporary Resin-Based Filling Materials. *J. Biomed. Mater. Res. Part B Appl. Biomater.* **2007**, *82*, 545–551. [CrossRef]
51. Al-Shekhli, A.A.R. Solubility of Nanofilled versus Conventional Composites. *Pak. Oral Dent. J.* **2014**, *34*, 118–121.
52. Langalia, A.K.; Pgdhhm, M.; Mds, A.B.; Khamar, M.; Patel, P. Polymerization Shrinkage of Composite Resins: A Review. *J. Maedical Dent. Sci. Res.* **2015**, *2*, 23–27.
53. Satterthwaite, J.D.; Maisuria, A.; Vogel, K.; Watts, D.C. Effect of Resin-Composite Filler Particle Size and Shape on Shrinkage-Stress. *Dent. Mater.* **2012**, *28*, 609–614. [CrossRef] [PubMed]
54. Kelly, P.; Akelah, A.; Qutubuddin, S.; Moet, A. Reduction of Residual Stress in Montmorillonite/Epoxy Compounds. *J. Mater. Sci.* **1994**, *29*, 2274–2280. [CrossRef]
55. Salahuddin, N.; Shehata, M. Polymethylmethacrylate–Montmorillonite Composites: Preparation, Characterization and Properties. *Polymer* **2001**, *42*, 8379–8385. [CrossRef]
56. Yılmaz Atalı, P.; Doğu Kaya, B.; Manav Özen, A.; Tarçın, B.; Şenol, A.A.; Tüter Bayraktar, E.; Korkut, B.; Bilgin Göçmen, G.; Tağtekin, D.; Türkmen, C. Assessment of Micro-Hardness, Degree of Conversion, and Flexural Strength for Single-Shade Universal Resin Composites. *Polymers* **2022**, *14*, 4987. [CrossRef]
57. Ferracane, J.L.; Greener, E.H. The Effect of Resin Formulation on the Degree of Conversion and Mechanical Properties of Dental Restorative Resins. *J. Biomed. Mater. Res.* **1986**, *20*, 121–131. [CrossRef]
58. Wilson, K.S.; Allen, A.J.; Washburn, N.R.; Antonucci, J.M. Interphase Effects in Dental Nanocomposites Investigated by Small-Angle Neutron Scattering. *J. Biomed. Mater. Res. Part A* **2007**, *81*, 113–123. [CrossRef]

Disclaimer/Publisher's Note: The statements, opinions and data contained in all publications are solely those of the individual author(s) and contributor(s) and not of MDPI and/or the editor(s). MDPI and/or the editor(s) disclaim responsibility for any injury to people or property resulting from any ideas, methods, instructions or products referred to in the content.

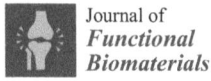

Article

Bactericidal Activity of Silver Nanoparticles on Oral Biofilms Related to Patients with and without Periodontal Disease

Perla Alejandra Hernández-Venegas [1], Rita Elizabeth Martínez-Martínez [2], Erasto Armando Zaragoza-Contreras [3], Rubén Abraham Domínguez-Pérez [4], Simón Yobanny Reyes-López [5], Alejandro Donohue-Cornejo [6], Juan Carlos Cuevas-González [6], Nelly Molina-Frechero [7] and León Francisco Espinosa-Cristóbal [6,*]

1. Chemical Biological Department, Institute of Biomedical Sciences, Autonomous University of Juarez City (UACJ), Envolvente del PRONAF and Estocolmo s/n, Ciudad Juárez 32310, Chihuahua, Mexico; al136416@alumnos.uacj.mx
2. Master Program in Advanced Dentistry, Faculty of Dentistry, Autonomous University of San Luis Potosi, Manuel Nava Avenue, Universitary Campus, San Luis Potosí 78290, San Luis Potosi, Mexico; ritae_martinez@hotmail.com
3. Department of Engineering and Materials Chemistry, Centro de Investigación en Materiales Avanzados, S. C., Miguel de Cervantes No. 120, Chihuahua 31109, Chihuahua, Mexico; armando.zaragoza@cimav.edu.mx
4. Laboratory of Multidisciplinary Dental Research, Faculty of Medicine, Autonomous University of Queretaro, Clavel Street, Prados de La Capilla, Santiago de Querétaro 76176, Queretaro, Mexico; dominguez.ra@uaq.mx
5. Institute of Biomedical Sciences, Autonomous University of Juarez City (UACJ), Envolvente del PRONAF and Estocolmo s/n, Ciudad Juárez 32310, Chihuahua, Mexico; simon.reyes@uacj.mx
6. Master Program in Dental Sciences, Stomatology Department, Institute of Biomedical Sciences, Autonomous University of Juarez City (UACJ), Envolvente del PRONAF and Estocolmo s/n, Ciudad Juárez 32310, Chihuahua, Mexico; adonohue@uacj.mx (A.D.-C.); juan.cuevas@uacj.mx (J.C.C.-G.)
7. Division of Biological and Health Sciences, Autonomous Metropolitan University Xochimilco (UAM), Mexico City 04960, Mexico; nmolinaf@hotmail.com
* Correspondence: leohamet@hotmail.com; Tel./Fax: +55-656-688-1823

Abstract: Background and Objectives: Periodontal disease (PD) is a multifactorial oral disease regularly caused by bacterial biofilms. Silver nanoparticles (AgNP) have offered good antimicrobial activity; moreover, there is no available scientific information related to their antimicrobial effects in biofilms from patients with PD. This study reports the bactericidal activity of AgNP against oral biofilms related to PD. Materials and Methods: AgNP of two average particle sizes were prepared and characterized. Sixty biofilms were collected from patients with (30 subjects) and without PD (30 subjects). Minimal inhibitory concentrations of AgNP were calculated and the distribution of bacterial species was defined by polymerase chain reaction. Results: Well-dispersed sizes of AgNP were obtained (5.4 ± 1.3 and 17.5 ± 3.4 nm) with an adequate electrical stability (−38.2 ± 5.8 and −32.6 ± 5.4 mV, respectively). AgNP showed antimicrobial activities for all oral samples; however, the smaller AgNP had significantly the most increased bactericidal effects (71.7 ± 39.1 µg/mL). The most resistant bacteria were found in biofilms from PD subjects ($p < 0.05$). *P. gingivalis, T. denticola,* and *T. forsythia* were present in all PD biofilms (100%). Conclusions: The AgNP showed efficient bactericidal properties as an alternative therapy for the control or progression of PD.

Keywords: metal nanoparticles; silver; biofilms; periodontal diseases; anti-bacterial agents; humans

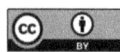

1. Introduction

Periodontal diseases (PD) are alterations that affect the supportive apparatus surrounding teeth, including gingival tissue, alveolar bone, periodontal ligament and cementum [1,2]. The PD involves inflammatory reactions induced basically by bacteria included in an oral biofilm in the periodontium [3,4], which is still a severe oral problem globally [3,5]. The initial stage of PD is called gingivitis, which is identified as an inflammation of the gingiva by the accumulation of bacteria or debris in a biofilm, which is a reactive and reversible condition [1,2]. However, periodontitis is presented in more severe stages of PD, which is a progressive periodontal condition, appearing as a chronic, destructive, irreversible inflammatory state [1,2,6]. The oral biofilm constituted by periodontal pathogens has been widely studied, determining that the interaction of specific species into the biofilm, the host response, and the development of PD, basically periodontitis, is a challenge [4,7]. The dysbiosis of the microbiota could alter bacterial ecology, facilitating the host's inflammatory and immune response, ending in tissue destruction [8]. Among the bacteria that have been more directly involved in the pathogenesis of PD are *Actinobacillus actinomycetemcomitans* (*A. actinomycetemcomitans*), *Porphyromonas gingivalis* (*P. gingivalis*), *Prevotella intermedia* (*P. intermedia*), *Bacteroides forsythus* (*B. forsythus*), and *Treponema denticola* (*T. denticola*). Other bacterial species such as *Prevotella nigrescens* (*P. nigrescens*), *Campylobacter rectus* (*C. rectus*), *Peptostreptococcus micros* (*P. micros*), *Eikenella corroden* (*E. corroden*), and *Fusobacterium nucleatum* (*F. nucleatum*) have a less relevant role, although they have occasionally been related to some forms of PD [4,7]. Particularly, the more prevalent bacteria in healthy oral biofilms could be mentioned, i.e., the Gram-positive bacteria such as *Streptococcus sanguinis* (*S. sanguinis*), *Streptococcus oralis* (*S. oralis*), *Streptococcus intermedius* (*S. intermedius*), *Streptococcus gordonii* (*S. gordonii*), *Peptostreptococcus micros* (*P. micros*), *Gemella morbillorum* (*G. morbillorum*), and others. In contrast, the Gram-negative bacteria more frequently found are *Veillonella parvula*, *V. atypica*, *Capnocytophaga ochracea*, and others [4,7,9,10]. In periodontal disease biofilms, the microorganisms more frequently distributed in gingivitis belong to Gram-negative bacteria such as *Prevotella* spp., *Selenomonas* spp., and *Fusobacterium nucleatum* ss. *polymorphum*, among others. For a more severe conditions of PD, such as periodontitis, the main bacteria are classically described in the red-complex triad, including Gram-negative bacteria such as *T. denticola*, *P. gingivalis*, and *T. forsythia* [4,7,10,11].

The main treatments of PD are the control of bacterial growth immersed into the oral biofilm, divided into mechanical and chemical procedures [12]. The mechanical treatments of supra and subgingival biofilms are based on the control of bacterial growth proliferation, using mechanical instruments such as daily oral hygiene habits (cleaning devices, toothbrushes, dental floss, dental toothpicks, and others) [13,14] and specific professional therapeutics (surgical and non-surgical mechanical debridement) [12,15]. In the case of chemical therapeutics, some antimicrobial solutions have been demonstrated to help the action of mechanical procedures, permitting more effective antimicrobial controls against periodontopathogenic species [12]. The most common antimicrobial agents used for periodontal treatments are present in toothpaste and mouthwashes, which are accompanied, after mechanical debridement, by particular concentrations of the agent, according to the periodontal diagnosis and treatment [12,14]. Chlorhexidine gluconate (CHX) is the gold standard antimicrobial solution in the PD treatment used after surgical and non-surgical periodontal procedures, inhibiting bacterial proliferation consistently in the supra and subgingival dental sites during long-term periods, even in low contents [12,16,17]. Moreover, the solution of CHX has shown several adverse effects related to the pigmentation of hard dental tissues and tongue, mucosal irritation, taste disturbances, numbness and pain in mouth and tongue, xerostomia, and calculus, to name a few [18–20].

Even though CHX has been the best antimicrobial agent for treating PD, other alternatives have been studied. Some works have reported that antibiotics systemically administrated, such as amoxicillin/clavulanic acid, clindamycin, metronidazole, and the combination therapy metronidazole/amoxicillin, have demonstrated positive responses against various periodontal bacteria associated with destructive PD [21,22]. However, at the same time, the increase in antimicrobial resistance is a significant limitation in long-term administration [22,23], including periodontal microbial affections [24]. In this sense, it is necessary to explore new and more effective antimicrobial agents [25–27] with properties that improve periodontal therapy through bacterial growth inhibition and the reduction of antibiotic resistance. The literature has recommended the use of silver nanoparticles (AgNP) for the control of bacterial proliferation, due to their excellent bacteriostatic and bactericidal properties in many microbial species, including oral microorganisms [28–33]. A significant number of researchers report the evaluation of the bactericidal effect of the AgNP against specific bacterial species using standard bacterial stocks provided by Microbial Type Culture Collection (MTCC) [34] or American Type Culture Collections (ATCC) [35,36] catalogs. Therefore, there are limited investigations that have determined the antimicrobial activity of AgNP using exclusively clinical bacterial oral biofilms, focused specifically on individual periodontal pathogens [34,37–39]. The purpose of this study was to evaluate the antimicrobial activity of AgNP against several oral biofilms isolated from patients with and without PD and to explore the associations of the antimicrobial activity of AgNP with the sociodemographic and clinical characteristics of the subjects under study. The results of this study will contribute both to a better understanding and the safe use of these metallic nanomaterials as an alternative approach for the prevention and control of PD.

2. Materials and Methods

2.1. Materials

Silver nitrate ($AgNO_3$, CTR Scientific, Monterrey, Nuevo León, Mexico), gallic acid ($C_7H_6O_5$, Sigma Aldrich, Saint Louis, MO, USA), sodium hydroxide (NaOH, Jalmek Scientific, San Nicolás de los Garza, Mexico), ammonia hydroxide (NH_4OH, Jalmek Scientific), Müller-Hinton broth (MH, BD™ Difco™, Rockville, MD, USA), 2.0% chlorhexidine gluconate (Consepsis, Ultradent Products Inc, South Jordan, UT, USA), were used and stored according to manufacturer's recommendations.

2.2. Preparation and Characterization of AgNP

AgNP of two average particle sizes were prepared using the synthesis method previously reported [40]. First, 0.169 g of silver nitrate ($AgNO_3$, CTR Scientific, Monterrey, Mexico), as a precursor agent, was dissolved in 100 mL of deionized water with magnetic stirring. Afterward, 10 mL of deionized water with 0.1 g of gallic acid ($C_7H_6O_5$, Sigma Aldrich, St. Louis, MI, USA), used as a reducing agent, was immediately added to the first solution. Finally, the pH was adjusted to 11 with a 1 M solution of sodium hydroxide (NaOH, Jalmek Scientific, San Nicolás de los Garza, Mexico) for the particle size stabilization. For the second particle size, 10 mL of deionized water with 0.5 g of gallic acid was incorporated into $AgNO_3$ solution, prepared as mentioned above, adjusting the pH to 11 using a solution of ammonium hydroxide (NH_4OH, Jalmek Scientific, San Nicolás de los Garza, Mexico) under magnetic stirring. Both solutions were stirred for 10 min under laboratory conditions. The characterization of the two samples of AgNP was carried out by dynamic light scattering (DLS) for the determination of average particle size and particle size distribution. The zeta potential of particles was analyzed using a nanoparticle analyzer (DLS, Nanoparticle Analyzer, Nano Partica SZ-100 series, HORIBA Scientific Ltd., Irvine, CA, USA), while transmission electron microscopy (TEM, Phillips CM-200) was used for the determination of particle shape using a voltage accelerating of 25 kV.

2.3. Patient Recruitment

A consecutive nonprobabilistic sampling was carried out to select patients from the Dental Admission Clinic belonging to the Stomatology Department at the Autonomous University of Ciudad Juárez (UACJ), Mexico. All recruited patients voluntarily signed an informed consent before taking the clinical samples regarding the ethical guidelines of the Helsinki Declaration (2008). The study was approved by the Biomedical Sciences Institute Research Committee (ICB), UACJ (project ID RIPI2019ICB5). The study involved 60 subjects between 30 to 50 years old, who were divided into two groups: (a) 30 subjects with PD and (b) 30 subjects without PD (healthy). The presence of PD was defined by evident partial or total gingival inflammation, with induced or spontaneous blood bleeding, up to the presence of apical migration of the periodontal attachment tissue in at least one single tooth during the oral examination. Clinical intern experts of the Dental Social Services of the Dentistry program at ICB-UACJ diagnosed the PD.

2.4. Sampling of Oral Biofilms

The oral biofilms were collected from subgingival and supragingival oral sites from the teeth of patients with or without PD, using a sterile wooden toothpick to create a mechanical scraping in the interproximal, vestibular, lingual, or palatal surface in a single direction. The toothpicks with the biofilm samples were immediately placed in a tube containing 5 mL of Müller–Hinton broth (MH, BD™ Difco™, Rockville, MD, USA), and incubated for anaerobic bacteria at 37 °C for 24 h.

2.5. Initial Bacterial Growth and Standard Microbial Suspension

The initial bacterial growth was measured using the optical density (OD) for each oral biofilm before antimicrobial activity tests. Once microbiological samples were incubated, 100 µL of each bacterial sample were added to 3 mL of phosphate buffer solution (PBS). The absorbance level was analyzed using a spectrophotometer (Eppendorf, BioPhotometer Plus, München, Germany) at a wavelength of 550 nm by triplicate. Then, the concentration of microbial samples was standardized at 1.3×10^8 colony-forming units per milliliter (CFU/mL), obtained when the bacterial suspensions reached an absorption of 0.126 at 550 nm of wavelength, according to the McFarland scale. Finally, all bacterial suspensions were diluted with PBS and homogenized in a concentration of 1.3×10^6 CFU/mL, which was used for all microbiological tests.

2.6. Antimicrobial Test

The antimicrobial assay was carried out according to the method previously reported [41]. The minimal inhibitory concentration (MIC) of AgNP, through microdilution plates with 96 wells, was used to determine the antimicrobial activity. From the second column to the twelfth, 100 µL of MH broth was placed in each well. After that, 200 mL of each antimicrobial solution was placed in the first column. Then, serial dilutions in a 1:1 proportion were made up to column eleven. Thus, 100 µL of the standardized bacterial suspensions (1.3×10^6 CFU/mL) were added to all wells. Finally, each plate was incubated in anaerobic conditions for 24 h at 37 °C. The MIC values were identified in the last well with no bacterial growth determined by visual and stereomicroscopic comparisons using turbidity parameters. This procedure was carried out for each oral biofilm related to PD and healthy (no PD) subjects in triplicate. Columns one and twelve were assigned as positive (no bacterial growth) and negative (bacterial growth) controls, respectively. The CHX solutions were identified as a gold antimicrobial standard reference.

2.7. Identification of Bacteria by Polymerase Chain Reaction (PCR)

Six samples of oral biofilms from patients with and without PD were randomly selected to identify periodontal bacteria using a polymerase chain reaction (PCR) assay. The presence of *P. gingivalis*, *T. forsythia*, *T. denticola*, *P. intermedia*, *F. nucleatum*, and *A. actinomycetemcomitans* was determined according to previously reported methods [42,43]. Specific primers for the detection of periodontal bacterial species were used according to previous methods by Tran and Rudney [44], Stubbs et al. [45], Watanabe and Frommel [46], Ashimoto et al. [47], and Poulsen et al. [48]. Positive and negative controls were included in each PCR set. All PCR products were submitted to electrophoresis in 2% agarose gels, stained with ethidium bromide, and analyzed under UV light (E-Gel Imager System with UV Base, Thermo Fisher Scientific, Life Technologies, Waltham, MA, USA).

2.8. Statistical Analysis

The general distribution of patients with and without PD, according to gender and bacterial identifications by PCR, was expressed in frequencies and percentages. The homogeneity of the study groups was examined using Pearson´s chi-square test. The values of age from patients, OD of initial bacterial growth, and MIC values from the antimicrobial activity of treatments were presented in means and standard deviations. The normality of variables was analyzed using the Shapiro–Wilks test. The independent comparisons according to treatments, gender, and type of oral biofilm were calculated using the Mann–Whitney U statistical test for nonparametric variables. In addition, Spearman´s rho analysis was used to identify correlations of age among OD, and MIC values from patients with and without PD. All statistical analyses were performed using IBM-SPSS software (SPSS, version 25, Chicago, CA, USA) considering statistical significance when $p < 0.05$.

3. Results

3.1. Characterization of AgNP

Table 1 reports the physical characteristics of AgNP determined by DLS and TEM. In the DLS analysis, single peaks and well-defined sizes were determined from the two colloidal solutions of AgNP (5.4 ± 1.3 and 17.5 ± 3.4 nm), which indicates that both samples of Ag had a narrow and uniform particle size distribution (Figure 1b,d), identifying spherical shapes for smaller and larger Ag particles, respectively (Figure 1a,c). The zeta potential results showed negative electrical charge values for smaller and larger sizes, with different electrical intensities that suggest good electrical stability (-38.2 ± 5.8 and -32.6 ± 5.4 mV, respectively), preventing particle agglomeration. These results support that the particles of both families have adequate size distribution and good superficial electrical properties.

Table 1. Physical characteristics of AgNP families.

AgNP	DLS (nm)	Shape	Concentration (µg/mL)	Zeta Potential (mV)
5.4 nm	5.4 ± 1.3	Spherical	1070	-38.2 ± 5.8
17.5 nm	17.5 ± 3.4	Spherical	1070	-32.6 ± 5.4

DLS = dynamic light scattering. DLS and zeta potential results are expressed in mean, standard, and zeta deviation, respectively.

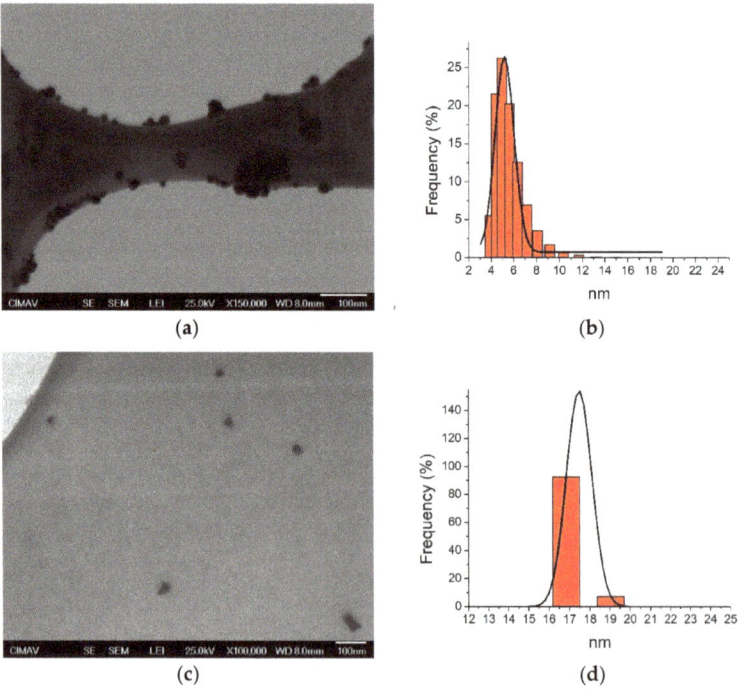

Figure 1. Transmission electron microscopy (TEM) and dynamic light scattering (DLS) analysis of silver nanoparticles (AgNP). (**a**,**b**) 5.4 nm; (**c**,**d**) 17.5 nm.

3.2. Distribution of Patients

Table 2 shows the general distribution of patients in the two study groups. In general, the subjects included in the PD and healthy groups were young adult patients. The subjects with PD (39 ± 6.9 years old), including women (37 ± 7.7 years old) and men (40.5 ± 5.8 years old), were older compared to the total of healthy patients (28 ± 8.9 years old) and both genders (28.3 ± 9.4 and 27.5 ± 8.6 years old, respectively); however, no statistical differences were identified ($p > 0.05$). Additionally, the subjects included in the PD and healthy groups had similar distribution (47% for women and 53% for men), determining no significant differences between both groups according to gender ($p > 0.05$). Those results suggest that the age and gender of patients had a similar distribution in the PD and healthy groups.

Table 2. General sociodemographic distribution of study groups.

	Periodontal Disease n = 30 Subjects (%)	Control (Healthy) n = 30 Subjects (%)
Age (years old)	39 ± 6.9	28 ± 8.9
Women	37 ± 7.7	28.3 ± 9.4
Men	40.5 ± 5.8	27.5 ± 8.6
Gender		
Women	14 (47)	14 (47)
Men	16 (53)	16 (53)

Values from age are expressed in mean and standard deviation. There were no statistical differences between periodontal disease and healthy patients according to age and gender ($p > 0.05$).

3.3. Bacterial Growth of Biofilms

Figure 2 illustrates the initial bacterial growth for each biofilm sample. As noted, the oral biofilms from men and women subjects with PD showed statistically increased bacterial growth compared to healthy patients (Figure 2a,d). Therefore, the biofilms from women and men patients had similar bacterial growth activity, with no statistical differences (Figure 2b,c). These results indicate that the bacterial growth capacity of microorganisms included in the oral biofilms is associated with the presence of PD.

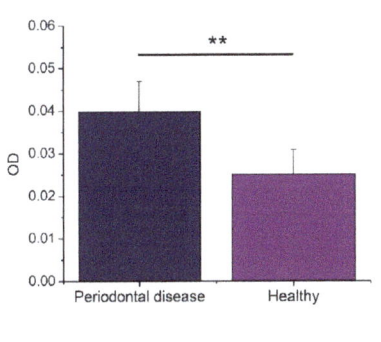

Figure 2. Cont.

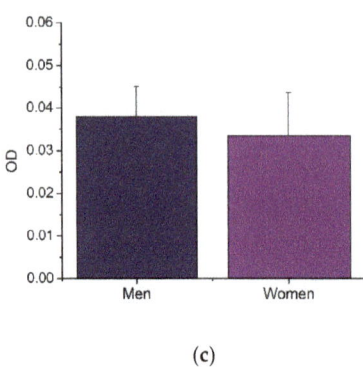
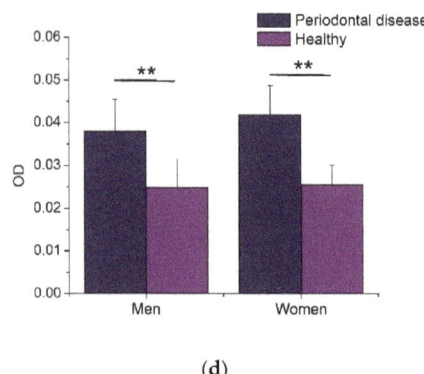

(c)   (d)

Figure 2. Initial growth of biofilm samples from subjects with and without periodontal disease. All values are expressed in mean and standard deviation. Asterisks indicate statistical differences ($p < 0.01$).

3.4. Antimicrobial Activity of AgNP

Figures 3 and 4 show the antimicrobial activity of AgNP in oral biofilms of periodontal disease and healthy patients. As seen, smaller (5.4 nm) and larger (17.5 nm) AgNP, as well as CHX, had good bacterial inhibition activity for all oral biofilms from PD and healthy subjects (Figures 3 and 4). The smaller AgNP showed significantly better antimicrobial activity (71.7 ± 39.1 µg/mL) compared to larger particles (146.9 ± 67.3 µg/mL). However, the CHX had the highest bacterial inhibition of dental biofilms (Figure 3a), even for oral biofilms from PD and healthy subjects (Figure 3d). Moreover, the microorganisms involved in periodontal disease samples demonstrated, statistically, more resistance activity (141.0 ± 69.9 µg/mL) compared to non-PD biofilms (77.7 ± 65.5 µg/mL) for any antimicrobial solution (Figure 3c), including CHX (Figure 3b). These results suggest that both families of AgNP had good antibacterial activity in all samples of oral biofilms from patients with and without PD, associating this activity with the particle size and the type of oral biofilm.

Figure 5 shows the antimicrobial activity of AgNP in oral biofilms from patients with and without PD according to gender. Women showed a tendency to higher resistance to any AgNP sample or CHX solution compared to men; consequently, no significant differences were determined (Figure 5a,b). On the other hand, the oral biofilms from periodontal disease patients and smaller AgNP (5.4 nm) demonstrated, statistically, that for both genders, there was more increased bactericidal activity than biofilms from healthy patients and larger Ag particles, respectively (Figure 5c,d). For all cases, the CHX solution had the best antimicrobial effects (Figure 5d). These results illustrate that gender is not associated with the antimicrobial effect of AgNP, acting similarly for oral biofilm from women and men patients.

The Spearman correlation results of OD and MIC, according to age from oral biofilms of patients with and without PD, are summarized in Table 3. In general, positive correlations were identified at the initial growth of biofilms ($rho = 0.501$), smaller ($rho = 0.223$), and larger ($rho = 0.223$) Ag particles for both groups (periodontal disease and healthy samples). Thus, the initial bacterial growth demonstrated only a significant correlation among the age of patients ($p < 0.05$). Furthermore, specific positive correlations were determined at the initial growth of oral biofilms from periodontal disease ($rho = 0.179$) and non-periodontal ($rho = 0.087$) disease patients, identifying no significant correlations ($p > 0.05$). Although PD biofilms showed positive correlations for smaller ($rho = 0.021$) and larger ($rho = 0.122$) AgNP, negative correlations for healthy biofilm samples were also determined for both particle families ($rho = -0.248$ and -0.042, respectively); however, no statistical correlations were found for any particle sample ($p > 0.05$). These results suggest that the initial bacterial growth capacity of both oral biofilms increases gradually with age ($p < 0.05$), demonstrating a particularly high tendency for periodontal disease biofilms. On the other hand, the concentration of AgNP for both particle sizes acts similarly at any age. However, the PD biofilms had a trend to need higher contents of AgNP according to age, while biofilms from patients with no PD showed an opposite tendency, requiring gradually lower concentrations of nanoparticles with respect to age.

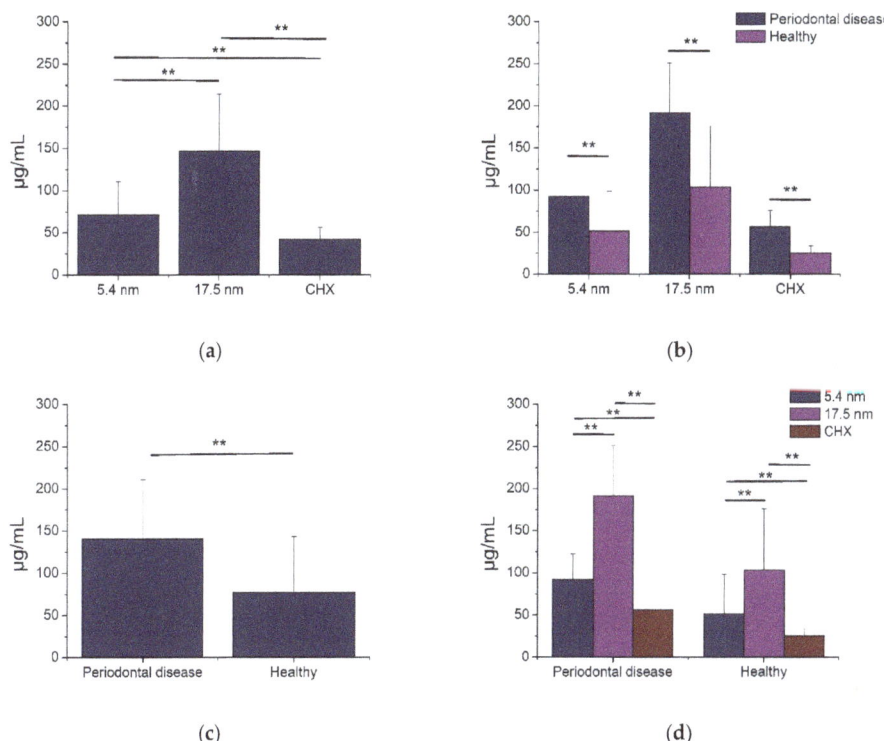

Figure 3. Antimicrobial activity of AgNP against biofilms associated with periodontal disease. All values are expressed in mean and standard deviation. Asterisks indicate statistical differences ($p < 0.01$).

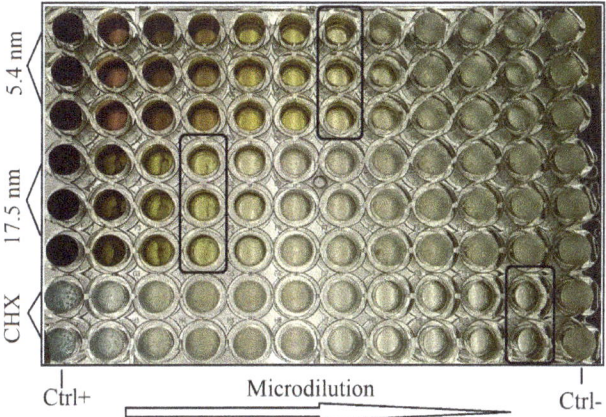

Figure 4. Representative microdilution plate with MIC values of AgNP and CHX in oral biofilm from PD subject. Black squares represent MIC values.

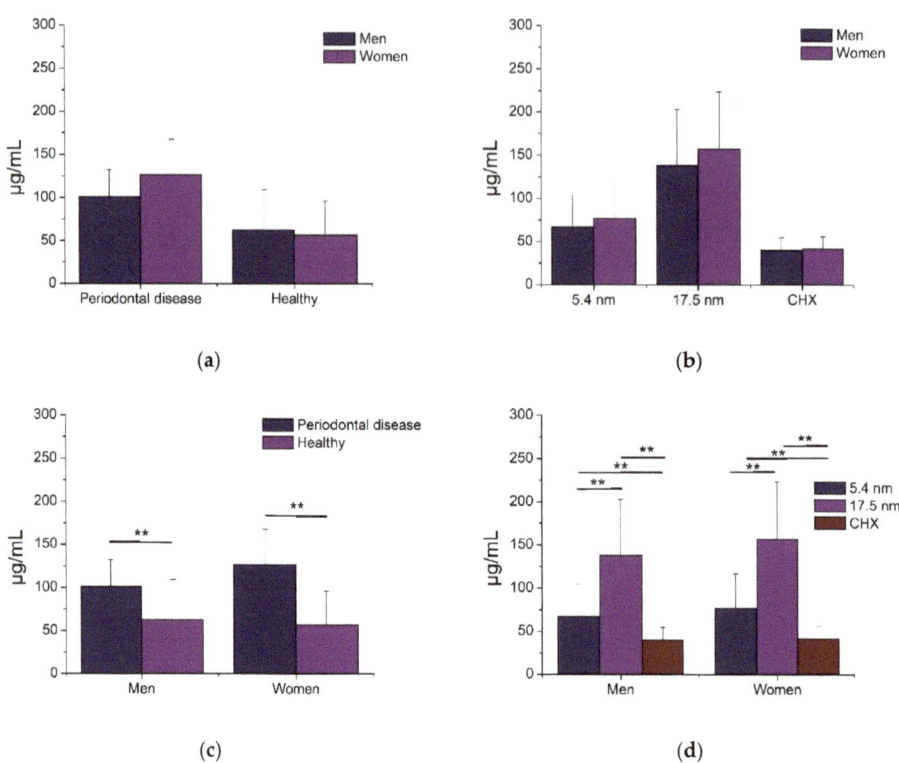

Figure 5. Antimicrobial activity of AgNP against biofilms associated with periodontal disease and gender. All values are expressed in mean and standard deviation. Asterisks indicate statistical differences ($p < 0.01$).

Table 3. Spearman's rho correlation of OD and MIC, according to age from periodontal disease and healthy patients.

Variable	Periodontal Disease (r)	p-Value	Healthy (r)	p-Value	Total (r)	p-Value
OD	0.179	0.345	0.087	0.647	0.501	0.000 **
AgNP 5.4 nm	0.021	0.914	−0.248	0.186	0.223	0.087
AgNP 17.5 nm	0.122	0.521	−0.042	0.825	0.223	0.074

** indicate significant correlations ($p < 0.01$).

3.5. Distribution of Periodontal Bacteria by PCR Assay

Periodontal bacteria profiles, identified by PCR, are shown in Table 4. As observed, the distribution of the population was represented by young adult patients with ages from 31 to 35 years old (32.5 ± 1.6 years old), in which females were more frequent (66.7%) compared to male subjects (33.3%). The identification of periodontal bacteria was represented mainly by *P. intermedia* (100%) and *F. nucleatum* (100%), followed by *P. gingivalis* (83.3%), *T. denticola* (83.3%), *T. forsythia* (66.7%) and, finally, *A. actinomycetemcomitans* (16.7%). Notably, the *P. gingivalis*, *T. denticola*, and *T. forsythia* strains were present in all oral biofilms from subjects with PD (100%). In contrast, the patients with no PD had less frequency of these bacteria in the biofilms (66.7, 66.7, and 33.3%, respectively). The *A. actinomycetemcomitans* was only present in one oral biofilm from subjects with PD (33.3%).

Table 4. Periodontal bacterial profiles detected by PCR.

Groups	No Periodontal Disease			Periodontal Disease		
Subjects	1	2	3	4	5	6
Age (years)	32	31	34	32	35	31
Gender	F	M	F	F	M	F
Bacterial strains						
P. gingivalis	+	−	+	+	+	+
T. forsythia	−	−	+	+	+	+
T. denticola	+	−	+	+	+	+
P. intermedia	+	+	+	+	+	+
F. nucleatum	+	+	+	+	+	+
A. actinomycetemcomitans	−	−	−	−	−	+

PCR: polymerase chain reaction. Gender is expressed in female (F) and male (M); + indicates the presence of bacteria; − indicates the absence of bacteria.

4. Discussion

This study identified that the AgNP significantly inhibits the bacterial growth of oral biofilms related to PD and healthy patients. The particle size and specific oral biofilms were associated with intervening in the antimicrobial activity of AgNP. Although gender tended to offer more bacterial resistance to both AgNP families and CHX solution, particularly for women, no significant associations were found. Additionally, significant correlations were located for the initial bacterial growth activity for PD and healthy oral biofilms, indicating that the growth of microorganisms involved for each biofilm was directly proportional to the age of the subjects. Although there was a tendency for PD biofilms to increase their antimicrobial resistance to both AgNP samples, no significant correlations were determined, suggesting that smaller and larger AgNP had statistically similar bacterial inhibition capacities for any age. To the best of our knowledge, this is the first study that evaluated the antimicrobial activity of two sizes of AgNP against representative oral biofilm samples taken from patients with and without active PD. Those results offer more precise and reliable information about the bactericidal effects of AgNP and oral biofilms obtained directly from patients, where complex microbiological interactions in different bacterial species with particular metabolic and microbiological characteristics were involved.

Various studies have reported synthesis methods for the preparation of AgNP using similar characteristics to this work, obtaining almost similar sizes and shapes of AgNP [31,41]. In this study, the synthesis of the AgNP included silver nitrate as a precursor and gallic acid as a reducing and stabilizing agent, which promoted the oxidation reaction of the phenol groups, facilitating the reduction of the silver ions [49]. The reaction was carried out at pH 10 for 17.5 nm and at pH 11 for 5.4 nm. At these pHs, the reaction is very fast and allows spherical morphology [31,50]. In the synthesis of the larger AgNPs, ammonium hydroxide caused faster reaction kinetics, having a promotion of hydrolysis, favoring the formation of particles of larger size [51] with more stable sizes [50,52]. As for 5.4 nm AgNP, the addition of sodium hydroxide promoted a sudden temperature gradient that resulted in rapid nucleation, thus inhibiting the growth of the particles [53,54] and limiting the particle agglomeration associated with the electrical charge [41,55]. Despite those reports, some variations might occur during the synthesis process. The results from this study showed that smaller and larger AgNP had narrow sizes with low standard deviations, which suggests adequate reproducibility of the synthesis technique for both particle sizes. Additionally, it is known that specific intervals of electrical charge particle surface of AgNP (from +31 to −30 mV) and high pH (>7) promote better conditions in colloid Ag dispersions to prevent particle agglomeration [30,56–58]. The zeta potential values support adequate electrical charges on the particle surface, facilitating the monodispersing and preventing particle agglomeration due to well-defined and distributed electrical surface energies on the Ag particles (-38.2 ± 5.8 mV for smaller and -32.6 ± 5.4 mV for larger particles). Results from the physical characterization of the particles indicate the improvement of the bactericidal activity of both AgNP samples, maintaining a colloid with more monodisperse particle dispersion, increasing the surface area and contact, limiting the agglomeration activity, resulting in more efficient bacterial inhibition behaviors against the oral biofilms [56,58].

The literature reports that the AgNP showed significantly higher bacteriostatic and bactericidal effects against five oral pathogenic microorganisms (*S. mutans, S. oralis, L. acidophilus, L. fermentum,* and *C. albicans*) compared to CHX, at less than five-fold concentration [34]. Additionally, another work reported that the AgNP had effective antibacterial activity against different microbial strains, including *P. gingivalis* and *Enterococcus faecalis*, which are bacterial species that have been strongly associated with PD and drug-resistant endodontic infectious, respectively [37]. Other works used various types of AgNP to evaluate the antimicrobial effect, using glutathione-stabilized AgNP [38] and AgNPs synthesized with *Ocimum Sanctum* leaf extract [59] against different oral pathogens associated with dental caries (*S. mutans*) and PD (*F. nucleatum*), particularly periodontitis (*P. gingivalis, P. intermedia,* and *A. actinomycetemcomitens*). It was determined that those AgNP exerted strong antibacterial functions in a concentration-dependent manner on the different microbial strains, suggesting the application of these nanomaterials for antibacterial treatments for the prevention of dental caries, periodontal conditions, or any other dental application related to oral biofilms [38,59]. A more recent study evaluated the antimicrobial and anti-inflammatory responses of polymeric PVA/chitosan thin films, containing AgNP and ibuprofen for the treatment of PD against Gram-positive (*Staphylococcus aureus*, ATCC 25, 923) and negative (*Pseudomonas aeruginosa* ATCC 27, 853; *Klebsiella pneumoniae* ATCC BAA-1705; and *P. gingivalis* ATCC 33, 377) bacteria. This resulted in biocomposite films with good bactericidal and biocompatible properties in representative oral pathogens, including microbial strains associated with PD (*P. gingivalis*) [39]. Our results agree with those previously reported, suggesting the great bactericidal effectiveness of AgNP against all bacterial biofilms from patients with periodontal and non-PD, determining better antimicrobial activities for smaller AgNP (Figure 3a,d) with significant microbial resistance to AgNP from microorganisms included in oral biofilms of patients with PD biofilms (Figure 3b,c). The evaluation of initial bacterial growth was made to determine the bacterial growth rate before the antimicrobial assay and defined differences in proliferation speed between different types of biofilms. This exploration determined differences among metabolic characteristics from various biofilms. We used multispecies cell suspensions initially from clinical oral biofilms, in which the presence of particular microbial species was confirmed by the PCR assay. Although the results from correlations indicated that the microorganisms included particularly in PD biofilms had more predispositions to accelerate the initial bacterial growth and, although no significant correlations were identified among AgNP samples, a strong tendency to resist the antimicrobial activity of the nanoparticles was determined (Table 3). The difference in the inhibitory effect between both sizes of AgNP was possibly due to their physical characteristics, which are observed in Table 1 and Figure 1. These findings suggest that the inhibitory effect of AgNP is inversely proportional to the size of the nanoparticle, with relevant participation of the PD biofilms to create more difficult conditions to facilitate the adequate bactericidal activities of AgNP.

Additionally, the female gender plays an important role in limiting the antimicrobial action of these nanostructured materials. In this sense, the small size of the AgNP can probably increase the ratio between the surface area and the volume in a very important way, which leads to significant modifications in their physical, chemical, and biological properties, including potentiated bacterial inhibitory effects [60,61]. The fact that the inhibitory effect with both sizes of AgNP was lower in dental plaque samples from patients with PD is possibly due to the bacterial species present in dental plaque. In the etiology of PD, there is not a single bacterial species involved. Rather, it is considered a polymicrobial infection, in which various microorganisms are involved, either in combination in the same period or in a sequential way [4,62,63]. Some investigations support the existence of the microbiota resistant to conventional antimicrobials in the dental plaque of patients with PD [64,65]. This capacity of the bacteria could explain the decrease in the inhibitory effect of AgNP mainly in biofilms associated with PD bacteria.

It is well known that in oral biofilms from patients without PD, a lower bacterial number exists than PD in subgingival biofilms, due to the control of bacterial growth and waste sub-products derived from metabolic activities in oral biofilms during regular oral hygiene habits [4,7,10]. Some authors have previously reported that in the oral dental plaque in patients with PD, the number of bacteria is greater [66]. This indicates that the first microbial colonizers adhere to the acquired film by specific molecules called adhesins, which are present on the bacterial surface [67]. Through the proliferation of attached species, the colonization and growth of other bacteria can also occur. In this microbiological succession, there is a transition from an aerobic environment, characterized by facultative microorganisms, to an anaerobic one, due to the consumption of oxygen by those first colonizers that favors the predominance of anaerobic microorganisms [66,67]. This information suggests that the antimicrobial resistance of oral biofilms from subjects with PD conditions are strongly associated with the specific distribution and type of microbial species in the oral biofilms, which is, at the same time, related to the oral hygiene habits of each patient and not only to the physical and chemical properties of AgNP.

On the other hand, immunological investigations have also reported that the innate immune response is more regulated in women than men, which limits the presence and progression of PD by the control of the growth of bacterial pathogens [68]. Additionally, the presence of estrogens (female hormone related to the reproductive system) increases gamma interferon (INF-γ) production, which represents an important role in the development of PD, principally periodontitis [69], suggesting an association with bone resorption. However, authors have also reported opposite approaches through in vitro and in vivo studies about sexual dimorphisms in oral bacterial infectious related to alveolar bone loss, resulting in increased inflammatory responses in males, which might create better biochemical conditions for the presence of more severe PD stages in comparison to females [70]. Although the relationship between gender and PD is not still clear, some studies have revealed interesting predispositions, according to gender, to increase the presence and severity of PD, including more antimicrobial resistance to certain microbial agents. Consequently, such specific hormonal factors, identified exclusively in women subjects, could alter the immune response in the PD, leading to the homeostasis loss from periodontal tissues and facilitating the development of gingivitis and periodontitis [71,72]. Results from this research regarding the characteristics of female patients show that there is a need for a greater concentration of AgNP and CHX treatments compared to males and, although no significant differences were found according to gender, an interesting tendency among females to be more resistant to all antimicrobial agents was identified. A possible explanation is that the concentrations of AgNP and CHX solutions needed to generate antimicrobial activity in women patients were greater than in men due to certain physiological and metabolic stages that can alter the hormonal conditions exclusively for women, such as puberty, menstrual cycle, pregnancy, menopause, postmenopause, and the use of contraceptive agents, promoting the modification of the immune response to periodontal disease, which leads to the homeostasis loss of periodontium tissue, facilitating the development of gingivitis and periodontitis [72–74].

The action mechanism of AgNP is still a controversial issue, but it is suggested that AgNP might gradually release silver ions that inhibit the production of adenosine triphosphate (ATP) and deoxyribonucleic acid (DNA) replication, which are fundamental elements for cell survival, but at the same time, promote the production of reactive oxygen species (ROS) and, subsequently, cell death [75–77]. This effect could be explained because silver ions have a strong affinity for the electron-donating groups present in various bacterial cells that contain sulfur, oxygen, or nitrogen [78], facilitating internalized particles into the bacterium due to their narrow size [79–81]. Then, AgNP releases silver ions and simultaneously joins to sulfhydryl groups of biomolecules and with phosphorosulfur compounds such as DNA, inactivating and altering the bacteria and cytoplasm leading to cell death [75–77]. In this sense, the action mechanism of AgNP might synergistically involve particular physical and chemical conditions such as silver release, chemical affinity with the cell wall, shape, size, electrical charge on the surface, concentration, distribution, and others [75,81,82]. Yet, specific microbiological and sociodemographic characteristics related to biofilms and patients such as type of oral infectious disease, particular microbial species, drug-resistance bacteria, type of cell wall, gender, oral hygiene habits, systemic disease, genetic, age, as well as immunological and metabolic conditions, among others, may be factors as well [41,73,83,84].

Additionally, the potential damage offered by nanomaterials, exclusively AgNP, to organs and systems of the body has been considered to promote the safe use of these metallic nanomaterials in biomedical uses. Studies have reported that AgNP can be distributed to specific organs according to a wide variety of routes, including inhalation, ingestion, skin contact, subcutaneous, or intravenous injection [85]. These routes will determine the specific organs where the AgNP will penetrate and accumulate. The absorbed AgNP are distributed in various organs and tissues such as the spleen, liver, stomach, lung, heart, brain, small intestine, and muscles, even in teeth and bones [86,87]; promoting cytotoxicity in dermal, ocular, respiratory, hepatobiliary, neural, or reproductive systems, limiting the application of these nanomaterials [86–88]. In addition, experiments have revealed that cytotoxicity is related to the chemical transformation of AgNP into silver ions (Ag+), facilitating the induction of cellular biochemical changes [89]. On the other hand, investigations have reported that AgNP could play an important anti-inflammatory role to reduce wound inflammation, modulation of fibrogenic and proinflammatory cytokines, and apoptosis in inflammatory cells [90]. Moreover, various studies have determined that in specific conditions, AgNP did not produce significant hepatotoxicity or immunotoxicity during in vivo studies with rats [87,91]. Additionally, an in vivo human oral time-exposure study reported that the commercial nanoscale silver particle solutions administrated to humans did not promote clinically important changes in the metabolic, hematologic, urine, or physical findings [92]. This means that it is very necessary to investigate the toxicity mechanisms of AgNP to elucidate the potential cytotoxicity, long-term adverse effects, routes of administration, doses, and other physical and biochemical properties to determine a well-defined and safe therapeutic with AgNP.

Although this study determined that AgNP exerts an inhibitory effect on oral biofilms in patients with PD, it is necessary to identify more realistic conditions from antimicrobial evaluations in future investigations, thus determining the antimicrobial particularities of AgNP among specific and well-controlled bacterial distributions from oral biofilms. This perspective will permit us to understand the relationship between the antimicrobial effects of AgNP related to particular microbiological conditions of biofilms, as well as to clinical and sociodemographic conditions from sampled patients such as oral or systemic disease, medical conditions, oral hygiene or eating habits, pharmacological treatment, race, genetics, gender, age, or any other particular conditions derived from patients. This will undoubtedly generate a better understanding, allowing for the recommendation of the safe use of AgNP as a potential antimicrobial alternative to control the presence and severity of PD in humans.

5. Conclusions

AgNP exerted a statistically significant growth inhibitory effect against clinically isolated oral biofilms from patients with and without PD. The primary antimicrobial associations of AgNP were determined according to particle size from AgNP and type of oral biofilm, determining a higher inhibitory effect for the smaller particles, while the most resistant antimicrobial activity was presented for microorganisms involved in PD biofilms. On the other hand, although no significant differences among the antimicrobial activity of AgNP were defined according to gender, an interesting tendency was shown for female subjects, having the predisposition to demonstrate a more resistant bactericidal activity to AgNP compared to males. Additionally, significant correlations were found among the initial bacterial growth, in particular, a trend for the PD group to increase the growth capacity, while the antimicrobial activity of both AgNP samples acted similarly in any age for any oral biofilm. Despite the fact that AgNP showed latent antimicrobial properties suggesting its potential for application as a complementary therapy for the prevention and control of PD, new investigations on AgNP using novel methodological approaches with more clinical and sociodemographic information from clinical oral biofilms, as well as other oral biofilms related to infectious diseases in the oral cavity, are strongly recommended.

Author Contributions: P.A.H.-V. and L.F.E.-C., conceptualization, methodological design, sample collection, interpretation of data, and writing of the protocol and manuscript. L.F.E.-C., R.E.M.-M., S.Y.R.-L., E.A.Z.-C. and A.D.-C. supervised the workflow and reviewed the paper. R.A.D.-P. and N.M.-F. participated in the concept design and reviewed the paper. J.C.C.-G. and A.D.-C. participated in the statistical analysis and reviewed the paper. All authors have read and agreed to the published version of the manuscript.

Funding: This research was funded by the National Council of Science and Technology (Fondo Mixto-CONACYT Gobierno del Estado de Chihuahua 2018-02), grant number CHIH-2018-02-01-1167 and the Stomatology Department at the Autonomous University of Ciudad Juarez (UACJ), grant number RIPI2019ICB5 and RIPI2022ICB10.

Data Availability Statement: All data obtained from this study can be found in the research archives of the Master's Program in Dental Sciences of the Autonomous University of Ciudad Juarez and can be requested through the corresponding author.

Conflicts of Interest: The authors declare no conflict of interest. The funders had no role in the design of the study; in the collection, analyses, or interpretation of data; in the writing of the manuscript, or in the decision to publish the results.

References

1. Chapple, I.L.C.; Mealey, B.L.; Van Dyke, T.E.; Bartold, P.M.; Dommisch, H.; Eickholz, P.; Geisinger, M.L.; Genco, R.J.; Glogauer, M.; Goldstein, M.; et al. Periodontal Health and Gingival Diseases and Conditions on an Intact and a Reduced Periodontium: Consensus Report of Workgroup 1 of the 2017 World Workshop on the Classification of Periodontal and Peri-Implant Diseases and Conditions. *J. Periodontol.* **2018**, *89* (Suppl. S1), S74–S84. [CrossRef]
2. Gasner, N.; Schure, R. Periodontal Disease—StatPearls—NCBI Bookshelf. Available online: https://www.ncbi.nlm.nih.gov/books/NBK554590/ (accessed on 19 May 2023).
3. Bárcena García, M.; Cobo Plana, J.M.; Arcos González, P.I. Prevalence and Severity of Periodontal Disease among Spanish Military Personnel. *BMJ Mil. Health* **2022**, *168*, 132–135. [CrossRef]
4. Curtis, M.A.; Diaz, P.I.; Van Dyke, T.E. The Role of the Microbiota in Periodontal Disease. *Periodontol. 2000* **2020**, *83*, 14–25. [CrossRef] [PubMed]
5. Mills, A.; Levin, L. Inequities in Periodontal Disease Prevalence, Prevention, and Management. *Quintessence Int.* **2022**, *53*, 122–132. [CrossRef] [PubMed]
6. Berglundh, T.; Armitage, G.; Araujo, M.G.; Avila-Ortiz, G.; Blanco, J.; Camargo, P.M.; Chen, S.; Cochran, D.; Derks, J.; Figuero, E.; et al. Peri-Implant Diseases and Conditions: Consensus Report of Workgroup 4 of the 2017 World Workshop on the Classification of Periodontal and Peri-Implant Diseases and Conditions. *J. Clin. Periodontol.* **2018**, *45* (Suppl. S2), S286–S291. [CrossRef]
7. Abusleme, L.; Dupuy, A.K.; Dutzan, N.; Silva, N.; Burleson, J.A.; Strausbaugh, L.D.; Gamonal, J.; Diaz, P.I. The Subgingival Microbiome in Health and Periodontitis and Its Relationship with Community Biomass and Inflammation. *ISME J.* **2013**, *7*, 1016–1025. [CrossRef]
8. Marsh, P.D. Microbial Ecology of Dental Plaque and Its Significance in Health and Disease. *Adv. Dent. Res.* **1994**, *8*, 263–271. [CrossRef] [PubMed]
9. Moore, W.E.C.; Moore, L.V.H. The Bacteria of Periodontal Diseases. *Periodontol. 2000* **1994**, *5*, 66–77. [CrossRef]
10. Hong, B.-Y.; Furtado Araujo, M.V.; Strausbaugh, L.D.; Terzi, E.; Ioannidou, E.; Diaz, P.I. Microbiome Profiles in Periodontitis in Relation to Host and Disease Characteristics. *PLoS ONE* **2015**, *10*, e0127077. [CrossRef]
11. Socransky, S.S.; Haffajee, A.D. Periodontal Microbial Ecology. *Periodontol. 2000* **2005**, *38*, 135–187. [CrossRef]
12. Chackartchi, T.; Hamzani, Y.; Shapira, L.; Polak, D. Effect of Subgingival Mechanical Debridement and Local Delivery of Chlorhexidine Gluconate Chip or Minocycline Hydrochloride Microspheres in Patients Enrolled in Supportive Periodontal Therapy: A Retrospective Analysis. *Oral Health Prev. Dent.* **2019**, *17*, 167–171. [CrossRef] [PubMed]
13. Poklepovic, T.; Worthington, H.V.; Johnson, T.M.; Sambunjak, D.; Imai, P.; Clarkson, J.E.; Tugwell, P. Interdental Brushing for the Prevention and Control of Periodontal Diseases and Dental Caries in Adults. *Cochrane Database Syst. Rev.* **2013**, *2013*, CD009857. [CrossRef] [PubMed]
14. Sälzer, S.; Graetz, C.; Dörfer, C.E.; Slot, D.E.; Van der Weijden, F.A. Contemporary Practices for Mechanical Oral Hygiene to Prevent Periodontal Disease. *Periodontol. 2000* **2020**, *84*, 35–44. [CrossRef]
15. Worthington, H.V.; MacDonald, L.; Poklepovic Pericic, T.; Sambunjak, D.; Johnson, T.M.; Imai, P.; Clarkson, J.E. Home Use of Interdental Cleaning Devices, in Addition to Toothbrushing, for Preventing and Controlling Periodontal Diseases and Dental Caries. *Cochrane Database Syst. Rev.* **2019**, *4*, CD012018. [CrossRef]

16. Chandra, S.S.; Miglani, R.; Srinivasan, M.R.; Indira, R. Antifungal Efficacy of 5.25% Sodium Hypochlorite, 2% Chlorhexidine Gluconate, and 17% EDTA With and Without an Antifungal Agent. *J. Endod.* **2010**, *36*, 675–678. [CrossRef] [PubMed]
17. Solderer, A.; Kaufmann, M.; Hofer, D.; Wiedemeier, D.; Attin, T.; Schmidlin, P.R. Efficacy of Chlorhexidine Rinses after Periodontal or Implant Surgery: A Systematic Review. *Clin. Oral Investig.* **2019**, *23*, 21–32. [CrossRef]
18. Haydari, M.; Bardakci, A.G.; Koldsland, O.C.; Aass, A.M.; Sandvik, L.; Preus, H.R. Comparing the Effect of 0.06% -, 0.12% and 0.2% Chlorhexidine on Plaque, Bleeding and Side Effects in an Experimental Gingivitis Model: A Parallel Group, Double Masked Randomized Clinical Trial. *BMC Oral Health* **2017**, *17*, 118. [CrossRef]
19. Brookes, Z.L.S.; Bescos, R.; Belfield, L.A.; Ali, K.; Roberts, A. Current Uses of Chlorhexidine for Management of Oral Disease: A Narrative Review. *J. Dent.* **2020**, *103*, 103497. [CrossRef]
20. Poppolo Deus, F.; Ouanounou, A. Chlorhexidine in Dentistry: Pharmacology, Uses, and Adverse Effects. *Int. Dent. J.* **2022**, *72*, 269–277. [CrossRef]
21. Feres, M.; Figueiredo, L.C.; Soares, G.M.S.; Faveri, M. Systemic Antibiotics in the Treatment of Periodontitis. *Periodontol. 2000* **2015**, *67*, 131–186. [CrossRef]
22. Walker, C.; Karpinia, K. Rationale for Use of Antibiotics in Periodontics. *J. Periodontol.* **2002**, *73*, 1188–1196. [CrossRef]
23. Blair, F.M.; Chapple, I.L.C. Prescribing for Periodontal Disease. *Prim. Dent. J.* **2014**, *3*, 38–43. [CrossRef]
24. Rams, T.E.; Degener, J.E.; van Winkelhoff, A.J. Antibiotic Resistance in Human Chronic Periodontitis Microbiota. *J. Periodontol.* **2014**, *85*, 160–169. [CrossRef] [PubMed]
25. Gowda, B.H.J.; Ahmed, M.G.; Chinnam, S.; Paul, K.; Ashrafuzzaman, M.; Chavali, M.; Gahtori, R.; Pandit, S.; Kesari, K.K.; Gupta, P.K. Current Trends in Bio-Waste Mediated Metal/Metal Oxide Nanoparticles for Drug Delivery. *J. Drug Deliv. Sci. Technol.* **2022**, *71*, 103305. [CrossRef]
26. Nizami, M.Z.I.; Xu, V.W.; Yin, I.X.; Yu, O.Y.; Chu, C.-H. Metal and Metal Oxide Nanoparticles in Caries Prevention: A Review. *Nanomaterials* **2021**, *11*, 3446. [CrossRef] [PubMed]
27. Ahmed, O.; Sibuyi, N.R.S.; Fadaka, A.O.; Madiehe, M.A.; Maboza, E.; Meyer, M.; Geerts, G. Plant Extract-Synthesized Silver Nanoparticles for Application in Dental Therapy. *Pharmaceutics* **2022**, *14*, 380. [CrossRef]
28. Wan, C.; Jiao, Y.; Sun, Q.; Li, J. Preparation, Characterization, and Antibacterial Properties of Silver Nanoparticles Embedded into Cellulose Aerogels. *Polym. Compos.* **2016**, *37*, 1137–1142. [CrossRef]
29. de Almeida, J.; Cechella, B.; Bernardi, A.; de Lima Pimenta, A.; Felippe, W. Effectiveness of Nanoparticles Solutions and Conventional Endodontic Irrigants against Enterococcus Faecalis Biofilm. *Indian J. Dent. Res.* **2018**, *29*, 347. [CrossRef]
30. Vanitha, G.; Rajavel, K.; Boopathy, G.; Veeravazhuthi, V.; Neelamegam, P. Physiochemical Charge Stabilization of Silver Nanoparticles and Its Antibacterial Applications. *Chem. Phys. Lett.* **2017**, *669*, 71–79. [CrossRef]
31. Hernández-Sierra, J.F.; Ruiz, F.; Cruz Pena, D.C.; Martínez-Gutiérrez, F.; Martínez, A.E.; de Jesús Pozos Guillén, A.; Tapia-Pérez, H.; Martínez Castañón, G. The Antimicrobial Sensitivity of Streptococcus Mutans to Nanoparticles of Silver, Zinc Oxide, and Gold. *Nanomed. Nanotechnol. Biol. Med.* **2008**, *4*, 237–240. [CrossRef]
32. Espinosa-Cristóbal, L.F.; Martínez-Castañón, G.A.; Martínez-Martínez, R.E.; Loyola-Rodríguez, J.P.; Patiño-Marín, N.; Reyes-Macías, J.F.; Ruiz, F. Antibacterial Effect of Silver Nanoparticles against Streptococcus Mutans. *Mater. Lett.* **2009**, *63*, 2603–2606. [CrossRef]
33. May, A.; Kopecki, Z.; Carney, B.; Cowin, A. Practical Extended Use of Antimicrobial Silver (PExUS). *ANZ J. Surg.* **2022**, *92*, 1199–1205. [CrossRef]
34. Panpaliya, N.P.; Dahake, P.T.; Kale, Y.J.; Dadpe, M.V.; Kendre, S.B.; Siddiqi, A.G.; Maggavi, U.R. In Vitro Evaluation of Antimicrobial Property of Silver Nanoparticles and Chlorhexidine against Five Different Oral Pathogenic Bacteria. *Saudi Dent. J.* **2019**, *31*, 76–83. [CrossRef]
35. Yin, I.X.; Yu, O.Y.; Zhao, I.S.; Mei, M.L.; Li, Q.-L.; Tang, J.; Chu, C.-H. Developing Biocompatible Silver Nanoparticles Using Epigallocatechin Gallate for Dental Use. *Arch. Oral Biol.* **2019**, *102*, 106–112. [CrossRef]
36. Lu, Z.; Rong, K.; Li, J.; Yang, H.; Chen, R. Size-Dependent Antibacterial Activities of Silver Nanoparticles against Oral Anaerobic Pathogenic Bacteria. *J. Mater. Sci. Mater. Med.* **2013**, *24*, 1465–1471. [CrossRef] [PubMed]
37. Halkai, K.; Halkai, R.; Mudda, J.; Shivanna, V.; Rathod, V. Antibiofilm Efficacy of Biosynthesized Silver Nanoparticles against Endodontic-Periodontal Pathogens: An in Vitro Study. *J. Conserv. Dent.* **2018**, *21*, 662. [CrossRef] [PubMed]
38. Zorraquín-Peña, I.; Cueva, C.; González de Llano, D.; Bartolomé, B.; Moreno-Arribas, M.V. Glutathione-Stabilized Silver Nanoparticles: Antibacterial Activity against Periodontal Bacteria, and Cytotoxicity and Inflammatory Response in Oral Cells. *Biomedicines* **2020**, *8*, 375. [CrossRef]
39. Constantin, M.; Lupei, M.; Bucatariu, S.-M.; Pelin, I.M.; Doroftei, F.; Ichim, D.L.; Daraba, O.M.; Fundueanu, G. PVA/Chitosan Thin Films Containing Silver Nanoparticles and Ibuprofen for the Treatment of Periodontal Disease. *Polymers* **2022**, *15*, 4. [CrossRef] [PubMed]
40. Espinosa-Cristóbal, L.F.; López-Ruiz, N.; Cabada-Tarín, D.; Reyes-López, S.Y.; Zaragoza-Contreras, A.; Constandse-Cortéz, D.; Donohué-Cornejo, A.; Tovar-Carrillo, K.; Cuevas-González, J.C.; Kobayashi, T. Antiadherence and Antimicrobial Properties of Silver Nanoparticles against Streptococcus Mutans on Brackets and Wires Used for Orthodontic Treatments. *J. Nanomater.* **2018**, *2018*, 9248527. [CrossRef]
41. Jiménez-Ramírez, A.J.; Martínez-Martínez, R.E.; Ayala-Herrera, J.L.; Zaragoza-Contreras, E.A.; Domínguez-Pérez, R.A.; Reyes-López, S.Y.; Donohue-Cornejo, A.; Cuevas-González, J.C.; Silva-Benítez, E.L.; Espinosa-Cristóbal, L.F. Antimicrobial Activity of Silver Nanoparticles against Clinical Biofilms from Patients with and without Dental Caries. *J. Nanomater.* **2021**, *2021*, 5587455. [CrossRef]

42. Martinez-Martinez, R.E.; Abud-Mendoza, C.; Patiño-Marin, N.; Rizo-Rodríguez, J.C.; Little, J.W.; Loyola-Rodríguez, J.P. Detection of Periodontal Bacterial DNA in Serum and Synovial Fluid in Refractory Rheumatoid Arthritis Patients. *J. Clin. Periodontol.* **2009**, *36*, 1004–1010. [CrossRef] [PubMed]
43. Martínez-Martínez, R.E.; Moreno-Castillo, D.F.; Loyola-Rodríguez, J.P.; Sánchez-Medrano, A.G.; Miguel-Hernández, J.H.S.; Olvera-Delgado, J.H.; Domínguez-Pérez, R.A. Association between Periodontitis, Periodontopathogens and Preterm Birth: Is It Real? *Arch. Gynecol. Obstet.* **2016**, *294*, 47–54. [CrossRef]
44. Tran, S.D.; Rudney, J.D. Multiplex PCR Using Conserved and Species-Specific 16S RRNA Gene Primers for Simultaneous Detection of Actinobacillus Actinomycetemcomitans and Porphyromonas Gingivalis. *J. Clin. Microbiol.* **1996**, *34*, 2674–2678. [CrossRef]
45. Stubbs, S.; Park, S.F.; Bishop, P.A.; Lewis, M.A.O. Direct Detection of Prevotella Intermedia and P. Nigrescens in Suppurative Oral Infection by Amplification of 16S RRNA Gene. *J. Med. Microbiol.* **1999**, *48*, 1017–1022. [CrossRef]
46. Watanabe, K.; Frommel, T.O. Porphyromonas Gingivalis, Actinobacillus Actinomycetemcomitans and Treponema Denticola Detection in Oral Plaque Samples Using the Polymerase Chain Reaction. *J. Clin. Periodontol.* **1996**, *23*, 212–219. [CrossRef] [PubMed]
47. Ashimoto, A.; Chen, C.; Bakker, I.; Slots, J. Polymerase Chain Reaction Detection of 8 Putative Periodontal Pathogens in Subgingival Plaque of Gingivitis and Advanced Periodontitis Lesions. *Oral Microbiol. Immunol.* **1996**, *11*, 266–273. [CrossRef]
48. Poulsen, K.; Ennibi, O.-K.; Haubek, D. Improved PCR for Detection of the Highly Leukotoxic JP2 Clone of Actinobacillus Actinomycetemcomitans in Subgingival Plaque Samples. *J. Clin. Microbiol.* **2003**, *41*, 4829–4832. [CrossRef]
49. Wang, W.; Chen, Q.; Jiang, C.; Yang, D.; Liu, X.; Xu, S. One-Step Synthesis of Biocompatible Gold Nanoparticles Using Gallic Acid in the Presence of Poly-(N-Vinyl-2-Pyrrolidone). *Colloids Surf. A Physicochem. Eng. Asp.* **2007**, *301*, 73–79. [CrossRef]
50. Martínez-Castañón, G.A.; Niño-Martínez, N.; Martínez-Gutierrez, F.; Martínez-Mendoza, J.R.; Ruiz, F. Synthesis and Antibacterial Activity of Silver Nanoparticles with Different Sizes. *J. Nanopart. Res.* **2008**, *10*, 1343–1348. [CrossRef]
51. Huong, P.T.L.; Van Son, T.; Phan, V.N.; Tam, L.T.; Le, A.-T. Microstructure and Chemo-Physical Characterizations of Functional Graphene Oxide-Iron Oxide-Silver Ternary Nanocomposite Synthesized by One-Pot Hydrothermal Method. *J. Nanosci. Nanotechnol.* **2018**, *18*, 5591–5599. [CrossRef]
52. Rodríguez-González, B.; Sánchez-Iglesias, A.; Giersig, M.; Liz-Marzán, L.M. AuAg Bimetallic Nanoparticles: Formation, Silica-Coating and Selective Etching. *Faraday Discuss.* **2004**, *125*, 133–144. [CrossRef]
53. Lee, H.K.; Talib, Z.A.; Mamat @ Mat Nazira, M.S.; Wang, E.; Lim, H.N.; Mahdi, M.A.; Ng, E.K.; Yusoff, N.M.; AL-Jumaili, B.E.; Liew, J.Y.C. Effect of Sodium Hydroxide Concentration in Synthesizing Zinc Selenide/Graphene Oxide Composite via Microwave-Assisted Hydrothermal Method. *Materials* **2019**, *12*, 2295. [CrossRef] [PubMed]
54. Abdel-Halim, E.S.; Al-Deyab, S.S. Antimicrobial Activity of Silver/Starch/Polyacrylamide Nanocomposite. *Int. J. Biol. Macromol.* **2014**, *68*, 33–38. [CrossRef] [PubMed]
55. Espinosa-Cristóbal, L.F.; Martínez-Castañón, G.A.; Loyola-Rodríguez, J.P.; Niño-Martínez, N.; Ruiz, F.; Zavala-Alonso, N.V.; Lara, R.H.; Reyes-López, S.Y. Bovine Serum Albumin and Chitosan Coated Silver Nanoparticles and Its Antimicrobial Activity against Oral and Nonoral Bacteria. *J. Nanomater.* **2015**, *2015*, 420853. [CrossRef]
56. Tuan, T.Q.; Van Son, N.; Dung, H.T.K.; Luong, N.H.; Thuy, B.T.; Van Anh, N.T.; Hoa, N.D.; Hai, N.H. Preparation and Properties of Silver Nanoparticles Loaded in Activated Carbon for Biological and Environmental Applications. *J. Hazard. Mater.* **2011**, *192*, 1321–1329. [CrossRef] [PubMed]
57. Kaler, A.; Jain, S.; Banerjee, U.C. Green and Rapid Synthesis of Anticancerous Silver Nanoparticles by Saccharomyces Boulardii and Insight into Mechanism of Nanoparticle Synthesis. *BioMed Res. Int.* **2013**, *2013*, 872940. [CrossRef]
58. Prema, P.; Veeramanikandan, V.; Rameshkumar, K.; Gatasheh, M.K.; Hatamleh, A.A.; Balasubramani, R.; Balaji, P. Statistical Optimization of Silver Nanoparticle Synthesis by Green Tea Extract and Its Efficacy on Colorimetric Detection of Mercury from Industrial Waste Water. *Environ. Res.* **2022**, *204*, 111915. [CrossRef]
59. Sirisha, P.; Gayathri, G.; Dhoom, S.; Amulya, K. Antimicrobial Effect of Silver Nanoparticles Synthesised with Ocimum Sanctum Leaf Extract on Periodontal Pathogens. *J. Oral Health Dent. Sci.* **2017**, *1*, 106.
60. Feng, Q.L.; Wu, J.; Chen, G.Q.; Cui, F.Z.; Kim, T.N.; Kim, J.O. A Mechanistic Study of the Antibacterial Effect of Silver Ions OnEscherichia Coli AndStaphylococcus Aureus. *J. Biomed. Mater. Res.* **2000**, *52*, 662–668. [CrossRef]
61. Qing, Y.; Cheng, L.; Li, R.; Liu, G.; Zhang, Y.; Tang, X.; Wang, J.; Liu, H.; Qin, Y. Potential Antibacterial Mechanism of Silver Nanoparticles and the Optimization of Orthopedic Implants by Advanced Modification Technologies. *Int. J. Nanomed.* **2018**, *13*, 3311–3327. [CrossRef]
62. Dewhirst, F.E.; Chen, T.; Izard, J.; Paster, B.J.; Tanner, A.C.R.; Yu, W.-H.; Lakshmanan, A.; Wade, W.G. The Human Oral Microbiome. *J. Bacteriol.* **2010**, *192*, 5002–5017. [CrossRef]
63. Arweiler, N.B.; Netuschil, L. The Oral Microbiota. *Adv. Exp. Med. Biol.* **2016**, *902*, 45–60. [CrossRef]
64. Soares, G.M.S.; Figueiredo, L.C.; Faveri, M.; Cortelli, S.C.; Duarte, P.M.; Feres, M. Mechanisms of Action of Systemic Antibiotics Used in Periodontal Treatment and Mechanisms of Bacterial Resistance to These Drugs. *J. Appl. Oral Sci.* **2012**, *20*, 295–309. [CrossRef]
65. Rams, T.E.; Feik, D.; Mortensen, J.E.; Degener, J.E.; van Winkelhoff, A.J. Antibiotic Susceptibility of Periodontal Enterococcus Faecalis. *J. Periodontol.* **2013**, *84*, 1026–1033. [CrossRef] [PubMed]
66. Zijnge, V.; van Leeuwen, M.B.M.; Degener, J.E.; Abbas, F.; Thurnheer, T.; Gmür, R.; Harmsen, H.J.M. Oral Biofilm Architecture on Natural Teeth. *PLoS ONE* **2010**, *5*, e9321. [CrossRef]
67. Zarco, M.F.; Vess, T.J.; Ginsburg, G.S. The Oral Microbiome in Health and Disease and the Potential Impact on Personalized Dental Medicine. *Oral Dis.* **2012**, *18*, 109–120. [CrossRef] [PubMed]

68. Ghazeeri, G.; Abdullah, L.; Abbas, O. Immunological Differences in Women Compared with Men: Overview and Contributing Factors. *Am. J. Reprod. Immunol.* **2011**, *66*, 163–169. [CrossRef]
69. Nakaya, M.; Tachibana, H.; Yamada, K. Effect of Estrogens on the Interferon-Gamma Producing Cell Population of Mouse Splenocytes. *Biosci. Biotechnol. Biochem.* **2006**, *70*, 47–53. [CrossRef]
70. Valerio, M.S.; Basilakos, D.S.; Kirkpatrick, J.E.; Chavez, M.; Hathaway-Schrader, J.; Herbert, B.A.; Kirkwood, K.L. Sex-Based Differential Regulation of Bacterial-Induced Bone Resorption. *J. Periodontal Res.* **2017**, *52*, 377–387. [CrossRef]
71. Bhardwaj, A.; Bhardwaj, S. Effect of Menopause on Women's Periodontium. *J. Midlife Health* **2012**, *3*, 5. [CrossRef] [PubMed]
72. Machtei, E.E.; Mahler, D.; Sanduri, H.; Peled, M. The Effect of Menstrual Cycle on Periodontal Health. *J. Periodontol.* **2004**, *75*, 408–412. [CrossRef] [PubMed]
73. Lipsky, M.S.; Su, S.; Crespo, C.J.; Hung, M. Men and Oral Health: A Review of Sex and Gender Differences. *Am. J. Mens. Health* **2021**, *15*, 155798832110163. [CrossRef] [PubMed]
74. Krejci, C.B.; Bissada, N.F. Women's Health Issues and Their Relationship to Periodontitis. *J. Am. Dent. Assoc.* **2002**, *133*, 323–329. [CrossRef] [PubMed]
75. Yin, I.X.; Zhang, J.; Zhao, I.S.; Mei, M.L.; Li, Q.; Chu, C.H. The Antibacterial Mechanism of Silver Nanoparticles and Its Application in Dentistry. *Int. J. Nanomed.* **2020**, *15*, 2555–2562. [CrossRef]
76. Lee, W.; Kim, K.-J.; Lee, D.G. A Novel Mechanism for the Antibacterial Effect of Silver Nanoparticles on Escherichia Coli. *BioMetals* **2014**, *27*, 1191–1201. [CrossRef]
77. Qin, G.; Tang, S.; Li, S.; Lu, H.; Wang, Y.; Zhao, P.; Li, B.; Zhang, J.; Peng, L. Toxicological Evaluation of Silver Nanoparticles and Silver Nitrate in Rats Following 28 Days of Repeated Oral Exposure. *Environ. Toxicol.* **2017**, *32*, 609–618. [CrossRef]
78. Venugopal, A.; Muthuchamy, N.; Tejani, H.; Gopalan, A.-I.; Lee, K.-P.; Lee, H.-J.; Kyung, H.M. Incorporation of Silver Nanoparticles on the Surface of Orthodontic Microimplants to Achieve Antimicrobial Properties. *Korean J. Orthod.* **2017**, *47*, 3. [CrossRef]
79. Sweet, M.J.; Chessher, A.; Singleton, I. Review: Metal-Based Nanoparticles; Size, Function, and Areas for Advancement in Applied Microbiology. In *Advances in Applied Microbiology*; Academic Press: Cambridge, MA, USA, 2012; pp. 113–142. ISBN 9780123943811.
80. Durán, N.; Marcato, P.D.; Durán, M.; Yadav, A.; Gade, A.; Rai, M. Mechanistic Aspects in the Biogenic Synthesis of Extracellular Metal Nanoparticles by Peptides, Bacteria, Fungi, and Plants. *Appl. Microbiol. Biotechnol.* **2011**, *90*, 1609–1624. [CrossRef]
81. Prabhu, S.; Poulose, E.K. Silver Nanoparticles: Mechanism of Antimicrobial Action, Synthesis, Medical Applications, and Toxicity Effects. *Int. Nano Lett.* **2012**, *2*, 32. [CrossRef]
82. Kailasa, S.K.; Park, T.-J.; Rohit, J.V.; Koduru, J.R. Antimicrobial Activity of Silver Nanoparticles. In *Nanoparticles in Pharmacotherapy*; Elsevier: Amsterdam, The Netherlands, 2019; ISBN 9780128165041.
83. Loyola-Rodriguez, J.P.; Ponce-Diaz, M.E.; Loyola-Leyva, A.; Garcia-Cortes, J.O.; Medina-Solis, C.E.; Contreras-Ramire, A.A.; Serena-Gomez, E. Determination and Identification of Antibiotic-Resistant Oral Streptococci Isolated from Active Dental Infections in Adults. *Acta Odontol. Scand.* **2018**, *76*, 229–235. [CrossRef]
84. Espinosa-Cristóbal, L.F.; Holguín-Meráz, C.; Zaragoza-Contreras, E.A.; Martínez-Martínez, R.E.; Donohue-Cornejo, A.; Loyola-Rodríguez, J.P.; Cuevas-González, J.C.; Reyes-López, S.Y. Antimicrobial and Substantivity Properties of Silver Nanoparticles against Oral Microbiomes Clinically Isolated from Young and Young-Adult Patients. *J. Nanomater.* **2019**, *2019*, 3205971. [CrossRef]
85. Xu, L.; Wang, Y.-Y.; Huang, J.; Chen, C.-Y.; Wang, Z.-X.; Xie, H. Silver Nanoparticles: Synthesis, Medical Applications and Biosafety. *Theranostics* **2020**, *10*, 8996–9031. [CrossRef]
86. Dos Santos, C.A.; Seckler, M.M.; Ingle, A.P.; Gupta, I.; Galdiero, S.; Galdiero, M.; Gade, A.; Rai, M. Silver Nanoparticles: Therapeutical Uses, Toxicity, and Safety Issues. *J. Pharm. Sci.* **2014**, *103*, 1931–1944. [CrossRef]
87. Espinosa-Cristobal, L.F.; Martinez-Castañon, G.A.; Loyola-Rodriguez, J.P.; Patiño-Marin, N.; Reyes-Macías, J.F.; Vargas-Morales, J.M.; Ruiz, F. Toxicity, Distribution, and Accumulation of Silver Nanoparticles in Wistar Rats. *J. Nanopart. Res.* **2013**, *15*, 1702. [CrossRef]
88. Ferdous, Z.; Nemmar, A. Health Impact of Silver Nanoparticles: A Review of the Biodistribution and Toxicity Following Various Routes of Exposure. *Int. J. Mol. Sci.* **2020**, *21*, 2375. [CrossRef] [PubMed]
89. Wang, L.; Zhang, T.; Li, P.; Huang, W.; Tang, J.; Wang, P.; Liu, J.; Yuan, Q.; Bai, R.; Li, B.; et al. Use of Synchrotron Radiation-Analytical Techniques To Reveal Chemical Origin of Silver-Nanoparticle Cytotoxicity. *ACS Nano* **2015**, *9*, 6532–6547. [CrossRef] [PubMed]
90. Hebeish, A.; El-Rafie, M.H.; EL-Sheikh, M.A.; Seleem, A.A.; El-Naggar, M.E. Antimicrobial Wound Dressing and Anti-Inflammatory Efficacy of Silver Nanoparticles. *Int. J. Biol. Macromol.* **2014**, *65*, 509–515. [CrossRef] [PubMed]
91. van der Zande, M.; Vandebriel, R.J.; Van Doren, E.; Kramer, E.; Herrera Rivera, Z.; Serrano-Rojero, C.S.; Gremmer, E.R.; Mast, J.; Peters, R.J.B.; Hollman, P.C.H.; et al. Distribution, Elimination, and Toxicity of Silver Nanoparticles and Silver Ions in Rats after 28-Day Oral Exposure. *ACS Nano* **2012**, *6*, 7427–7442. [CrossRef] [PubMed]
92. Munger, M.A.; Radwanski, P.; Hadlock, G.C.; Stoddard, G.; Shaaban, A.; Falconer, J.; Grainger, D.W.; Deering-Rice, C.E. In Vivo Human Time-Exposure Study of Orally Dosed Commercial Silver Nanoparticles. *Nanomedicine* **2014**, *10*, 1–9. [CrossRef]

Disclaimer/Publisher's Note: The statements, opinions and data contained in all publications are solely those of the individual author(s) and contributor(s) and not of MDPI and/or the editor(s). MDPI and/or the editor(s) disclaim responsibility for any injury to people or property resulting from any ideas, methods, instructions or products referred to in the content.

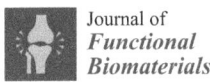

Article

Effects of Polishing and Artificial Aging on Mechanical Properties of Dental LT Clear® Resin

Anna Paradowska-Stolarz [1,*], Joanna Wezgowiec [2], Andrzej Malysa [2] and Mieszko Wieckiewicz [2,*]

[1] Division of Dentofacial Anomalies, Department of Maxillofacial Orthopedics and Orthodontics, Wroclaw Medical University, 50-425 Wroclaw, Poland
[2] Department of Experimental Dentistry, Wroclaw Medical University, 50-425 Wroclaw, Poland; joanna.wezgowiec@umw.edu.pl (J.W.); andrzej.malysa@umw.edu.pl (A.M.)
* Correspondence: anna.paradowska-stolarz@umw.edu.pl (A.P.-S.); m.wieckiewicz@onet.pl (M.W.)

Abstract: Three-dimensional printing has become incorporated into various aspects of everyday life, including dentistry. Novel materials are being introduced rapidly. One such material is Dental LT Clear by Formlabs, a resin used for manufacturing occlusal splints, aligners, and orthodontic retainers. In this study, a total of 240 specimens, comprising two shapes (dumbbell and rectangular), were evaluated through compression and tensile tests. The compression tests revealed that the specimens were neither polished nor aged. However, after polishing, the compression modulus values decreased significantly. Specifically, the unpolished and nonaged specimens measured 0.87 ± 0.02, whereas the polished group measured 0.086 ± 0.03. The results were significantly affected by artificial aging. The polished group measured 0.73 ± 0.05, while the unpolished group measured 0.73 ± 0.03. In contrast, the tensile test proved that the specimens showed the highest resistance when the polishing was applied. The artificial aging influenced the tensile test and reduced the force needed to damage the specimens. The tensile modulus had the highest value when polishing was applied (3.00 ± 0.11). The conclusions drawn from these findings are as follows: 1. Polishing does not change the properties of the examined resin. 2. Artificial aging reduces resistance in both compression and tensile tests. 3. Polishing reduces the damage to the specimens in the aging process.

Keywords: 3D print; resin; dental LT clear; polishing; artificial aging; compression; tensile modulus

Citation: Paradowska-Stolarz, A.; Wezgowiec, J.; Malysa, A.; Wieckiewicz, M. Effects of Polishing and Artificial Aging on Mechanical Properties of Dental LT Clear® Resin. *J. Funct. Biomater.* **2023**, *14*, 295. https://doi.org/10.3390/jfb14060295

Academic Editors: Lavinia Cosmina Ardelean and Laura-Cristina Rusu

Received: 1 May 2023
Revised: 22 May 2023
Accepted: 23 May 2023
Published: 25 May 2023

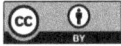

Copyright: © 2023 by the authors. Licensee MDPI, Basel, Switzerland. This article is an open access article distributed under the terms and conditions of the Creative Commons Attribution (CC BY) license (https://creativecommons.org/licenses/by/4.0/).

1. Introduction

Three-dimensional (3D) printing is becoming one of the most popular methods for fabricating customized dental elements in contemporary dentistry. It is widely employed for various applications, including dental restorations, personalized orthodontic and prosthetic appliances, as well as precise components such as surgical guides [1,2]. The ability to create precise and individualized elements has propelled 3D printing materials to the forefront of modern dentistry, enabling in-house treatment planning [3].

Clear aligners have emerged as a popular trend in modern orthodontics, affecting various branches of dentistry. While thermoformed plates have traditionally been used for their fabrication, there is a growing preference for 3D printed materials due to their enhanced accuracy and precision. The integration of digital technologies has prompted dentists and dental companies to explore novel materials, among which Dental LT Clear resin (Formlabs) stands out. This material is classified as a IIa biocompatible resin, making it suitable for long-term use on the skin and mucosal surfaces. In addition to its high translucency, Dental LT Clear resin exhibits nonlinear compression resistance of up to 600 N, comparable to the biting force. This value is comparable to other popular materials commonly used for fabricating clear aligners, such as Duran and Durasoft [4].

Biocompatibility is a critical feature of dental materials, particularly when they come into contact with tissues for extended periods. Technical tests are employed to assess the biocompatibility of materials and ensure their safety for human use [5]. According to the manufacturer [6], Dental LT Clear resin is a new-generation, biocompatible material specifically designed for long-term applications. It is composed of several chemical components, including 7,7,9-(or 7,9,9)-trimethyl-4,13-dioxo-3,14-dioxa-5,12-diazahexadecane-1,16-diyl bismethacrylate, 2-hydroxyethyl methacrylate, a reaction mass of Bis(1,2,2,6,6-pentamethyl-4-piperidyl) sebacate and methyl 1,2,2,6,6-pentamethyl-4-piperidyl sebacate, diphenyl(2,4,6-trimethylbenzoyl)phosphine oxide, acrylic acid, monoester with propane-1,2-diol, ethylene dimethacrylate, 2-hydroxyethyl acrylate, mequinol, 4-methoxyphenol, and hydroquinone monomethyl ether. The material possesses translucency, rigidity, and strength, making it an ideal choice for esthetically pleasing individual appliances, including dental aligners. Additionally, the resin is used for fabricating occlusal guards, splints, and orthodontic retainers. It is important to note that food and beverages can affect the properties of intraoral appliances, diminishing their esthetics and compromising their structural integrity [7,8]. The properties of materials are also influenced by intraoral conditions. Originally, CAD/CAM materials were used for dental restorations (temporary and permanent ones) and the purpose of the use is longitudinal—which means that the pieces of material stay in contact with the oral cavity for a long time. Consequently, the properties of the materials are examined in terms of color stability and durability [8,9]. Recently, more materials have been introduced, and therefore doctors and laboratories are able to prepare more customized pieces, such as individual face masks or individual appliances for cleft patients [10–12].

Dental LT Clear is a relatively new material that has not yet been fully investigated [3,13]. Therefore, the study we have designed is among the first of its kind in our opinion. Apart from its intended use in intraoral splints, Dental LT Clear may also have potential applications in the fabrication of precise individual and orthopedic appliance components, such as nasal–alveolar molding plates for patients with clefts [13]. A similar rigid material, BioMed Amber, produced by the same manufacturer (Formlabs), has shown greater resistance to compression but lower resistance to tensile forces. This makes BioMed Amber more suitable for the fabrication of mouth guards and occlusal splints. However, it should be noted that BioMed Amber is not designed for long-term use and should only remain in contact with the human body for a short period [6].

In another study [14], a comparison of three dental 3D printed materials revealed that Dental LT Clear exhibited the greatest stability following compression and tensile tests. Fractal dimension and texture analyses showed minimal changes in the material's properties. However, bone index analysis of BioMed Amber indicated a decline in material quality because of the performed tests. It should be noted that according to the information provided by the manufacturer [6], Dental LT Clear material is not recommended for sterilization. Nonetheless, a recent study [15] revealed the benefits of sterilization in terms of reducing monomer elution, and autoclaving at 132 °C for 4 min improved the microhardness of the resin. Therefore, sterilization should be considered during the prefabrication of occlusal splints.

The aim of this study was to examine the mechanical resistance properties of a selected 3D printable resin, specifically Dental LT Clear from Formlabs, with regard to the effects of specimen polishing and aging. To evaluate the material, we formulated the following hypotheses:

- There is no influence of polishing on the material's durability.
- There is no influence of artificial aging on the material's durability.
- There is no relation between application of polishing and artificial aging regarding the material's durability.
- Polishing does not change the properties of the material in terms of artificial aging.

2. Materials and Methods

2.1. Materials

In this study, we examined the properties of Dental LT Clear, a 3D printable biocompatible resin provided by Formlabs, located in Milbury, OH, USA. The specimens were prepared using the Form 2 printer from Formlabs, specifically designed for this resin. The printer is a self-adjusting device, which automatically sets the print settings once the cartridge is inserted. The printing process was carried out using violet light (405 nm) with a power output of 250 mW. The print layer thickness was set to 100 microns, and the temperature was maintained at 35 °C. The manufacturer's recommendations regarding potential applications and properties of Dental LT Clear are summarized in Table 1.

Table 1. A brief description of Dental LT Clear applications recommended by the producer.

Resin	Application
Dental LT Clear Resin	Characteristics: • Long-term use • Biocompatible • Suitable for mucosal and skin contact • Highly esthetic • Transparent, translucent • Strong, rigid Use: • Hard splints • Occlusal guards • Retainers • Aligners • Other direct-printed long-term orthodon-tic appliances

2.2. Specimens' Preparation and Artificial Aging

For this research, two types of specimens were prepared. The rectangular specimens were designed for the compression test following the ISO 604:2003 standard [16]. The dumbbell-shaped specimens (type 1BA) were prepared for the tensile test according to the ISO 527-1:2019(E) standard [17]. While the standards required a minimum of five samples, the authors decided to expand the test to 30 specimens for each test. In total, 240 specimens of Dental LT Clear resin were printed using the Form 2 printer by Formlabs, following the ISO standards and the manufacturer's instructions. Of these, 120 were rectangular-shaped and 120 were dumbbell-shaped.

After printing, the specimens were rinsed twice for 10 min each in 99% isopropanol alcohol (Stanlab, Lublin, Poland). Following a 30 min drying period at room temperature, the specimens were postcured using Form Cure from Formlabs at 80 °C for 20 min, as recommended by the manufacturer for Dental LT Clear resin. Once the specimens were prepared, the supports were removed. All specimens were then ground using sandpaper, but only half of them (60 rectangular and 60 dumbbell-shaped) underwent further polishing on one side using 0.2 pumice (Everall 7, Warsaw, Poland) and polishing paste (Everall 7) with the Reiter Poliret Mini Feinwerktechnik (GmbH, Bad Essen, Germany). The polishing process involved a rotational range of 1000–4500 rotations per minute and an average speed of 2250 rpm.

Following preparation, the specimens were stored at room temperature and 50% humidity for 24 h (for the tensile test) or 4 days (for the compression test). Half of the specimens were tested immediately after the storage period, while the other half (60 of each shape) underwent artificial aging for 90 days in distilled water at 37 °C. The water was changed weekly, based on the scheme used in a previous study on conventional dental restorative materials [18]. The decision to change the water every 7 days was made to prevent any potential alteration of properties while ensuring that the water did not evaporate.

2.3. Compression Test

According to the ISO 604:2003 [15] standard, specimens measuring (10.0 ± 0.2) mm × (10.0 ± 0.2) mm × (4 ± 0.2) mm were selected for testing. Prior to the test, the specimens were conditioned for 4 days at 23 °C/50% relative humidity (RH) in ambient air. The height and width of the specimens were then measured at five points using a Magnusson digital caliper (150 mm) (Limit, Wroclaw, Poland). The mean values of these measurements were calculated.

Axial compression tests were conducted using the Z10-X700 universal testing machine from AML Instruments in Lincoln, UK. The tests were performed at a constant speed of 1 mm/min (Figure 1). By recording the uniaxial stress–strain curve, the compressive modulus (E [MPa]) of each specimen was determined using the slope of the curve. The changes in width and height during the compression test were compared to the measurements taken before and after compression, as shown in Table 2.

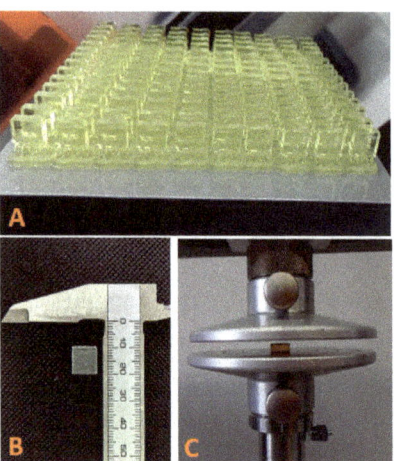

Figure 1. Compression test: (**A**) set of specimens after printing; (**B**) a finished specimen before compression; (**C**) resin specimen between the compression plates.

Table 2. The formulas for calculation of the compression and tensile modulus.

	Formula	Explanations
Compressive modulus	Compressive stress $\sigma = \frac{F}{A}$ [MPa] Nominal strain $\varepsilon = \frac{\Delta L}{L}$	F—force [N] A—initial cross sectional area measurement [mm^2] L—the initial distance between the compression plates [mm] ΔL—the decrease in the distance between the plates after the test [mm]
Tensile modulus	Tensile stress $\sigma = \frac{F}{A}$ [MPa] Nominal strain $\varepsilon = \frac{\Delta L}{L}$ $E_t = \frac{\sigma_2 - \sigma_1}{\varepsilon_2 - \varepsilon_1}$ [MPa]	F—force [N] A—initial cross sectional area measurement [mm^2] L—the initial distance between the grips [mm] ΔL—the increase in the distance between the grips after the test [mm] σ_1—the stress in MPa measured at a strain of 0.0005 (ε_1) σ_2—the stress in MPa measured at a strain of 0.0025 (ε_2)

2.4. Tensile Test

The dumbbell-shaped specimens (type 1BA) were 3D printed with a length of 75 mm and an end width of 10 mm, while the thickness was 2 mm. These measurements adhered to the ISO 527-2:2019 standard [17]. Prior to the tensile test, the specimens were conditioned at room temperature (23 °C) and 50% RH for 24 h. Using a Magnusson digital caliper

(150 mm) (Limit, Wroclaw, Poland), the width and height of the specimens were measured at the test length, with measurements taken at five points. The mean values of these measurements were then calculated.

To perform the tensile test, a universal testing machine (Z10-X700, AML Instruments, Lincoln, UK) was utilized. The test was conducted at a constant speed of 5 mm/min, as shown in Figure 2. If any of the specimens broke outside of the test length, they were discarded. Based on the measurements obtained during the test, the stress and strain of the specimens were determined. The formulas for these calculations are presented in Table 2.

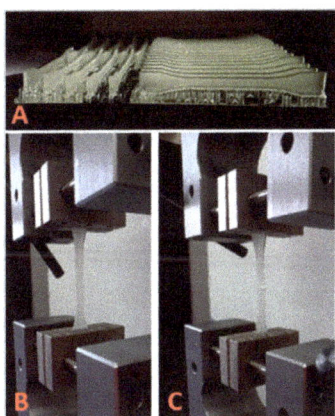

Figure 2. Tensile test: (**A**) set of specimens after printing; (**B**) a finished specimen mounted between grips before tensile force application; (**C**) a specimen broken by tensile force.

2.5. Statistical Analysis

The statistical analysis was conducted using Statistica c. 13 software (TIBCO Software Inc., Palo Alto, CA, USA).

The analysis involved calculating the mean values, along with their corresponding standard deviations, for both the compression and tensile modulus of the specimens. To assess any potential statistical differences between the specimens, the Kruskal–Wallis test by rank was employed, with a p-value threshold set at the range of $p < 0.001$. To compare the results obtained from the four tests for each trial, a multivariate analysis of variance (MANOVA) test was conducted. Finally, to determine the significance of the presented results, the Mann–Whitney U test was performed.

3. Results

The results of the conducted tests are summarized and presented in three tables and four figures. Table 3 provides an overview of the elasticity modulus measurements of Dental LT Clear resin. It was found that the highest compression modulus values were observed in specimens that had not undergone polishing or aging. On the other hand, specimens subjected to aging or both polishing and aging exhibited lower mean compression modulus values. It is worth noting that the tensile test results showed the widest ranges when polishing was applied without aging, while the narrowest ranges were observed after the application of aging.

Figures 3 and 4 depict the comparisons of the elasticity modulus. Figure 3 illustrates that the impact of polishing on compression resistance is minimal, while artificial aging noticeably weakens the material properties by reducing the force required to damage the specimens. This difference is statistically significant ($p < 0.001$). In Figure 4, the largest disparity is observed when comparing the nonpolished and nonaged group with the group of specimens that underwent both polishing and aging.

Table 3. The measurements of elasticity module of Dental LT Clear resin after the compression (E_c) and tensile (E_t) tests.

E (GPa)	Polishing	Aging	N	M ± SD	Me [Q1–Q3]	Min–Max
Compression E_c	No	No	30	0.87 ± 0.02	0.87 [0.86–0.88]	0.81–0.89
	No	Yes	30	0.73 ± 0.03	0.73 [0.71–0.74]	0.67–0.80
	Yes	No	32	0.86 ± 0.03	0.87 [0.85–0.88]	0.74–0.90
	Yes	Yes	30	0.73 ± 0.05	0.73 [0.69–0.77]	0.62–0.81
Tensile E_t	No	No	32	2.96 ± 0.20	2.97 [2.84–3.07]	2.31–3.33
	No	Yes	32	2.20 ± 0.10	2.23 [2.13–2.26]	2.01–2.39
	Yes	No	28	3.00 ± 0.11	3.00 [2.93–3.08]	2.77–3.23
	Yes	Yes	36	2.38 ± 0.16	2.43 [2.25–2.51]	1.95–2.62

M—mean, SD—standard deviation, Me—median (50th percentile), Q1—lower quartile (25th percentile), Q3—upper quartile (75th percentile), Min—smallest value, Max—greatest value.

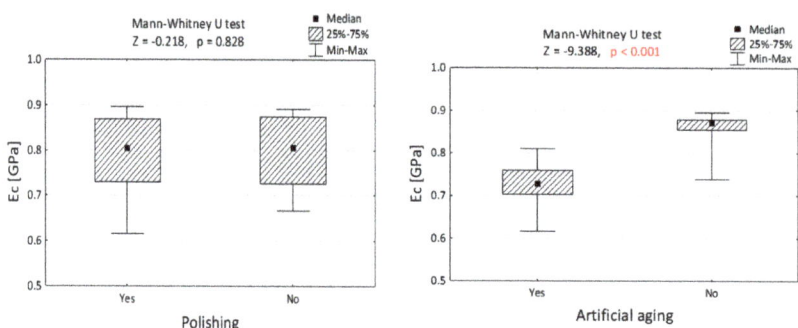

Figure 3. Module of elasticity in compression (E_c) of Dental LT Clear resins, differing in polishing and artificial aging. The Mann–Whitney U test was performed to validate the importance of the result. *p* value lower than 0.001 is presented in red.

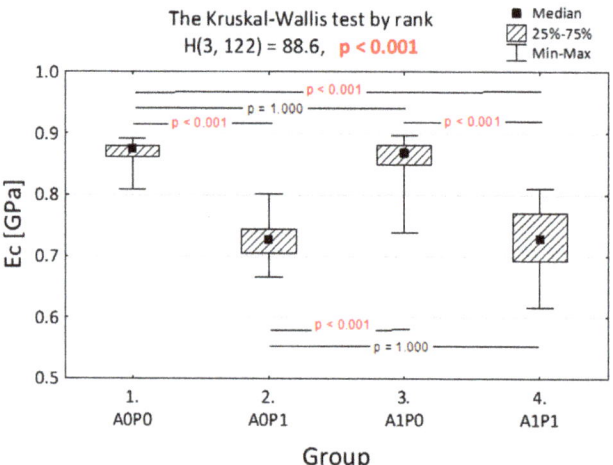

Figure 4. Module of elasticity in compression (E_c) of the Dental LT Clear specimens after different technological treatments (A0P0—no artificial aging and polishing, A0P1—no artificial aging, after polishing, A1P0—artificial aging applied without polishing, and A1P1—both polishing and artificial aging). The Kruskal–Wallis and post hoc tests were applied. *p* value lower than 0.001 is presented in red.

Figure 4 displays the variance analysis conducted to determine the influence of artificial aging and polishing on the module of elasticity in compression (E_c). The mean values of the elastic modulus varied depending on whether artificial aging was applied with or without polishing. Polishing had an impact on the nonaged specimens, but when comparing the aged specimens, polishing itself did not influence the material's properties.

Additionally, Table 4 shows the results of the MANOVA test, indicating that there were statistically significant differences among the results obtained from all the processes performed on the specimens.

Table 4. MANOVA test for elasticity module for Dental LT Clear resin in compression test. p value lower than 0.001 is presented in red.

Effect	SS	df	MS	F	p
Constant	731.1	1	731.1	60901	<0.001
Direct	210.1	1	210.1	17502	<0.001
Polishing	0.166	1	0.166	13.8	<0.001
Artificial aging	10.60	1	10.60	883	<0.001
Direct Polishing	0.213	1	0.213	17.7	<0.001
Polishing + Artificial aging	4.773	1	4.773	398	<0.001
Artificial aging + Polishing	0.078	1	0.078	6.49	0.011
Direct Polishing + Artificial aging	0.060	1	0.060	5.02	0.026
Error	2.9052	242	0.012		

In contrast to the previous results, Table 5 presents the MANOVA test results for the module of elasticity in applied tension. It shows that the only significant influence observed was due to artificial aging. There was no observed influence of the interaction between polishing and artificial aging.

Table 5. MANOVA test for module of elasticity in tension of Dental LT Clear resin. p value lower than 0.001 is presented in red.

Effect	SS	df	MS	F	p
Constant	77.10	1	77.10	62136	0.000
Polishing	0.001	1	0.001	1.16	0.283
Artificial aging	0.562	1	0.562	452.6	0.000
Artificial aging + Polishing	0.001	1	0.001	0.44	0.506
Error	0.146	118	0.001		

The results depicted in Figure 5 demonstrate that polishing had no significant influence on the tensile properties of the examined resin. However, artificial aging was found to reduce the resistance to breakage during the tensile test.

Figure 6 provides a summary of the previous findings, indicating that polishing has a slight positive effect on the resistance to tension, but it does not affect the resistance to compression. In contrast, artificial aging decreases the force required to damage the specimens in both the compression and tensile tests, although the impact is less noticeable in compression. Additionally, the tensile modulus value significantly decreases with the application of artificial aging.

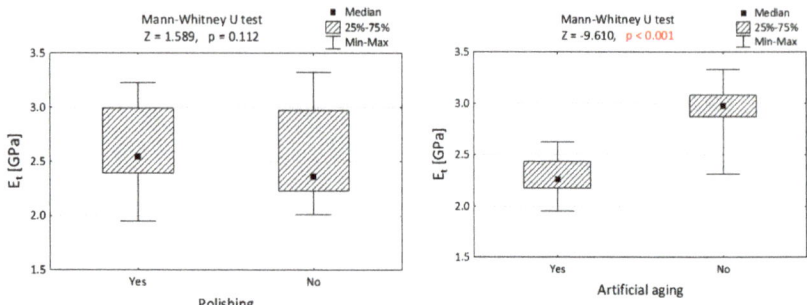

Figure 5. Module of elasticity in tension (E_t) of specimens made of Dental LT Clear resin, differing with polishing and artificial aging. Results presented in the form of Mann–Whitney U test. *p* value lower than 0.001 is presented in red.

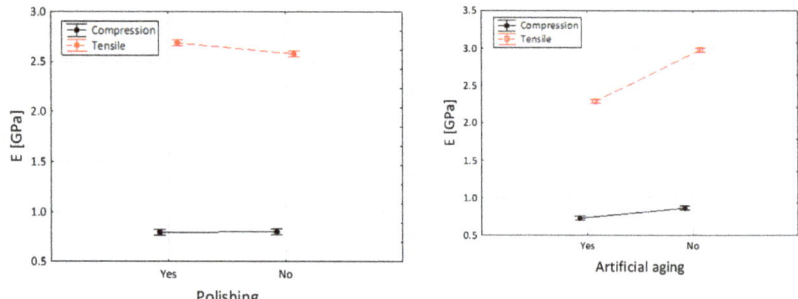

Figure 6. The influence of polishing and artificial aging on the compression and tensile modulus of Dental LT Clear.

4. Discussion

Dental LT Clear, as a class IIa biocompatible resin, is specifically designed for long-term use and contact with tissues, including oral mucosa. It is commonly utilized in the production of clear aligners and dental guards, which are intended for extended wear by patients [4,19]. These splints are designed for long-term use and stay in the patient's mouth for several hours per day and should not be used while eating and drinking due to the potential loss of color stability and mechanical properties [7,20]. With this in mind, we conducted this study to evaluate the mechanical properties of Dental LT Clear resin when subjected to two technological activities: polishing and artificial aging.

Considering that the examined material is designed for long-term use, such as in splints, aligners, and retainers [6], we decided to assess its resistance to artificial aging to simulate this condition. We chose to use water for artificial aging to mimic the humid environment of the oral cavity. Thermocycling, which involves temperature variations during eating, was not considered in our study [19]. Water storage provides valuable information on hydrolytic degradation [21]. Patient appliances should be polished to create smoother surfaces and prevent irritations. The results we obtained supported the notion that polishing helps protect the resin from unfavorable conditions, thereby confirming the durability of its mechanical properties. However, it is important to note that Dental LT Clear is a transparent, clear resin and is not intended for dental fillings. Therefore, thermocycling was not included as a method of material aging. We found a study [22] that examined the influence of artificial aging on the material's properties. Although their study had a similar design to ours, they assessed the resistance to mechanical forces after 2 and 4 weeks. The two-week period, presented by Reymus and Stawarczyk [22], provides insights into the material's durability within a clear aligner treatment timeframe. In contrast, our study was conducted over a period of 3 months, which is a more appropriate timeframe for assessing the long-term use of Dental LT Clear as an occlusal splint or retainer. It is also worth mentioning that other resins, such as Tera Harz TC-85 (Graphy), have been studied in more detail in the context of artificial aging [3]. Dental LT Clear is a relatively new resin and, therefore, the available studies on this specific topic are limited.

Dental LT Clear is indeed a relatively new material, and during our literature search, we did not come across articles specifically examining the features presented in this research. Existing studies on resin use in dentistry often focus on color changes, which is a primary concern for researchers [23–26]. Our study demonstrates that polishing has minimal impact on the mechanical resistance of Dental LT Clear, while artificial aging significantly weakens these properties. Therefore, we believe that our paper holds value and importance, especially for clinicians. Over time, splints may become less precise and show signs of wear. Another interesting study revealed that printed splints tend to be thicker than the designed file, suggesting potential loss of precision during use [27]. Scanning, which replaces traditional intraoral impressions, can also introduce errors and distortions [28]. Additionally, the properties of impressions may change during disinfection. Silicone materials are known to be more resistant to disinfecting agents and sterilization, whereas commonly used alginate materials are less stable and accurate, losing their precision after undergoing antibacterial procedures [29–31].

An interesting observation is that the angle of printing is crucial in the context of polishing, as the layers of material used for occlusal splint preparation can result in irregularities and reduced precision in the structure of the splint [32]. However, this aspect was not the focus of our study, as we did not plan to print the specimens at different angles.

In a comparative study, it was found that Dental LT Clear has the highest fracture rate among other resins used for occlusal splints [33]. This finding highlights the importance of considering the properties of different materials when planning any type of splint. It also emphasizes the need for further research and the development of new materials with more stable properties for similar applications.

Furthermore, a study by Paradowska-Stolarz et al. [14] demonstrated that the application of external forces does not significantly alter the fractal dimension and texture analysis reveals only resistance to compression—the study shows that Dental LT Clear remains stable in its mechanical features, which indicates that the microscopic structure of the material remains relatively unchanged after undergoing the tested conditions. The study also revealed the high stability of Dental LT Clear against mechanical action, as indicated by its resistance to compression.

It is worth mentioning that 3D composite materials may absorb water and undergo changes in weight. Although this feature was not evaluated in our study, it is an interesting finding that warrants further investigation [34].

We acknowledge that our research has certain limitations. One of the main limitations is that we only focused on one resin, Dental LT Clear, without comparing it to other materials. However, we believe that our study is a novel contribution to this field and was designed with this specific material in mind. It is worth noting that other papers in the literature tend to concentrate on restorative and prosthetic materials [23–26], whereas our study specifically examines a material used for occlusal splints and clear aligners.

ISO standards typically suggest using five samples for this type of research. However, by expanding our sample size to 30 specimens, we believe that our study gains a significant advantage in terms of statistical analysis and the reliability of our findings. Furthermore, the scarcity of references on this particular topic underscores the novelty and originality of our research.

5. Conclusions

Based on the obtained results, we can draw several conclusions. Firstly, polishing has minimal influence on the properties of Dental LT Clear resin. However, artificial aging significantly affects both the compressive modulus and tension of the material. Secondly, polishing increases the resistance of the specimens to artificial aging, as evidenced by the higher force required to damage the specimens. Therefore, it is recommended to polish appliances made from Dental LT Clear resin after printing to enhance their durability and resistance to wear during use.

Author Contributions: Conceptualization: A.P.-S., M.W., and J.W.; methodology: A.P.-S., A.M., and J.W.; validation: A.P.-S.; investigation: J.W.; writing—original draft preparation: A.P.-S., A.M., and J.W.; writing—review and editing: M.W.; visualization: J.W. and A.P.-S.; supervision: A.P.-S.; project administration: J.W. and A.P.-S.; and funding acquisition: M.W. All authors have read and agreed to the published version of the manuscript.

Funding: This research was funded by Wroclaw Medical University, grant number SUBK.B032.22.023 (A.P.-S.), according to records in the Simple System.

Institutional Review Board Statement: Not applicable.

Informed Consent Statement: Not applicable.

Data Availability Statement: The data presented in this study are available on request from the corresponding author. The data are not publicly available due to privacy.

Conflicts of Interest: The authors declare that they have no conflict of interest.

References

1. Malysa, A.; Wezgowiec, J.; Danel, D.; Boening, K.; Walczak, K.; Wieckiewicz, M. Bond strength of modern self-adhesive resin cements to human dentin and different CAD/CAM ceramics. *Acta Bioeng. Biomech.* **2020**, *22*, 25–34. [CrossRef] [PubMed]
2. Karatas, O.; Gul, P.; Akgul, N.; Celik, N.; Gundogdu, M.; Duymus, Z.; Seven, N. Effect of staining and bleaching on the microhardness, surface roughness and color of different composite resins. *Dent. Med. Probl.* **2021**, *58*, 369–376. [CrossRef]
3. Goracci, C.; Juloski, J.; D'Amico, C.; Balestra, D.; Volpe, A.; Juloski, J.; Vichi, A. Clinically Relevant Properties of 3D Printable Materials for Intraoral Use in Orthodontics: A Critical Review of the Literature. *Materials* **2023**, *16*, 2166. [CrossRef] [PubMed]
4. Jindal, P.; Worcester, F.; Siena, F.L.; Forbes, C.; Juneja, M.; Breedon, P. Mechanical behaviour of 3D printed vs thermoformed clear dental aligner materials under non-linear compressive loading using FEM. *J. Mech. Behav. Biomed. Mater.* **2020**, *112*, 104045. [CrossRef] [PubMed]
5. Skośkiewicz-Malinowska, K.; Mysior, M.; Rusak, A.; Kuropka, P.; Kozakiewicz, M.; Jurczyszyn, K. Application of Texture and Fractal Dimension Analysis to Evaluate Subgingival Cement Surfaces in Terms of Biocompatibility. *Materials* **2021**, *14*, 5857. [CrossRef]
6. Paradowska-Stolarz, A.; Malysa, A.; Mikulewicz, M. Comparison of the Compression and Tensile Modulus of Two Chosen Resins Used in Dentistry for 3D Printing. *Materials* **2022**, *15*, 8956. [CrossRef]
7. Warnecki, M.; Sarul, M.; Kozakiewicz, M.; Zięty, A.; Babiarczuk, B.; Kawala, B.; Jurczyszyn, K. Surface Evaluation of Aligners after Immersion in Coca-Cola and Orange Juice. *Materials* **2022**, *15*, 6341. [CrossRef]
8. Memè, L.; Notarstefano, V.; Sampalmieri, F.; Orilisi, G.; Quinzi, V. ATR-FTIR Analysis of Orthodontic Invisalign® Aligners Subjected to Various In Vitro Aging Treatments. *Materials* **2021**, *14*, 818. [CrossRef]
9. Kul, E.; Abdulrahim, R.; Bayındır, F.; Matori, K.A.; Gül, P. Evaluation of the color stability of temporary materials produced with CAD/CAM. *Dent. Med. Probl.* **2021**, *58*, 187–191. [CrossRef]
10. Paradowska-Stolarz, A.; Wezgowiec, J.; Mikulewicz, M. Comparison of Two Chosen 3D Printing Resins Designed for Orthodontic Use: An In Vitro Study. *Materials* **2023**, *16*, 2237. [CrossRef]
11. Vichi, A.; Balestra, D.; Scotti, N.; Louca, C.; Paolone, G. Translucency of CAD/CAM and 3D Printable Composite Materials for Permanent Dental Restorations. *Polymers* **2023**, *15*, 1443. [CrossRef] [PubMed]
12. Franchi, L.; Vichi, A.; Marti, P.; Lampus, F.; Guercio, S.; Recupero, A.; Giuntini, V.; Goracci, C. 3D Printed Customized Facemask for Maxillary Protraction in the Early Treatment of a Class III Malocclusion: Proof-of-Concept Clinical Case. *Materials* **2022**, *15*, 3747. [CrossRef] [PubMed]
13. Thurzo, A.; Šufliarsky, B.; Urbanová, W.; Čverha, M.; Strunga, M.; Varga, I. Pierre Robin Sequence and 3D Printed Personalized Composite Appliances in Interdisciplinary Approach. *Polymers* **2022**, *14*, 3858. [CrossRef] [PubMed]
14. Paradowska-Stolarz, A.; Wieckiewicz, M.; Kozakiewicz, M.; Jurczyszyn, K. Mechanical Properties, Fractal Dimension, and Texture Analysis of Selected 3D-Printed Resins Used in Dentistry That Underwent the Compression Test. *Polymers* **2023**, *15*, 1772. [CrossRef]
15. Tangpothitham, S.; Pongprueksa, P.; Inokoshi, M.; Mitrirattanakul, S. Effect of post-polymerization with autoclaving treatment on monomer elution and mechanical properties of 3D-printing acrylic resin for splint fabrication. *J. Mech. Behav. Biomed. Mater.* **2022**, *126*, 105015. [CrossRef]

16. *ISO 604:2003*; Plastics—Determination of Compressive Properties. International Organization for Standardization: Geneva, Switzerland, 2003.
17. *ISO 527-1:2019*; Plastics—Determination of Tensile Properties—Part 1: General Principles. International Organization for Standardization: Geneva, Switzerland, 2019.
18. Drummond, J.L.; Savers, E.E. In vitro aging of a heat/pressure-cured composite. *Dent. Mater.* **1993**, *9*, 214–216. [CrossRef] [PubMed]
19. Malysa, A.; Wezgowiec, J.; Grzebieluch, W.; Danel, D.P.; Wieckiewicz, M. Effect of Thermocycling on the Bond Strength of Self-Adhesive Resin Cements Used for Luting CAD/CAM Ceramics to Human Dentin. *Int. J. Mol. Sci.* **2022**, *23*, 745. [CrossRef]
20. Riley, P.; Glenny, A.M.; Worthington, H.V.; Jacobsen, E.; Robertson, C.; Durham, J.; Davies, S.; Petersen, H.; Boyers, D. Oral splints for patients with temporomandibular disorders or bruxism: A systematic review and economic evaluation. *Health Technol. Assess* **2020**, *24*, 1–224. [CrossRef] [PubMed]
21. Comino-Garayoa, R.; Peláez, J.; Tobar, C.; Rodríguez, V.; Suárez, M.J. Adhesion to Zirconia: A Systematic Review of Surface Pretreatments and Resin Cements. *Materials* **2021**, *14*, 2751. [CrossRef]
22. Reymus, M.; Stawarczyk, B. In vitro study on the influence of postpolymerization and aging on the Martens parameters of 3D-printed occlusal devices. *J. Prosthet. Dent.* **2021**, *125*, 817–823. [CrossRef]
23. Miletic, V.; Trifković, B.; Stamenković, D.; Tango, R.N.; Paravina, R.D. Effects of staining and artificial aging on optical properties of gingiva-colored resin-based restorative materials. *Clin. Oral. Investig.* **2022**, *26*, 6817–6827. [CrossRef] [PubMed]
24. Valizadeh, S.; Asiaie, Z.; Kiomarsi, N.; Kharazifard, M.J. Color stability of self-adhering composite resins in different solutions. *Dent. Med. Probl.* **2020**, *57*, 31–38. [CrossRef] [PubMed]
25. El-Rashidy, A.A.; Abdelraouf, R.M.; Habib, N.A. Effect of two artificial aging protocols on color and gloss of single-shade versus multi-shade resin composites. *BMC Oral. Health* **2022**, *22*, 321. [CrossRef] [PubMed]
26. Gómez-Polo, C.; Martín Casado, A.M.; Quispe, N.; Gallardo, E.R.; Montero, J. Colour Changes of Acetal Resins (CAD-CAM) In Vivo. *Appl. Sci.* **2023**, *13*, 181. [CrossRef]
27. Edelmann, A.; English, J.D.; Chen, S.J.; Kasper, F.K. Analysis of the thickness of 3-dimensional printed orthodontic aligners. *Am. J. Orthod. Dentofac. Orthop.* **2020**, *158*, e91–e98. [CrossRef]
28. Emam, M.; Ghanem, L.; Abdel Sadek, H.M. Effect of different intraoral scanners and post-space depths on the trueness of digital impressions. *Dent. Med. Probl.* **2023**, *ahead of print*. [CrossRef]
29. Wezgowiec, J.; Paradowska-Stolarz, A.; Malysa, A.; Orzeszek, S.; Seweryn, P.; Wieckiewicz, M. Effects of Various Disinfection Methods on the Material Properties of Silicone Dental Impressions of Different Types and Viscosities. *Int. J. Mol. Sci.* **2022**, *23*, 10859. [CrossRef]
30. Iwasaki, Y.; Hiraguchi, H.; Iwasaki, E.; Yoneyama, T. Effects of immersion disinfection of agar-alginate combined impressions on the surface properties of stone casts. *Dent. Mater. J.* **2016**, *35*, 45–50. [CrossRef]
31. Al Mortadi, N.; Al-Khatib, A.; Alzoubi, K.H.; Khabour, O.F. Disinfection of dental impressions: Knowledge and practice among dental technicians. *Clin. Cosmet. Investig. Dent.* **2019**, *11*, 103–108. [CrossRef]
32. Grymak, A.; Aarts, J.M.; Ma, S.; Waddell, J.N.; Choi, J.J.E. Comparison of hardness and polishability of various occlusal splint materials. *J. Mech. Behav. Biomed. Mater.* **2021**, *115*, 104270. [CrossRef]
33. Aretxabaleta, M.; Xepapadeas, A.B.; Poets, C.F.; Koos, B.; Spintzyk, S. Fracture Load of an Orthodontic Appliance for Robin Sequence Treatment in a Digital Workflow. *Materials* **2021**, *14*, 344. [CrossRef] [PubMed]
34. Islam, M.S.; Nassar, M.; Elsayed, M.A.; Jameel, D.B.; Ahmad, T.T.; Rahman, M.M. In Vitro Optical and Physical Stability of Resin Composite Materials with Different Filler Characteristics. *Polymers* **2023**, *15*, 2121. [CrossRef] [PubMed]

Disclaimer/Publisher's Note: The statements, opinions and data contained in all publications are solely those of the individual author(s) and contributor(s) and not of MDPI and/or the editor(s). MDPI and/or the editor(s) disclaim responsibility for any injury to people or property resulting from any ideas, methods, instructions or products referred to in the content.

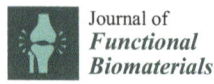

Review

Surface Coatings of Dental Implants: A Review

Angelo Michele Inchingolo [1,†], Giuseppina Malcangi [1,†], Laura Ferrante [1], Gaetano Del Vecchio [1], Fabio Viapiano [1], Alessio Danilo Inchingolo [1], Antonio Mancini [1], Ciro Annicchiarico [1], Francesco Inchingolo [1,*], Gianna Dipalma [1,*], Elio Minetti [2], Andrea Palermo [3,‡] and Assunta Patano [1,‡]

1. Department of Interdisciplinary Medicine, University of Bari "Aldo Moro", 70124 Bari, Italy; angeloinchingolo@gmail.com (A.M.I.); giuseppinamalcangi@libero.it (G.M.); lauraferrante79@virgilio.it (L.F.); dr.gdelvecchio96@gmail.com (G.D.V.); viapianofabio96@gmail.com (F.V.); ad.inchingolo@libero.it (A.D.I.); dr.antonio.mancini@gmail.com (A.M.); annicchiarico.ciro63@gmail.com (C.A.); assuntapatano@gmail.com (A.P.)
2. Department of Biomedical, Surgical, and Dental Science, University of Milan, 20122 Milan, Italy; elio.minetti@gmail.com
3. College of Medicine and Dentistry Birmingham, University of Birmingham, Birmingham B4 6BN, UK; andrea.palermo2004@libero.it
* Correspondence: francesco.inchingolo@uniba.it (F.I.); giannadipalma@tiscali.it (G.D.); Tel.: +39-331-211-1104 (F.I.); +39-339-698-9939 (G.D.)
† These authors contributed equally to this work as first authors.
‡ These authors contributed equally to this work as last authors.

Abstract: Replacement of missing teeth is possible using biocompatible devices such as endosseous implants. This study aims to analyze and recognize the best characteristics of different implant surfaces that ensure good peri-implant tissue healing and thus clinical success over time. The present review was performed on the recent literature concerning endosseous implants made of titanium, a material most frequently used because of its mechanical, physical, and chemical characteristics. Thanks to its low bioactivity, titanium exhibits slow osseointegration. Implant surfaces are treated so that cells do not reject the surface as a foreign material and accept it as fully biocompatible. Analysis of different types of implant surface coatings was performed in order to identify ideal surfaces that improve osseointegration, epithelial attachment to the implant site, and overall peri-implant health. This study shows that the implant surface, with different adhesion, proliferation, and spreading capabilities of osteoblastic and epithelial cells, influences the cells involved in anchorage. Implant surfaces must have antibacterial capabilities to prevent peri-implant disease. Research still needs to improve implant material to minimize clinical failure.

Keywords: osseointegration; surface; coating; dental implant; titanium; treatment surface; peri-implant health; implant stability; bacterial adhesion; marginal bone level

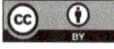

1. Introduction

Natural tooth loss has serious emotional, psychological, and social effects in addition to physical and functional effects on an individual [1]. Implantoloy is one of the most secure and effective surgical procedures [2]. The most common dental implant materials are titanium, zirconium, and polyetheretherketone (PEEK) [3,4].

Zirconium implants have good aesthetic qualities but a moderate rate of fracture, which leads to implant failure [5]. PEEK implants have demonstrated high fallibility rates; hence, long-term multicentric studies are required to confirm the reliability [6].

Titanium is the material that best complies with the requirements of dental implantology, including osseointegration, biocompability, mechanical resistance, and anti-bacterial properties [7,8]. The term "osseointegration" was first used by Albrektsson (1981) to refer to the functional and structural connection between a vulnerable structure's surface and its critical organs [9]. Accordingly, a number of critical factors for proper bone resorption have been identified: biocompatibility, implant design, implant surface characteristics, condition of the recipient bone site, surgical technique, operator's skill, and implant storage conditions [9].

The characteristics of the implants' surface and the quality of the recipient site bone determine the interface between the two: the bone–implant interface [10]. For instance, an implant positioned in a lamellar bone has 90% contact, whereas one positioned in a midollar bone has 50% contact [11,12].

Morphologically, dental and implant periodontal tissues have many common features, as both are marked by a well-keratinized oral epithelium and a portion of connective tissue in direct contact with the implant and tooth [13]. More collagen and fewer fibroblasts are found in the implantable connective tissue [13,14].

The physicochemical properties of the implant outermost layer and its interaction with the surrounding essential tissues play a role in determining whether osseointegration succeeds or fails [15].

A fundamental prerequisite for the long-term success of the implant is biological anchorage between the surface of the dental implant and the bone tissue [16,17]. Bone response is closely related to the implant surface [17].

Hydrophilic and hydrophobic implant surfaces can be distinguished [11,18]. Hydrophilic surfaces, compared with hydrophobic structures, favor interactions with biological fluids and cells allowing a good surface wettability [18,19]. Implant surfaces with the same chemical composition actually offer a different contact angle for biological fluids depending on the topography of the surface: rough surfaces, such as sandblasted and etched surfaces, are more likely to be wettable than surfaces considered to be smooth [18,20] (Figure 1).

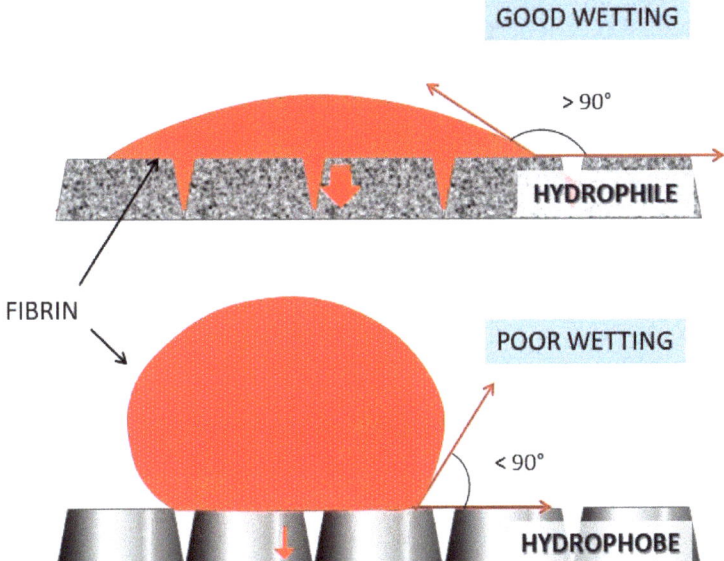

Figure 1. Fibrin implant wettability. The hydrophobe surface shows poor wettability, unlike the hydrophile one with good wettability. The red arrow indicates the magnitude of liquid permeability on the surface of the implant.

The hydrophilicity of the implant surface results in abrupt contact of the implant with the clot, favouring the osseointegration process [21,22]. Some surfaces have such hydrophilicity that mere contact of the first coils with blood results in suction along the entire implant surface [21,21] (Figure 2). Roughened surfaces increase blood clot retention [23].

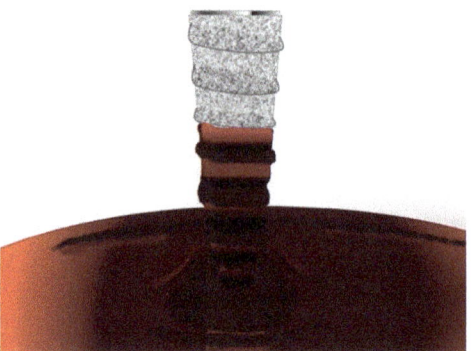

Figure 2. Good implant wettability: As soon as the implant is inserted into the bone, there is immediate blood–fixture contact. Blood is attracted to the implant surface.

The implant surface treated with rumination exhibits a double retraction of fibrin filaments and a double blood clotting compared with the smooth surface [24] (Figure 3).

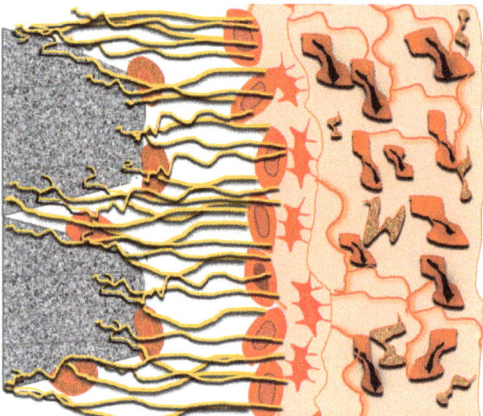

Figure 3. Fibrin adhesion to the implant surface.

During the wound healing phase, the following takes place:
- Fibrin formation that protects the wound and, together with platelets, plugs the wound and releases the repair factors;
- Fibrinolysis: reabsorption of the clot;
- Osteoclastic activity: migration of cells from the blood;
- Migration of mesenchymal cells, precursors of bone cells [25–27].

Implant stability is necessary for effective osseointegration and healing [3,13,24,28]. The features of the bone, the implant's design, and the procedure used to place it all affect primary stability [29]. Bone remodeling and bone production around the implant lead to secondary stability [30]. Growing research demonstrates that implant surface features also affect secondary stability [31,32].

Bone apposition on the implant surface begins first in trabecular bone, then in compact bone [24,33]. Peri-implant bone metabolism is at its peak 1–4 months after surgery [34,35].

The clinical success of the implant, in addition to osseointegration, depends on the health of the bone–implant–soft tissue interface [16] (Figure 4).

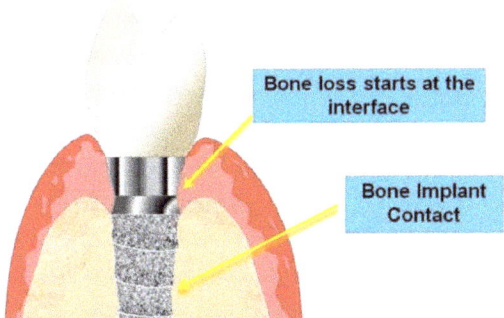

Figure 4. Schematic image of the implant–bone interface.

Implant failure may result from titanium's reduced ability to induce osseointegration, which causes poor or delayed osseointegration [36,37]. Furthermore, early titanium implants had a mechanically polished surface that was smooth, and research in recent years revealed that this surface is less stable over time than those with a rough surface [36,38]. In order to achieve a larger contact surface, treatment of the implant surface was performed in order to increase the osseointegration between the bone and the implant [36].

This review aimed to analyze different surfaces and, therefore, identify the ideal implant structure from a clinical and durability point of view, with the least post-surgical complications and the least discomfort to the body [17,39,40]. Research is extensive and challenging because of ongoing scientific discoveries and innovations [41].

In fact, an appropriate modification of titanium surface, which increases the percentage of BIC (bone implant contact), is still being studied to favor osseointegration, which has antibacterial properties to prevent peri-implant diseases and resists the stresses it will undergo with functionalization, such as chewing, thus guaranteeing healthy peri-implant tissue over time [30,39,42].

2. Materials and Methods

2.1. Search Processing

The present review was performed in accordance with the principles of PRISMA. PubMed, Scopus, and Web of Science were searched to find papers that matched our topic dating from 1 January 2019 up to 31 March 2023, with English-language restriction. The search strategy was built using a combination of words that matched the purpose of the investigation, whose primary focus is the difference of implant surface coatings on osseointegration; hence, the following Boolean keywords were used: different dental implant surface AND osseointegration (Table 1).

Table 1. Database search indicators.

Articles' Screening Strategy
KEYWORDS: A: different dental implant surface; B: osseointegration.
Boolean Indicators: A AND B.
Timespan: 2019–2023.
Electronic databases: Pubmed; Scopus; WOS.

2.2. Inclusion and Exclusion Criteria

The inclusion criteria were as follows: (1) human in vivo study; (2) English language; (3) open access studies; (4) clinical studies; (5) studies examining the variety of surfaces of titanium dental implants: implant surface treatments and coatings; and (6) in vitro studies concerning the analysis of implant surface coatings of great interest to our research.

The exclusion criteria were as follows: (1) animal; (2) other languages different from English; (3) not open access studies; (4) case report/series, reviews, editorials, book chapters; (5) research about zirconium and peek dental implant; and (6) in vitro studies far from the focus of our research.

The review was conducted using the PICO criteria:

- Population: Titanium endosseous implants;
- Intervention: Implant surface treatment;
- Comparisons: Different implant surfaces;
- Outcomes: Interaction with biological tissues;

2.3. Data Processing

Author disagreements on the choice of articles were discussed and settled.

3. Results

A total of 1262 publications were identified from the following databases, Pubmed (482), Scopus (344), and Web of Science (436), which led to 732 articles after removing duplicates (530). A total of 290 articles accessed the screening phase, while 442 items were removed because 3 were not found, 131 were in animal, 1 was a chapter in a book, 75 were not in vivo and far from the focus of this review, 66 were reviews and meta-analyses, and 166 were off topic. From these papers, 279 were additionally removed because of lack of interest and eligibility was assigned to 11 records that were finally included in the review for qualitative analysis, of which 5 were in vitro (Figure 5). The results of each study are reported in Tables 2 and 3.

Table 2. Characteristics of the in vivo studies included in the qualitative analysis.

Authors (Year)	Type of the Study	Aim of the Study	Materials	Results
Bielemann et al. (2022) [43]	Randomized controlled trial	Evaluate the clinical and radiological peri-implant parameters between hydrophilic and hydrophobic dental implants	For 2 types of surfaces, hydrophobic and hydrophilic, different peri-implant health indices were evaluated: (i) early healing index (EHI), visible plaque index (VPI), presence of tartar (CP), peri-implant inflammation (PI), probing depth (PD), and bleeding on probing (BOP); implant stability quotient (ISQ), crestal bone loss (CBL), and bone level change (BLC); and implant success and survival rates.	There were no differences in peri-implant healing, stability, and bone remodeling after 1 year.
Gursaytrak et al. (2020) [44]	Randomized controlled trial	Evaluate the stability of implants with different surfaces (alkali-modified or sandblasted) using resonance frequency analysis (RFA).	Immediately after implantation as well as at 2, 6, and 12 weeks, RFA was utilized to assess the stability quotient of implants with alkali-modified (bioactive) and sandblasted surfaces.	After placement, implants with alkali-modified surfaces were more stable than implants with sandblasted surfaces after, but the two types had similar clinical results at 12 weeks after surgery.

Table 2. Cont.

Authors (Year)	Type of the Study	Aim of the Study	Materials	Results
Hasegawa et al. (2020) [45]	Randomized controlled trial	Optimize the implant surface's biological potential for improved osseointegration.	The titanium surface was etched with sulfuric acid at different temperatures (120, 130, 140, and 150 °C).	The maximum capacity for osseous integration was reached when the surface of the implant was acidified at 140 °C, significantly increasing the capacity for osteoconductive and osteointegrative growth.
Ko et al. (2019) [46]	Randomized controlled trial	Comparing the peri-implant marginal bone level around CaP-coated and uncoated sandblasted, large-grit, acid-etched (SLA) surface implants 1 year after implantation.	Clinical and radiographic examinations were performed to assess initial stability and changes in marginal bone level after 3 months and after 12 months.	All of the implants were successful.
Kormoczi et al. (2021) [47]	Randomized controlled trial	Comparison of early loaded implants with different modified surface stability.	Implant success, implant stability, and periodontal parameters were evaluated after the placement of implants with SA (alumina blasting and acid etching), NH (bioabsorbable apatite nanocoating), or SLA (coarse-grain blasting and acid etching) surfaces.	No significant differences were found in the two groups and good periodontal parameters were found.
Velloso et al. (2019) [11]	Randomized controlled trial	Evaluating the effects of implant devices with the same brand, design, length, and diameter but with two different surface treatments: sandblasting and etching with acid (SAE) and SAE modified chemically (hydrophilic).	20 distinct patients received 20 implants with the same shape, size, and diameter but with two different surface treatments (10 SAE and 10 modified SAE). After six weeks, implant stability values were assessed.	Implants with a modified SAE surface showed superior and faster implant stability.

Table 3. Characteristics of the in vitro studies included in the qualitative analysis.

Authors (Year)	Type of the Study	Aim of the Study	Materials	Results
Chauhan et al. (2021) [48]	In vitro	To investigate the action of acid etching on the surface characteristics of titanium alloy implants and to optimize the process variables to produce micro- and nanotopography on the surface of dental implants.	Without heating the acid solution, the optimum implant surface was carefully examined and compared with the etched surface.	Titanium alloy had a very different surface topography than commercially pure titanium, and it had a distinct surface topography depending on whether the attachment was done at ambient temperature or at higher temperature, which has an impact on cells' behavior
Gavinho et al. (2019) [49]	In vitro	Analyze Bioglass 45S5 with CeO, evaluating whether its antioxidant effect reverses oxidative stress after implantation in bone.	The materials' morphological, structural, and biological properties (cytotoxicity, bioactivity, and antibacterial activity) were examined.	The addition of cerio did not lead to structural changes in the biocompatible glass, which did not exhibit cytotoxicity, but it prevent the growth of Escherichia coli and Streptococcus mutans, and all of the tests revealed the initial deposition of a CaP-rich layer on the material's surface after 24 h.
Rausch et al. (2021) [17]	In vitro	Evaluate the ability of human gingival cells to attach to and grow on differently treated titanium or zirconia implant surfaces	Zirconia and titanium implant surfaces were treated differently and subsequently had different roughness: some surfaces were machined and smooth, while other surfaces were sandblasted and rough.	Gingival cell behavior is mainly influenced by surface roughness, and no relevant difference was found between titanium and zirconia implants.
Schupbach et al. (2019) [50]	In vitro	Comparing several commercially available implant systems with SA-modified surfaces and their surface-level morphological and cleaning characteristics.	Six candidates from three different lots were chosen to be the installation team for each system. The average particulate counts for each project were calculated from three different interest regions and compared.	Not all manufacturers can create implant surfaces without contaminating them with particulates.
Zhang et al. (2021) [8]	In vitro	Reduce associated infection symptoms and improve early osseointegration of dental implant.	Anodic oxidation with hydrogen fluoride was performed on the Ti-Cu alloy implant surface.	Etching hydrogen fluoride + Ti-5Cu alloy revealed that it has high corrosion resistance, great biological compatibility, and extremely potent antibacterial characteristics.

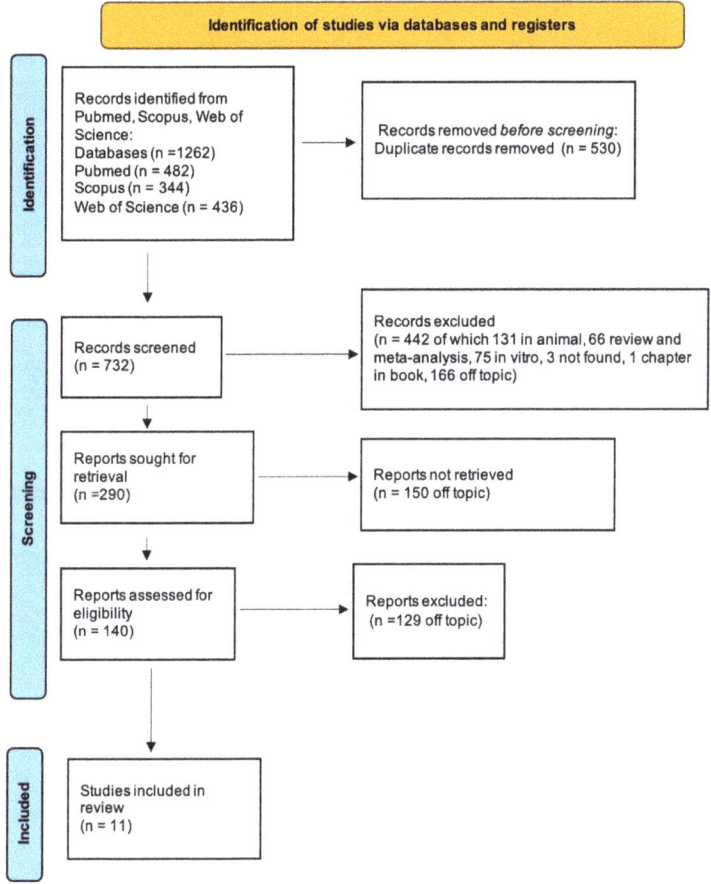

Figure 5. PRISMA flow chart.

4. Discussion

Thanks to its excellent mechanical properties, including biocompatibility, corrosion resistance, non-magnetism, and non-toxicity, titanium and its alloys are widely used to create body armor and dental implants, with success rates close to 95–97% [51].

It is also very reactive and forms an ossidic layer of about 5 nm in thickness, which, in contact with air and water, protects it from corrosion and improves its affinity for patient cells [8].

However, even if titanium is a biologically inert material, it lacks anti-bacterial properties [52]. As a result, bacteria tend to adhere to the collars of implants, and implant failure can be linked to peri-implant infections [51,53]. Once discovered, perimplantite must be treated with antibiotics, which not only increases the risk of developing antibiotic resistance but also causes discomfort and costs the patient money [54]. As a result, it is crucial that titanium implants have long-term anti-bacterial properties and improve early osseointegration capability [55,56]. To meet these clinical requirements, it is necessary to apply a treatment to change the surface of pure titanium, optimizing the surface's morphology and chemical composition [8].

Researchers are working to increase the capacity of the surfaces of titanium machinery [57]. The surface, shape, and structure of the implant affect the osseointegration process, which is necessary to provide implant stability [36]. The stability of the implant, both primary and secondary, is a factor that affects how well the implant itself will osseointegrate [58]. While the primary stability is a mechanical phenomenon that depends on both the implant's macroscopic and microscopic design and the surgical technique used to position it, numerous studies have found that the implant's surface is the key factor in achieving a high level of secondary stability [58,59].

Among the characteristics of implant surfaces, topography and chemical composition are those that have the most impact on the interaction between biomaterial and osseous tissue and, consequently, on secondary stability [17,29]. In particular, numerous studies have demonstrated that, compared with implant surfaces, textured surfaces exhibit a greater capacity for determining a biological response from some osseous cellular lines [60]. In fact, the roughness provides a larger area of contact and interconnection, leading to a greater number of cellular colonies that create strong adhesions to the implant site and enhancing osteoblast proliferation and adhesion processes while decreasing osteoclastic activity and promoting mineralization [61]. In addition, implant roughness aids in the differentiation of mesenchymal cells into the osteoblastic phenotype [29].

Physicochemical treatments of major implant surfaces give rise to different types of implants:

- machined;
- polished;
- treated;
- hybrid [17,62].

A significant advantage of treated and hybridized surfaces is the increased degree of hydrophilicity and wettability compared with untreated, machined, smooth surfaces, which are considered hydrophobic [19]. The only way to modify something on the surface is to add or reduce materials on a micro- or nanometric scale [50] (Figure 6).

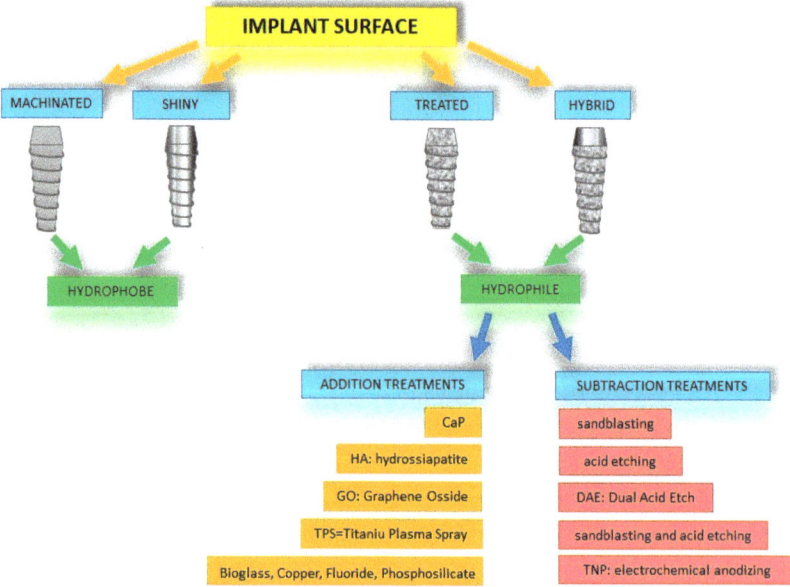

Figure 6. Summary diagram of implant surface treatments. The diagram shows how the hydrophilic property of the implant surfaces (treated and hybrid) lends itself better than the hydrophobic surfaces (machined and smooth) to further treatments to improve their general characteristics.

Bone-to-implant contact (BIC), early in the healing phase, is considerably increased by implants with a hydrophilic surface because these implants typically display more cell differentiation and aggregation [11] (Figure 7).

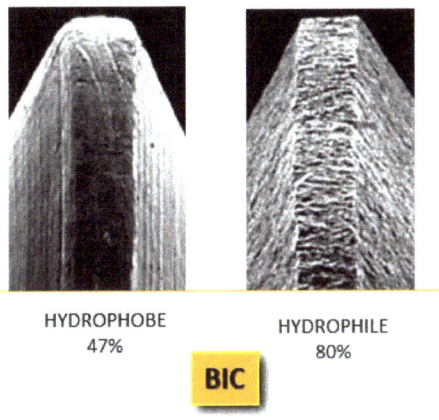

Figure 7. Electron microscopy detail of a smooth (hydrophobe) and a rough (hydrophile) implant surface, with re-wetting percentages. The hydrophilic surface has a higher BIC percentage than the hydrophobic surface.

The most significant advancement in implant dentistry has been the observation of direct bone-to-implant contact (BIC), which was verified with electron microscopy [47].

In comparison with freshly worked surfaces, titanium dental implants with moderately rough surfaces exhibit better osseointegration and faster osseous growth [50].

4.1. Implant Surface Treatments

4.1.1. Subtraction Treatments

A technique for creating moderately rough implant surfaces is sandblasting and acid mordantation (SA) [50,60,63]. According to some studies, the surface modification using the SA technique needs to be properly planned and managed in order to produce a final medical device that is clean and reliable [17]. This is because it has been observed that the majority of implant surface areas contain particulates, which are remnants of the sandblasting [64]. This causes a 15% reduction in tensile strength, which could lead to the beginning of a fracture process [9,11,17,65].

On the other hand, for the past ten years, a widely employed method of surface modification has been the combination of sandblasting and etching [66]. Sandblasting theoretically allows to achieve the ideal roughness for mechanical fixation, while additional etching, by raising the peak height of the roughness peaks, allows to enhance the protein adhesion mechanism, which is crucial in the early stages of bone healing [67]. In fact, these two techniques are used in succession [48].

Surface alteration techniques that use subtractive processes include sandblasting and acid etching [62]. Acid etching causes selective corrosion to occur, leaving holes or grooves on the metal surface [38,68].

Because of its hydrophilic qualities, sandblasted, coarse-grained, acid-etched (SLA) surface is a characteristic form of rough surface generated on a dental implant and has been employed on the newest commercial dental implants [68].

Dual Acid Etch, or DAE Technology, uses double acid etching without first sandblasting [69]. Using this method, the danger of ingesting sand particles is reduced, and surfaces are created that improve BIC, platelet retention, and the release of bone growth hormones [70–72].

By producing a special titanium surface with distinctive meso, micro, and nanoscale roughness features that ensure better osteoconductive and osseointegrative capacities than the more popular micro-rough titanium surface, a method for enhancing osseointegration has been devised [45]. Sulfuric acid was used to etch commercially pure titanium at four different temperatures (120, 130, 140, and 150 °C) [45]. Particularly when acid etching was carried out at 140 °C, the new surface considerably stimulated osteoblast development and, subsequently, osseointegration [17,45].

One of the nanoengineering methods for titanium implants is called electrochemical anodizing [73]. This method involves immersing the titanium implant, which serves as the anode, in an organic electrolyte containing water and fluoride in an electrochemical cell with appropriate voltage, such that titania nanopores (TNPs) are created on the implant surface in order to enhance soft tissue integration and wound healing [73,74]. Anodizing has emerged as a useful technique for changing the surface morphology of titanium or titanium alloys to enhance bone development because it is inexpensive, simple to apply, and easy to control [75,76]. Anodizing can provide a surface morphology with a pore structure on a micronano scale as well as increase the wear and corrosion resistance of pure titanium implants [8].

Further frontiers of research that deserve further investigation are 3D-printed implants and micro-ark oxidizing, which help improve biocompatibility. These are promising fields that will offer new possibilities in the future of clinical practice [77].

4.1.2. Addition Treatments

Biomaterials in implantology have been promoting bone response and biomechanical ability in recent years [78,79]. Many substances, including polyhydroxyalkanoates, calcium phosphate, carbon, bisphosphonates, hydroxyapatite, bone-stimulating agents, bioactive glass, bioactive ceramics, collagen, chitosan, metal and their alloys, fluoride, and titanium/titanium nitride, are known as promising candidates for dental implant coatings [78,80]. It is crucial that biomaterials degrade naturally; polyhydroxyalkanoates, for instance, degrade naturally and do not harm tissues or cells in the process [81,82].

Owing to the development of biofilms, which are thought to aid bacteria in evading antibiotics and the host defense mechanism, bacterial colonization of titanium results in implant loss. Pathogens cause deterioration of the bone surrounding the implant, necessitating surgery to repair the infected bone or to remove or replace infected implants. [37,78,83,84].

Although both implant types generated comparable clinical outcomes at 12 weeks following surgery, implants with alkali-modified surfaces were consistently more stable after implantation than implants with sandblasted surfaces [44,85].

Improved contact osteogenesis surrounding the dental implant was seen on surfaces coated with calcium phosphate (CaP), and early healing phase osseointegration was also seen to be enhanced [9,36]. Increasing the biocompatibility of titanium and encouraging osteogenesis were among the first goals to be achieved by researchers, and for this, some authors employed chemical modifications, such as the addition of fluoride to the implant surface [48].

The interaction of fluoride with hydroxyapatite in bone tissue creates fluorapatite followed by increased osteoblast proliferation and activation of alkaline phosphatase activity [86–88]. Because of its outstanding physical and chemical characteristics, particularly its potential for osteoinduction, graphene oxide (GO) is a promising nanomaterial [57,89,90]. The addition of inorganic bioactive elements confers the important and necessary osteogenic, angiogenic, and antibacterial capabilities [53].

Broad-spectrum antibacterial capabilities, high efficiency, and durability are all properties of copper (Cu) [86,91]. Copper-containing titanium alloy has been confirmed to have a constant precipitation of copper ions and long-lasting antibacterial activity [53,83,92]. It is a necessary trace element for the human body because it can prevent osteoporosis, promote osteogenic differentiation, and induce angiogenesis [93]. Ti-5Cu alloy has remarkable anti-infective efficacy, osteogenic potential, and biological compatibility, which have been amply demonstrated by laboratory investigations [8,91,94].

Implants are frequently vulnerable to infections like peri-implantitis, which affect the surrounding hard and soft tissues and result in implant loss and biocompatibility [95].

Peri-implantitis is an inflammatory condition that affects all surrounding tissues [96]. A deep pocket with hemorrhage, suppuration, and slight bone loss accompanies mucosal injury [33,97,98] (Figure 8).

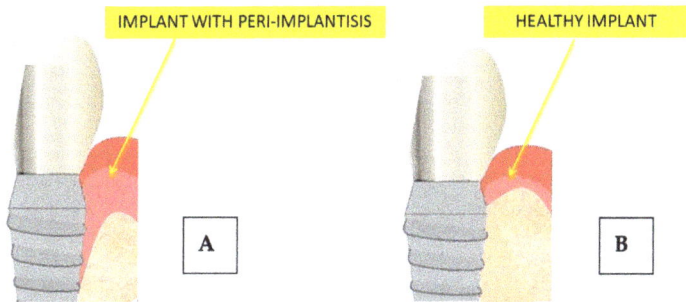

Figure 8. Difference in implant bone contact in conditions of implant good health (**B**) and during peri-implantitis disease (**A**).

Therefore, a recent scientific study has focused on the interface between the implant and the surrounding soft tissues, highlighting the significance of establishing a sufficient epithelial biological seal that is necessary to prevent bacterial contamination [17,97,99,100]. The underlying bone tissues are shielded from germs by the peri-implant tissues, which are made up of connective and epithelial components [101]. It has been claimed that coating the implant with bioactive materials will help to avoid the development of this disease [49].

A bioactive glass known as Bioglass 45S5 or calcium sodium phosphosilicate is made up of silica, calcium oxide, phosphorus pentoxide, and sodium oxide [102]. Biomaterials for bone grafts, periodontal defect repair, cranial and maxillofacial repair, wound care, blood loss management, stimulation of vascular regeneration, and nerve repair are among the typical uses of Bioglass 45S5 [49].

4.1.3. CGF Coated Dental Implants

More recent studies are focusing on the biological properties of growth factor concentrate (CGF), an autologous blood-derived biomaterial, in improving the osseointegration of dental implants [103,104]. The surface of CGF permeated dental implants is biocompatible and biologically active, significantly improving the adhesion of endothelial cells to the implants themselves [31]. All of this guarantees better results in terms of osseointegration and decline in post-surgical complications [31,103].

Some basic parameters are to be monitored during the osseointegration period and after loading to ascertain peri-implant health over time: early healing index, visible plaque index, tartar, peri-implant inflammation, probing depth and bleeding at probing, implant stability quotient, crestal bone loss, bone level variation, and implant success and survival rates [105]. Implant surface modifications can improve implant durability and health and thus ensure proper prosthetic rehabilitation [38,106]. This is also especially true in those patients in whom implant-prosthetic rehabilitation is not only cosmetic, but functional [107]. Sometimes, such patients have systemic diseases or have compromised bone conditions [108]. Implants with surface treatments that can improve bone–implant interactions, protein uptake, adhesion, differentiation, and cell proliferation have been used in these patients. In clinical trials with patients using anticoagulants, diabetics, people who had radiation therapy to the head and neck, and people who needed bone grafting, implants with hydrophilic surfaces displayed encouraging outcomes [109,110]. In comparison with other treated, coated implants, mandibular implant overdentures showed considerably higher 1-year survival rates in clinical trials using SLActive hydrophilic surfaces [43,110,111].

5. Conclusions

From the present study, it emerged that, although all surfaces allowed osseointegration and cell proliferation, the treated surfaces, owing to surface irradiation, had a better propensity for epithelial cell attachment and adhesion, proliferation, and differentiation of osteoblastic cells.

However, research must be directed not only to the osseointegration of the implant into the bone structure, to ensure primary and secondary stability, but also to the seal that the soft tissues provide superficially, which is essential to protect the peri-implant tissues and stability of the prosthesis.

Researchers in designing an implant must give equal importance to both osseointegration and mucointegration, key parameters for generating stability and creating a mucosal seal around the prosthesis. Research in micro and macro implant topography must be focused on designing successful medical devices, reducing clinical failure.

In summary, the primary objectives for the creation of implant surface changes are as follows:

- Enhance clinical effectiveness in regions with both qualitative and quantitative bone deficiencies;
- Speed up the osseointegration process so that immediate or early loading protocols can be addressed;
- Sncourage bone formation in areas where there is insufficient alveolar ridge to enable the implantation of implants;
- Properly seal the muco-gingival biological junction in order to prevent bacterial contamination.

Owing to continuous scientific discoveries and innovation, research is extensive and expanding. It is difficult to apply research in vivo; therefore, a long period of control is still necessary before being able to have certain results on patients.

Author Contributions: Conceptualization, A.M.I., L.F., G.D.V., F.I. and F.V.; methodology G.M., L.F., A.D.I., A.M., G.D., A.P. (Andrea Palermo) and A.P. (Assunta Patano); software, A.M.I., G.D.V., F.V., F.I., E.M. and A.P. (Andrea Palermo); validation, G.M., L.F., F.V. and A.M.; formal analysis, A.M.I., G.D.V., A.D.I., F.I. and A.P. (Assunta Patano); investigation, G.M., A.M., C.A. and A.P. (Andrea Palermo); resources, A.D.I., A.M., C.A., G.D., E.M. and A.P. (Andrea Palermo); data curation, G.M., A.D.I., C.A., G.D., E.M. and A.P. (Assunta Patano); writing—original draft preparation, A.M.I., G.M., A.D.I., G.D. and A.P. (Assunta Patano); writing—review and editing, L.F., G.D.V., F.I., E.M. and A.P. (Andrea Palermo); visualization, L.F., G.D.V., C.A. and G.D.; supervision, A.M.I., F.V., A.M., C.A. and F.I.; project administration, G.M., F.V., E.M. and A.P. (Assunta Patano); All authors have read and agreed to the published version of the manuscript.

Funding: This research received no external funding.

Data Availability Statement: Not applicable.

Conflicts of Interest: The authors declare no conflict of interest.

Abbreviations

BIC	Bone implant contact
BMMSC	Multipotent mesenchymal stem cells from bone marrow
CaP	Calcium phosphate
CGF	Concentrated growth factors
Cu	Copper
DAE	Dual acid etch
GO	Graphene oxide

HF	Hydrogen fluoride
PEEK	Polyetheretherketone
RFA	Resonance frequency analysis
SA	Sandblasting and acid etching
SEM	Scanning electron microscopy
SLA	Coarse-grain blasting and acid etching
Ti	Titanium
Ti-5Cu	Titanium-copper alloy
TPS	Titanium plasma spray
TNP	Titanium nano pores

References

1. Calabriso, N.; Stanca, E.; Rochira, A.; Damiano, F.; Giannotti, L.; Di Chiara Stanca, B.; Massaro, M.; Scoditti, E.; Demitri, C.; Nitti, P.; et al. Angiogenic Properties of Concentrated Growth Factors (CGFs): The Role of Soluble Factors and Cellular Components. *Pharmaceutics* **2021**, *13*, 635. [CrossRef] [PubMed]
2. Colombo, M.; Mangano, C.; Mijiritsky, E.; Krebs, M.; Hauschild, U.; Fortin, T. Clinical Applications and Effectiveness of Guided Implant Surgery: A Critical Review Based on Randomized Controlled Trials. *BMC Oral Health* **2017**, *17*, 150. [CrossRef]
3. Osman, R.B.; Swain, M.V. A Critical Review of Dental Implant Materials with an Emphasis on Titanium versus Zirconia. *Materials* **2015**, *8*, 932–958. [CrossRef]
4. Khurshid, Z.; Hafeji, S.; Tekin, S.; Habib, S.R.; Ullah, R.; Sefat, F.; Zafar, M.S. 2—Titanium, Zirconia, and Polyetheretherketone (PEEK) as a Dental Implant Material. In *Dental Implants*; Zafar, M.S., Khurshid, Z., Khan, A.S., Najeeb, S., Sefat, F., Eds.; Woodhead Publishing Series in Biomaterials; Woodhead Publishing: Cambridge, UK, 2020; pp. 5–35. ISBN 978-0-12-819586-4.
5. Gahlert, M.; Burtscher, D.; Grunert, I.; Kniha, H.; Steinhauser, E. Failure Analysis of Fractured Dental Zirconia Implants. *Clin. Oral Implant. Res.* **2012**, *23*, 287–293. [CrossRef] [PubMed]
6. Gowda, E.M.; Iyer, S.R.; Verma, K.; Murali Mohan, S. Evaluation of PEEK Composite Dental Implants: A Comparison of Two Different Loading Protocols. *J. Dent. Res. Rep.* **2018**, *1*. [CrossRef]
7. Safi, I.N.; Hussein, B.M.A.; Aljudy, H.J.; Tukmachi, M.S. Effects of Long Durations of RF–Magnetron Sputtering Deposition of Hydroxyapatite on Titanium Dental Implants. *Eur. J. Dent.* **2021**, *15*, 440–447. [CrossRef]
8. Zhang, W.; Zhang, S.; Liu, H.; Ren, L.; Wang, Q.; Zhang, Y. Effects of Surface Roughening on Antibacterial and Osteogenic Properties of Ti-Cu Alloys with Different Cu Contents. *J. Mater. Sci. Technol.* **2021**, *88*, 158–167. [CrossRef]
9. Gao, X.; Fraulob, M.; Haïat, G. Biomechanical Behaviours of the Bone–Implant Interface: A Review. *J. R. Soc. Interface* **2019**, *16*, 20190259. [CrossRef]
10. Jain, R.; Kapoor, D. The Dynamic Interface: A Review. *J. Int. Soc. Prev. Community Dent.* **2015**, *5*, 354. [CrossRef]
11. Velloso, G.; Moraschini, V.; Dos Santos Porto Barboza, E. Hydrophilic Modification of Sandblasted and Acid-Etched Implants Improves Stability during Early Healing: A Human Double-Blind Randomized Controlled Trial. *Int. J. Oral Maxillofac. Surg.* **2019**, *48*, 684–690. [CrossRef]
12. Elias, C.N. *Factors Affecting the Success of Dental Implants*; IntechOpen: London, UK, 2011; ISBN 978-953-307-658-4.
13. Silva, E.; Félix, S.; Rodriguez-Archilla, A.; Oliveira, P.; Martins dos Santos, J. Revisiting Peri-Implant Soft Tissue—Histopathological Study of the Peri-Implant Soft Tissue. *Int. J. Clin. Exp. Pathol.* **2014**, *7*, 611–618. [PubMed]
14. Moon, I.-S.; Berglundh, T.; Abrahamsson, I.; Linder, E.; Lindhe, J. The Barrier between the Keratinized Mucosa and the Dental Implant. *J. Clin. Periodontol.* **1999**, *26*, 658–663. [CrossRef] [PubMed]
15. Barberi, J.; Spriano, S. Titanium and Protein Adsorption: An Overview of Mechanisms and Effects of Surface Features. *Materials* **2021**, *14*, 1590. [CrossRef] [PubMed]
16. Parithimarkalaignan, S.; Padmanabhan, T.V. Osseointegration: An Update. *J. Indian Prosthodont. Soc.* **2013**, *13*, 2–6. [CrossRef] [PubMed]
17. Rausch, M.A.; Shokoohi-Tabrizi, H.; Wehner, C.; Pippenger, B.E.; Wagner, R.S.; Ulm, C.; Moritz, A.; Chen, J.; Andrukhov, O. Impact of Implant Surface Material and Microscale Roughness on the Initial Attachment and Proliferation of Primary Human Gingival Fibroblasts. *Biology* **2021**, *10*, 356. [CrossRef] [PubMed]
18. Gittens, R.A.; Scheideler, L.; Rupp, F.; Hyzy, S.L.; Geis-Gerstorfer, J.; Schwartz, Z.; Boyan, B.D. A Review on the Wettability of Dental Implant Surfaces II: Biological and Clinical Aspects. *Acta Biomater.* **2014**, *10*, 2907–2918. [CrossRef]
19. Webb, K.; Hlady, V.; Tresco, P.A. Relative Importance of Surface Wettability and Charged Functional Groups on NIH 3T3 Fibroblast Attachment, Spreading, and Cytoskeletal Organization. *J. Biomed. Mater. Res.* **1998**, *41*, 422–430. [CrossRef]
20. Nychka, J.; Gentleman, M. Implications of Wettability in Biological Materials Science. *JOM* **2010**, *62*, 39–48. [CrossRef]
21. Albertini, M.; Fernandez-Yague, M.; Lázaro, P.; Herrero-Climent, M.; Rios-Santos, J.-V.; Bullon, P.; Gil, F.-J. Advances in Surfaces and Osseointegration in Implantology. Biomimetic Surfaces. *Med. Oral Patol. Oral Cir. Bucal.* **2015**, *20*, e316–e325. [CrossRef]
22. Hong, J.; Kurt, S.; Thor, A. A Hydrophilic Dental Implant Surface Exhibit Thrombogenic Properties In Vitro. *Clin. Implant. Dent. Relat. Res.* **2013**, *15*, 105–112. [CrossRef]
23. Yu, Z.; Liu, L.; Deng, Y.; Zhang, X.; Yu, C. Study on the Blood Flow Characteristics of Venous Needle Retention with Different Super-Hydrophobic Surface Structures. *Med. Biol. Eng. Comput.* **2023**, *61*, 867–874. [CrossRef]

24. Traini, T.; Murmura, G.; Sinjari, B.; Perfetti, G.; Scarano, A.; D'Arcangelo, C.; Caputi, S. The Surface Anodization of Titanium Dental Implants Improves Blood Clot Formation Followed by Osseointegration. *Coatings* **2018**, *8*, 252. [CrossRef]
25. Lotz, E.M.; Berger, M.B.; Schwartz, Z.; Boyan, B.D. Regulation of Osteoclasts by Osteoblast Lineage Cells Depends on Titanium Implant Surface Properties. *Acta Biomater.* **2018**, *68*, 296–307. [CrossRef]
26. Inchingolo, F.; Tatullo, M.; Marrelli, M.; Inchingolo, A.M.; Scacco, S.; Inchingolo, A.; Dipalma, G.; Vermesan, D.; Abbinante, A.; Cagiano, R. Trial with Platelet-Rich Fibrin and Bio-Oss Used as Grafting Materials in the Treatment of the Severe Maxillar Bone Atrophy: Clinical and Radiological Evaluations. *Eur. Rev. Med. Pharmacol. Sci.* **2010**, *14*, 1075–1084.
27. Tatullo, M.; Marrelli, M.; Cassetta, M.; Pacifici, A.; Stefanelli, L.V.; Scacco, S.; Dipalma, G.; Pacifici, L.; Inchingolo, F. Platelet Rich Fibrin (P.R.F.) in Reconstructive Surgery of Atrophied Maxillary Bones: Clinical and Histological Evaluations. *Int. J. Med. Sci.* **2012**, *9*, 872–880. [CrossRef]
28. Minetti, E.; Gianfreda, F.; Palermo, A.; Bollero, P. Autogenous Dentin Particulate Graft for Alveolar Ridge Augmentation with and without Use of Collagen Membrane: Preliminary Histological Analysis on Humans. *Materials* **2022**, *15*, 4319. [CrossRef]
29. Redžepagić-Vražalica, L.; Mešić, E.; Pervan, N.; Hadžiabdić, V.; Delić, M.; Glušac, M. Impact of Implant Design and Bone Properties on the Primary Stability of Orthodontic Mini-Implants. *Appl. Sci.* **2021**, *11*, 1183. [CrossRef]
30. Ivanova, V.; Chenchev, I.; Zlatev, S.; Mijiritsky, E. Correlation between Primary, Secondary Stability, Bone Density, Percentage of Vital Bone Formation and Implant Size. *Int. J. Environ. Res. Public Health* **2021**, *18*, 6994. [CrossRef]
31. Palermo, A.; Giannotti, L.; Di Chiara Stanca, B.; Ferrante, F.; Gnoni, A.; Nitti, P.; Calabriso, N.; Demitri, C.; Damiano, F.; Batani, T.; et al. Use of CGF in Oral and Implant Surgery: From Laboratory Evidence to Clinical Evaluation. *Int. J. Mol. Sci.* **2022**, *23*, 15164. [CrossRef]
32. Simonpieri, A.; Del Corso, M.; Vervelle, A.; Jimbo, R.; Inchingolo, F.; Sammartino, G.; Dohan Ehrenfest, D.M. Current Knowledge and Perspectives for the Use of Platelet-Rich Plasma (PRP) and Platelet-Rich Fibrin (PRF) in Oral and Maxillofacial Surgery Part 2: Bone Graft, Implant and Reconstructive Surgery. *Curr. Pharm. Biotechnol.* **2012**, *13*, 1231–1256. [CrossRef]
33. Tchinda, A.P.; Pierson, G.; Kouitat-Njiwa, R.; Bravetti, P. The Surface Conditions and Composition of Titanium Alloys in Implantology: A Comparative Study of Dental Implants of Different Brands. *Materials* **2022**, *15*, 1018. [CrossRef] [PubMed]
34. Dimonte, M.; Inchingolo, F.; Dipalma, G.; Stefanelli, M. Maxillary sinus lift in conjunction with endosseous implants. A long-term follow-up scintigraphic study. *Minerva Stomatol.* **2002**, *51*, 161–165. [PubMed]
35. Matsuo, Y.; Ogawa, T.; Yamamoto, M.; Shibamoto, A.; Sáenz, J.R.V.; Yokoyama, M.; Kanda, Y.; Toyohara, J.; Sasaki, K. Evaluation of Peri-Implant Bone Metabolism under Immediate Loading Using High-Resolution Na18F-PET. *Clin. Oral Investig.* **2017**, *21*, 2029–2037. [CrossRef] [PubMed]
36. Jeon, J.-H.; Kim, M.-J.; Yun, P.-Y.; Jo, D.-W.; Kim, Y.-K. Randomized Clinical Trial to Evaluate the Efficacy and Safety of Two Types of Sandblasted with Large-Grit and Acid-Etched Surface Implants with Different Surface Roughness. *J. Korean Assoc. Oral Maxillofac. Surg.* **2022**, *48*, 225–231. [CrossRef] [PubMed]
37. Bavetta, G.; Bavetta, G.; Randazzo, V.; Cavataio, A.; Paderni, C.; Grassia, V.; Dipalma, G.; Isacco, C.G.; Scarano, A.; Vito, D.D.; et al. A Retrospective Study on Insertion Torque and Implant Stability Quotient (ISQ) as Stability Parameters for Immediate Loading of Implants in Fresh Extraction Sockets. *BioMed Res. Int.* **2019**, *2019*, 9720419. [CrossRef]
38. Bereznai, M.; Pelsöczi, I.; Tóth, Z.; Turzó, K.; Radnai, M.; Bor, Z.; Fazekas, A. Surface Modifications Induced by Ns and Sub-Ps Excimer Laser Pulses on Titanium Implant Material. *Biomaterials* **2003**, *24*, 4197–4203. [CrossRef]
39. Scarano, A.; Khater, A.G.A.; Gehrke, S.A.; Serra, P.; Francesco, I.; Di Carmine, M.; Tari, S.R.; Leo, L.; Lorusso, F. Current Status of Peri-Implant Diseases: A Clinical Review for Evidence-Based Decision Making. *J. Funct. Biomater.* **2023**, *14*, 210. [CrossRef]
40. Converti, I.; Palermo, A.; Mancini, A.; Maggiore, M.E.; Tartaglia, G.M.; Ferrara, E.; Vecchiet, F.; Lorusso, F.; Scarano, A.; Bordea, I.R.; et al. Chewing and Cognitive Performance: What We Know. *J. Biol. Regul. Homeost. Agents* **2022**, *36*, 193–204. [CrossRef]
41. Coccia, M. Probability of Discoveries between Research Fields to Explain Scientific and Technological Change. *Technol. Soc.* **2022**, *68*, 101874. [CrossRef]
42. Converti, I.; Palermo, A.; Mancini, A.; Maggiore, M.E.; Ferrara, E.; Vecchiet, F.; Sforza, C.; Maspero, C.; Farronato, M.; Cagetti, M.G.; et al. The Effects of Physical Exercise on the Brain and Oral Health. *J. Biol. Regul. Homeost. Agents* **2022**, *36*, 425–437.
43. Bielemann, A.M.; Schuster, A.J.; da Rosa Possebon, A.P.; Schinestsck, A.R.; Chagas-Junior, O.L.; Faot, F. Clinical Performance of Narrow-Diameter Implants with Hydrophobic and Hydrophilic Surfaces with Mandibular Implant Overdentures: 1-Year Results of a Randomized Clinical Trial. *Clin. Oral Implant. Res.* **2022**, *33*, 21–32. [CrossRef]
44. Gursoytrak, B.; Ataoglu, H. Use of Resonance Frequency Analysis to Evaluate the Effects of Surface Properties on the Stability of Different Implants. *Clin. Oral Implant. Res.* **2020**, *31*, 239–245. [CrossRef]
45. Hasegawa, M.; Saruta, J.; Hirota, M.; Taniyama, T.; Sugita, Y.; Kubo, K.; Ishijima, M.; Ikeda, T.; Maeda, H.; Ogawa, T. A Newly Created Meso-, Micro-, and Nano-Scale Rough Titanium Surface Promotes Bone-Implant Integration. *Int. J. Mol. Sci.* **2020**, *21*, 783. [CrossRef]
46. Ko, K.-A.; Kim, S.; Choi, S.-H.; Lee, J.-S. Randomized Controlled Clinical Trial on Calcium Phosphate Coated and Conventional SLA Surface Implants: 1-Year Study on Survival Rate and Marginal Bone Level. *Clin. Implant. Dent. Relat. Res.* **2019**, *21*, 995–1001. [CrossRef]

47. Körmöczi, K.; Komlós, G.; Papócsi, P.; Horváth, F.; Joób-Fancsaly, Á. The Early Loading of Different Surface-Modified Implants: A Randomized Clinical Trial. *BMC Oral Health* **2021**, *21*, 207. [CrossRef]
48. Chauhan, P.; Koul, V.; Bhatnagar, N. Critical Role of Etching Parameters in the Evolution of Nano Micro SLA Surface on the Ti6Al4V Alloy Dental Implants. *Materials* **2021**, *14*, 6344. [CrossRef]
49. Gavinho, S.R.; Pádua, A.S.; Sá-Nogueira, I.; Silva, J.C.; Borges, J.P.; Costa, L.C.; Graça, M.P.F. Biocompatibility, Bioactivity, and Antibacterial Behaviour of Cerium-Containing Bioglass®. *Nanomaterials* **2022**, *12*, 4479. [CrossRef]
50. Schupbach, P.; Glauser, R.; Bauer, S. Al_2O_3 Particles on Titanium Dental Implant Systems Following Sandblasting and Acid-Etching Process. *Int. J. Biomater.* **2019**, *2019*, e6318429. [CrossRef]
51. Lorusso, F.; Conte, R.; Inchingolo, F.; Festa, F.; Scarano, A. Survival Rate of Zygomatic Implants for Fixed Oral Maxillary Rehabilitations: A Systematic Review and Meta-Analysis Comparing Outcomes between Zygomatic and Regular Implants. *Dent. J.* **2021**, *9*, 38. [CrossRef]
52. Williams, J.C.; Boyer, R.R. Opportunities and Issues in the Application of Titanium Alloys for Aerospace Components. *Metals* **2020**, *10*, 705. [CrossRef]
53. Zhou, J.; Wang, X.; Zhao, L. Antibacterial, Angiogenic, and Osteogenic Activities of Ca, P, Co, F, and Sr Compound Doped Titania Coatings with Different Sr Content. *Sci. Rep.* **2019**, *9*, 14203. [CrossRef] [PubMed]
54. Llor, C.; Bjerrum, L. Antimicrobial Resistance: Risk Associated with Antibiotic Overuse and Initiatives to Reduce the Problem. *Ther. Adv. Drug. Saf.* **2014**, *5*, 229–241. [CrossRef]
55. López-Valverde, N.; Macedo-de-Sousa, B.; López-Valverde, A.; Ramírez, J.M. Effectiveness of Antibacterial Surfaces in Osseointegration of Titanium Dental Implants: A Systematic Review. *Antibiotics* **2021**, *10*, 360. [CrossRef] [PubMed]
56. Sindeeva, O.A.; Prikhozhdenko, E.S.; Schurov, I.; Sedykh, N.; Goriainov, S.; Karamyan, A.; Mordovina, E.A.; Inozemtseva, O.A.; Kudryavtseva, V.; Shchesnyak, L.E.; et al. Patterned Drug-Eluting Coatings for Tracheal Stents Based on PLA, PLGA, and PCL for the Granulation Formation Reduction: In Vivo Studies. *Pharmaceutics* **2021**, *13*, 1437. [CrossRef] [PubMed]
57. Inchingolo, A.M.; Malcangi, G.; Inchingolo, A.D.; Mancini, A.; Palmieri, G.; Di Pede, C.; Piras, F.; Inchingolo, F.; Dipalma, G.; Patano, A. Potential of Graphene-Functionalized Titanium Surfaces for Dental Implantology: Systematic Review. *Coatings* **2023**, *13*, 725. [CrossRef]
58. Inchingolo, A.D.; Inchingolo, A.M.; Bordea, I.R.; Xhajanka, E.; Romeo, D.M.; Romeo, M.; Zappone, C.M.F.; Malcangi, G.; Scarano, A.; Lorusso, F.; et al. The Effectiveness of Osseodensification Drilling Protocol for Implant Site Osteotomy: A Systematic Review of the Literature and Meta-Analysis. *Materials* **2021**, *14*, 1147. [CrossRef]
59. Hazballa, D.; Inchingolo, A.; Inchingolo, A.M.; Malcangi, G.; Santacroce, L.; Minetti, E.; Di Venere, D.; Limongelli, L.; Bordea, I.; Scarano, A.; et al. The Effectiveness of Autologous Demineralized Tooth Graft for the Bone Ridge Preservation: A Systematic Review of the Literature. *J. Biol. Regul. Homeost. Agents* **2021**, *35*, 283–294. [CrossRef]
60. Smeets, R.; Stadlinger, B.; Schwarz, F.; Beck-Broichsitter, B.; Jung, O.; Precht, C.; Kloss, F.; Gröbe, A.; Heiland, M.; Ebker, T. Impact of Dental Implant Surface Modifications on Osseointegration. *BioMed Res. Int.* **2016**, *2016*, 6285620. [CrossRef]
61. Asensio, G.; Vázquez-Lasa, B.; Rojo, L. Achievements in the Topographic Design of Commercial Titanium Dental Implants: Towards Anti-Peri-Implantitis Surfaces. *J. Clin. Med.* **2019**, *8*, 1982. [CrossRef]
62. Jemat, A.; Ghazali, M.J.; Razali, M.; Otsuka, Y. Surface Modifications and Their Effects on Titanium Dental Implants. *BioMed Res. Int.* **2015**, *2015*, 791725. [CrossRef]
63. Park, C.-J.; Lim, J.H.; Tallarico, M.; Hwang, K.-G.; Choi, H.; Cho, G.-J.; Kim, C.; Jang, I.-S.; Song, J.-D.; Kwon, A.M.; et al. Coating of a Sand-Blasted and Acid-Etched Implant Surface with a PH-Buffering Agent after Vacuum-UV Photofunctionalization. *Coatings* **2020**, *10*, 1040. [CrossRef]
64. Stavropoulos, A.; Bertl, K.; Winning, L.; Polyzois, I. What Is the Influence of Implant Surface Characteristics and/or Implant Material on the Incidence and Progression of Peri-Implantitis? A Systematic Literature Review. *Clin. Oral Implant. Res.* **2021**, *32*, 203–229. [CrossRef]
65. Lorusso, F.; Mastrangelo, F.; Inchingolo, F.; Mortellaro, C.; Scarano, A. In Vitro Interface Changes of Two vs Three Narrow-Diameter Dental Implants for Screw-Retained Bar under Fatigue Loading Test. *J. Biol. Regul. Homeost. Agents* **2019**, *33*, 115–120.
66. Medvedev, A.E.; Ng, H.P.; Lapovok, R.; Estrin, Y.; Lowe, T.C.; Anumalasetty, V.N. Effect of Bulk Microstructure of Commercially Pure Titanium on Surface Characteristics and Fatigue Properties after Surface Modification by Sand Blasting and Acid-Etching. *J. Mech. Behav. Biomed. Mater.* **2016**, *57*, 55–68. [CrossRef]
67. Finger, C.; Stiesch, M.; Eisenburger, M.; Breidenstein, B.; Busemann, S.; Greuling, A. Effect of Sandblasting on the Surface Roughness and Residual Stress of 3Y-TZP (Zirconia). *SN Appl. Sci.* **2020**, *2*, 1700. [CrossRef]
68. Velasco-Ortega, E.; Alfonso-Rodríguez, C.A.; Monsalve-Guil, L.; España-López, A.; Jiménez-Guerra, A.; Garzón, I.; Alaminos, M.; Gil, F.J. Relevant Aspects in the Surface Properties in Titanium Dental Implants for the Cellular Viability. *Mater. Sci. Eng. C* **2016**, *64*, 1–10. [CrossRef]
69. Giner, L.; Mercadé, M.; Torrent, S.; Punset, M.; Pérez, R.A.; Delgado, L.M.; Gil, F.J. Double Acid Etching Treatment of Dental Implants for Enhanced Biological Properties. *J. Appl. Biomater. Funct. Mater.* **2018**, *16*, 83–89. [CrossRef]
70. Rapone, B.; Inchingolo, A.D.; Trasarti, S.; Ferrara, E.; Qorri, E.; Mancini, A.; Montemurro, N.; Scarano, A.; Inchingolo, A.M.; Dipalma, G.; et al. Long-Term Outcomes of Implants Placed in Maxillary Sinus Floor Augmentation with Porous Fluorohydroxyapatite (Algipore® FRIOS®) in Comparison with Anorganic Bovine Bone (Bio-Oss®) and Platelet Rich Plasma (PRP): A Retrospective Study. *J. Clin. Med.* **2022**, *11*, 2491. [CrossRef]

71. Steller, D.; Simon, R.; Bialy, R.V.; Pries, R.; Hakim, S.G. Impact of Zoledronic Acid and Denosumab Treatment on Growth Factor Concentration in Platelet Rich Fibrin of Patients With Osteolytic Bone Metastases. *Anticancer Res.* **2021**, *41*, 3917–3923. [CrossRef]
72. Lazzara, R.J.; Testori, T.; Trisi, P.; Porter, S.S.; Weinstein, R.L. A Human Histologic Analysis of Osseotite and Machined Surfaces Using Implants with 2 Opposing Surfaces. *Int. J. Periodontics Restor. Dent.* **1999**, *19*, 117–129.
73. Gulati, K.; Moon, H.-J.; Li, T.; Sudheesh Kumar, P.T.; Ivanovski, S. Titania Nanopores with Dual Micro-/Nano-Topography for Selective Cellular Bioactivity. *Mater. Sci. Eng. C* **2018**, *91*, 624–630. [CrossRef] [PubMed]
74. Jayasree, A.; Raveendran, N.T.; Guo, T.; Ivanovski, S.; Gulati, K. Electrochemically Nano-Engineered Titanium: Influence of Dual Micro-Nanotopography of Anisotropic Nanopores on Bioactivity and Antimicrobial Activity. *Mater. Today Adv.* **2022**, *15*, 100256. [CrossRef]
75. Alipal, J.; Lee, T.C.; Koshy, P.; Abdullah, H.Z.; Idris, M.I. Evolution of Anodised Titanium for Implant Applications. *Heliyon* **2021**, *7*, e07408. [CrossRef] [PubMed]
76. Yao, C.; Webster, T. Anodization: A Promising Nano-Modification Technique of Titanium Implants for Orthopedic Applications. *J. Nanosci. Nanotechnol.* **2006**, *6*, 2682–2692. [CrossRef] [PubMed]
77. Kozelskaya, A.I.; Rutkowski, S.; Frueh, J.; Gogolev, A.S.; Chistyakov, S.G.; Gnedenkov, S.V.; Sinebryukhov, S.L.; Frueh, A.; Egorkin, V.S.; Choynzonov, E.L.; et al. Surface Modification of Additively Fabricated Titanium-Based Implants by Means of Bioactive Micro-Arc Oxidation Coatings for Bone Replacement. *J. Funct. Biomater.* **2022**, *13*, 285. [CrossRef]
78. Eftekhar Ashtiani, R.; Alam, M.; Tavakolizadeh, S.; Abbasi, K. The Role of Biomaterials and Biocompatible Materials in Implant-Supported Dental Prosthesis. *Evid. Based Complement. Altern. Med.* **2021**, *2021*, e3349433. [CrossRef]
79. Gauthier, O.; Müller, R.; von Stechow, D.; Lamy, B.; Weiss, P.; Bouler, J.-M.; Aguado, E.; Daculsi, G. In Vivo Bone Regeneration with Injectable Calcium Phosphate Biomaterial: A Three-Dimensional Micro-Computed Tomographic, Biomechanical and SEM Study. *Biomaterials* **2005**, *26*, 5444–5453. [CrossRef]
80. López-Valverde, N.; Aragoneses, J.; López-Valverde, A.; Rodríguez, C.; Sousa, B.; Aragoneses, J. Role of Chitosan in Titanium Coatings. Trends and New Generations of Coatings. *Front. Bioeng. Biotechnol.* **2022**, *10*, 907589. [CrossRef]
81. Thorat Gadgil, B.S.; Killi, N.; Rathna, G.V.N. Polyhydroxyalkanoates as Biomaterials. *MedChemComm* **2017**, *8*, 1774–1787. [CrossRef]
82. Dalton, B.; Bhagabati, P.; De Micco, J.; Padamati, R.B.; O'Connor, K. A Review on Biological Synthesis of the Biodegradable Polymers Polyhydroxyalkanoates and the Development of Multiple Applications. *Catalysts* **2022**, *12*, 319. [CrossRef]
83. Inchingolo, A.D.; Inchingolo, A.M.; Malcangi, G.; Avantario, P.; Azzollini, D.; Buongiorno, S.; Viapiano, F.; Campanelli, M.; Ciocia, A.M.; De Leonardis, N.; et al. Effects of Resveratrol, Curcumin and Quercetin Supplementation on Bone Metabolism—A Systematic Review. *Nutrients* **2022**, *14*, 3519. [CrossRef]
84. Scarano, A.; Assenza, B.; Inchingolo, F.; Mastrangelo, F.; Lorusso, F. New Implant Design with Midcrestal and Apical Wing Thread for Increased Implant Stability in Single Postextraction Maxillary Implant. *Case Rep. Dent.* **2019**, *2019*, 9529248. [CrossRef]
85. Comuzzi, L.; Tumedei, M.; Romasco, T.; Petrini, M.; Afrashtehfar, K.I.; Inchingolo, F.; Piattelli, A.; Di Pietro, N. Insertion Torque, Removal Torque, and Resonance Frequency Analysis Values of Ultrashort, Short, and Standard Dental Implants: An In Vitro Study on Polyurethane Foam Sheets. *J. Funct. Biomater.* **2023**, *14*, 10. [CrossRef]
86. Ciosek, Ż.; Kot, K.; Kosik-Bogacka, D.; Łanocha-Arendarczyk, N.; Rotter, I. The Effects of Calcium, Magnesium, Phosphorus, Fluoride, and Lead on Bone Tissue. *Biomolecules* **2021**, *11*, 506. [CrossRef]
87. Mavriqi, L.; Lorusso, F.; Tartaglia, G.; Inchingolo, F.; Scarano, A. Transinusal Pathway Removal of an Impacted Third Molar with an Unusual Approach: A Case Report and a Systematic Review of the Literature. *Antibiotics* **2022**, *11*, 658. [CrossRef]
88. Everett, E.T. Fluoride's Effects on the Formation of Teeth and Bones, and the Influence of Genetics. *J. Dent. Res.* **2011**, *90*, 552–560. [CrossRef]
89. Li, Q.; Wang, Z. Involvement of FAK/P38 Signaling Pathways in Mediating the Enhanced Osteogenesis Induced by Nano-Graphene Oxide Modification on Titanium Implant Surface. *Int. J. Nanomed.* **2020**, *15*, 4659–4676. [CrossRef]
90. Lorusso, F.; Inchingolo, F.; Greco Lucchina, A.; Scogna, G.; Scarano, A. Graphene-Doped Poly(Methyl-Methacrylate) as an Enhanced Biopolymer for Medical Device and Dental Implant. *J. Biol. Regul. Homeost. Agents* **2021**, *35*, 195–204. [CrossRef]
91. Ma, S.; Luo, X.; Ran, G.; Zhou, Z.; Xie, J.; Li, Y.; Li, X.; Yan, J.; Cai, W.; Wang, L. Copper Stabilized Bimetallic Alloy Cu–Bi by Convenient Strategy Fabrication: A Novel Fenton-like and Photothermal Synergistic Antibacterial Platform. *J. Clean. Prod.* **2022**, *336*, 130431. [CrossRef]
92. Liu, J.; Li, F.; Liu, C.; Wang, H.; Ren, B.; Yang, K.; Zhang, E. Effect of Cu Content on the Antibacterial Activity of Titanium–Copper Sintered Alloys. *Mater. Sci. Eng. C* **2014**, *35*, 392–400. [CrossRef]
93. Su, Y.; Cappock, M.; Dobres, S.; Kucine, A.J.; Waltzer, W.C.; Zhu, D. Supplemental Mineral Ions for Bone Regeneration and Osteoporosis Treatment. *Eng. Regen.* **2023**, *4*, 170–182. [CrossRef]
94. Zhao, X.; Zhou, X.; Sun, H.; Shi, H.; Song, Y.; Wang, Q.; Zhang, G.; Xu, D. 3D Printed Ti-5Cu Alloy Accelerates Osteogenic Differentiation of MC3T3-E1 Cells by Stimulating the M2 Phenotype Polarization of Macrophages. *Front. Immunol.* **2022**, *13*, 1001526. [CrossRef] [PubMed]
95. De Avila, E.D.; van Oirschot, B.A.; van den Beucken, J.J.J.P. Biomaterial-based Possibilities for Managing Peri-implantitis. *J. Periodontal Res.* **2020**, *55*, 165–173. [CrossRef] [PubMed]
96. Prathapachandran, J.; Suresh, N. Management of Peri-Implantitis. *Dent. Res. J.* **2012**, *9*, 516–521. [CrossRef]

97. Lorusso, F.; Tartaglia, G.; Inchingolo, F.; Scarano, A. Peri-Implant Mucositis Treatment with a Chlorexidine Gel with A.D.S. 0.5%, PVP-VA and Sodium DNA vs. a Placebo Gel: A Randomized Controlled Pilot Clinical Trial. *Front. Biosci.* **2022**, *14*, 30. [CrossRef]
98. Scarano, A.; Inchingolo, F.; Scogna, S.; Leo, L.; Greco Lucchina, A.; Mavriqi, L. Peri-Implant Disease Caused by Residual Cement around Implant-Supported Restorations: A Clinical Report. *J. Biol. Regul. Homeost. Agents* **2021**, *35*, 211–216. [CrossRef]
99. Osman, M.A.; Alamoush, R.A.; Kushnerev, E.; Seymour, K.G.; Watts, D.C.; Yates, J.M. Biological Response of Epithelial and Connective Tissue Cells to Titanium Surfaces with Different Ranges of Roughness: An in-Vitro Study. *Dent. Mater.* **2022**, *38*, 1777–1788. [CrossRef]
100. Libonati, A.; Marzo, G.; Klinger, F.G.; Farini, D.; Gallusi, G.; Tecco, S.; Mummolo, S.; De Felici, M.; Campanella, V. Embryotoxicity Assays for Leached Components from Dental Restorative Materials. *Reprod. Biol. Endocrinol.* **2011**, *9*, 136. [CrossRef]
101. Kim, J.-J.; Lee, J.-H.; Kim, J.C.; Lee, J.-B.; Yeo, I.-S.L. Biological Responses to the Transitional Area of Dental Implants: Material- and Structure-Dependent Responses of Peri-Implant Tissue to Abutments. *Materials* **2019**, *13*, 72. [CrossRef]
102. Schmitz, S.I.; Widholz, B.; Essers, C.; Becker, M.; Tulyaganov, D.U.; Moghaddam, A.; Gonzalo de Juan, I.; Westhauser, F. Superior Biocompatibility and Comparable Osteoinductive Properties: Sodium-Reduced Fluoride-Containing Bioactive Glass Belonging to the CaO–MgO–SiO2 System as a Promising Alternative to 45S5 Bioactive Glass. *Bioact. Mater.* **2020**, *5*, 55–65. [CrossRef]
103. Lokwani, B.V.; Gupta, D.; Agrawal, R.S.; Mehta, S.; Nirmal, N.J. The Use of Concentrated Growth Factor in Dental Implantology: A Systematic Review. *J. Indian Prosthodont. Soc.* **2020**, *20*, 3–10. [CrossRef]
104. Mummolo, S.; Mancini, L.; Quinzi, V.; D'Aquino, R.; Marzo, G.; Marchetti, E. Rigenera® Autologous Micrografts in Oral Regeneration: Clinical, Histological, and Radiographical Evaluations. *Appl. Sci.* **2020**, *10*, 5084. [CrossRef]
105. Bielemann, A.M.; Marcello-Machado, R.M.; Leite, F.R.M.; Martinho, F.C.; Chagas-Júnior, O.L.; Antoninha Del Bel Cury, A.; Faot, F. Comparison between Inflammation-Related Markers in Peri-Implant Crevicular Fluid and Clinical Parameters during Osseointegration in Edentulous Jaws. *Clin. Oral Investig.* **2018**, *22*, 531–543. [CrossRef]
106. Tranquillo, E.; Bollino, F. Surface Modifications for Implants Lifetime Extension: An Overview of Sol-Gel Coatings. *Coatings* **2020**, *10*, 589. [CrossRef]
107. Palermo, A.; Minetti, E.; Bellinvia, C.G.; Ferronato, D.; Conte, E. Full Arch Immediate Loading in the Upper Jaw. *Dent. Cadmos* **2010**, *78*, 89–98.
108. Yazici, H.; Fong, H.; Wilson, B.; Oren, E.E.; Amos, F.A.; Zhang, H.; Evans, J.S.; Snead, M.L.; Sarikaya, M.; Tamerler, C. Biological Response on a Titanium Implant-Grade Surface Functionalized with Modular Peptides. *Acta Biomater.* **2013**, *9*, 5341–5352. [CrossRef]
109. Tumedei, M.; Piattelli, A.; Degidi, M.; Mangano, C.; Iezzi, G. A Narrative Review of the Histological and Histomorphometrical Evaluation of the Peri-Implant Bone in Loaded and Unloaded Dental Implants. A 30-Year Experience (1988–2018). *Int. J. Environ. Res. Public Health* **2020**, *17*, 2088. [CrossRef]
110. Alla, I.; Lorusso, F.; Gehrke, S.A.; Inchingolo, F.; Di Carmine, M.; Scarano, A. Implant Survival in Patients with Chronic Kidney Disease: A Case Report and Systematic Review of the Literature. *Int. J. Environ. Res. Public Health* **2023**, *20*, 2401. [CrossRef]
111. DENTAL SUPPLEMENT; Minetti, E.; Palermo, A.; Savadori, P.; Barlattani, A.; Franco, R.; Michele, M.; Gianfreda, F.; Bollero, P. Autologous Tooth Graft: A Histological Comparison between Dentin Mixed with Xenograft and Dentin Alone Grafts in Socket Preservation. *J. Biol. Regul. Homeost. Agents* **2019**, *33*, 189–197.

Disclaimer/Publisher's Note: The statements, opinions and data contained in all publications are solely those of the individual author(s) and contributor(s) and not of MDPI and/or the editor(s). MDPI and/or the editor(s) disclaim responsibility for any injury to people or property resulting from any ideas, methods, instructions or products referred to in the content.

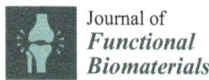 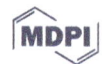

Article

Effects of Surface Preparation Methods on the Color Stability of 3D-Printed Dental Restorations

Zbigniew Raszewski [1], Katarzyna Chojnacka [2] and Marcin Mikulewicz [3,*]

[1] SpofaDental, Markova 238, 506-01 Jicin, Czech Republic; zbigniew.raszewski@envistaco.com
[2] Department of Advanced Material Technologies, Faculty of Chemistry, Wroclaw University of Science and Technology, Smoluchowskiego 25, 50-372 Wroclaw, Poland; katarzyna.chojnacka@pwr.edu.pl
[3] Department of Dentofacial Orthopaedics and Orthodontics, Division of Facial Abnormalities, Wroclaw Medical University, Krakowska 26, 50-425 Wroclaw, Poland
* Correspondence: marcin.mikulewicz@umw.edu.pl

Abstract: Background: Color stability is a crucial performance parameter for dental restorations, and limited research exists on how surface preparation methods affect it. The purpose of this study was to test the color stability of three resins intended for 3D printing, which can be used to make dentures or crowns in A2 and A3 colors. Materials and Methods: Samples were prepared in the form of incisors; the first group was not subjected to any treatment after curing and washing with alcohol, the second was covered with light-curing varnish, and the third was polished in a standard way. Then, the samples were placed in solutions of coffee, red wine, and distilled water and stored in the laboratory. After 14, 30, and 60 days, color changes were measured (presented as Delta E) compared to material stored in the dark. Results: The greatest changes were observed for samples that were not polished, then were placed in red wine dilutions (ΔE = 18.19 ± 0.16). Regarding the samples covered with varnish, during storage, some parts detached, and the dyes penetrated inside. Conclusions: 3D-printed material should be polished as thoroughly as possible to limit the adhesion of dyes from food to their surface. Applying varnish may be a temporary solution.

Keywords: 3D printing; dental restorations; color stability; surface preparation; polishing; varnishing; red wine; coffee

1. Introduction

The field of dentistry has seen rapid advancements in the development of dental materials over the past few decades. One of the most important aspects of dental materials is their ability to mimic the natural appearance of teeth. The esthetic expectations of patients have been continuously increasing, leading to a greater demand for dental restorations that can achieve a high level of color stability, biocompatibility, and mechanical properties.

The color stability of dental materials is crucial because it ensures that the restoration maintains its original color and appearance over time. When dental materials are exposed to staining agents, such as coffee or red wine, they can discolor and become unsightly. Patients expect their dental restorations to match the natural appearance of their teeth, and the development of dental materials with enhanced color stability can help achieve this goal.

Three-dimensional printing is increasingly utilized in healthcare due to its ability to create patient-specific restorations with the necessary accuracy and precision. Examples of 3D printing technology applications include implanted heart valves, elements of rib cages, bones, dentures, orthodontic appliances, and the first maxillofacial implants [1].

Three-dimensional printing technology has revolutionized various industries, including dentistry, by offering more efficient and precise methods for fabricating dental restorations [2]. Additive manufacturing techniques, such as stereolithography (SLA), digital light processing (DLP), and selective laser sintering (SLS), enable the production of dental prostheses with complex geometries and intricate structures that would be difficult to achieve through traditional manufacturing methods [3,4]. The use of resin materials in 3D printing has gained popularity in recent years due to their versatility, biocompatibility, and favorable mechanical properties [5,6]. Additionally, 3D printing has proven to be advantageous in terms of reduced chair time, customization, and waste compared to CAD CAM technology [7].

The decreasing cost of professional printers has led to a surge of interest in this technology among dental technicians, particularly in the use of SLA technology with light-curing resins. Three-dimensional printing technology can also be used in the dental office, especially when it comes to making temporary crowns and bridges. This has allowed for a reduction in the number of visits; during one chair time, the patient can have their dental arches scanned. Using databases from the computer, the design of the future temporary restoration is adjusted. While the dentist is grinding the teeth, the dental assistant can 3D-print a temporary crown or bridge. [8].

Loges and Tiberius address the implementation challenges of 3D printing in prosthodontics, highlighting the need for further research and development. Among the key advantages of this technique are the capacity to print multiple prosthetic elements simultaneously, such as crowns, bridges, and removable dentures, and the elimination of intermediate steps like wax modeling and plaster use [9].

Color stability is a critical aspect of dental restorations, as it directly impacts the esthetic outcome and patient satisfaction [10]. Factors such as staining solutions, surface treatments, and resin composition can affect the color stability of dental materials [11,12]. Dental restorations are frequently exposed to staining agents like coffee, tea, and red wine, which may cause discoloration over time [13]. To ensure the longevity and esthetic appearance of dental restorations, it is crucial to investigate the color stability of 3D-printed dental materials and evaluate the effects of different surface treatments.

Color stability is a crucial performance parameter for patients, and as such, new materials entering the market should be tested for this attribute. Studies have identified various beverages, including coffee, red wine, orange juice, and burqa juice, as agents that can alter the color of materials, including 3D-printed elements [8,14–16].

However, limited research exists on how surface preparation methods affect color stability and the geometry of printed objects [17,18]. There are various guidelines in the literature on how to cure samples after polymerization in the printer. For this purpose, you can cover the samples with glycerin, use resin, or raise the temperature during polymerization in the light oven.

A change in the color of printed restorations may also occur during their use in the mouth, as a result of changes in the temperature of the food eaten and tooth brushing with toothpastes and brushes [19].

The speed of printing and the thickness of individual layers affects the mechanical properties of the obtained product, which is very important from the point of view of materials used in medicine. Finite Element (FE) simulations are very useful for analyzing this phenomenon [20].

As each material can be cured in various ways, the obtained results may be significantly influenced by factors such as the thickness and shape of the element itself.

Dental technicians and dentists often question the proper method for finishing a prosthetic restoration. Should self-polishing suffice, or should surfaces be protected with varnishes? [21]. The aim of this study is to address this question by determining the color change of three types of resins designed for 3D printing when placed in different media: coffee, red wine, and distilled water, for two months. Based on previous in vitro tests described in the literature, it is assumed that 24 h in the staining solution simulates food intake for 30 days [22]. The 60-day period can successfully indicate how the material will behave throughout its entire service life, assuming that the use of one prosthesis lasts 2–3 years maximum.

The purpose of this study was to test the color stability of three resins intended for 3D printing, which can be used to make removable dentures or crowns and bridges in A2 and A3 colors. The hypothesis put forward at the beginning of this study is that there will be no separation between surfaces prepared in different ways or test solutions.

2. Materials and Methods

2.1. 3D Printing and Sample Preparation

Three commercial resins from NextDent were utilized for the tests: Denture 3D+ (dark pink color), Crowntec (color A3), and A2 (NextDent, Soesterberg, The Netherlands). The framework composition of the tested materials based on the available SDS is presented in Table 1. The materials were mixed prior to use with moving rollers for 1 h to ensure proper mixing of the dyes within the resin (according to the manufacturer's instructions). In total, 141 incisor tooth models were printed, with 47 models for each resin type (Figure 1). The specimens were designed using 3D Builder (10.1.9.0, Microsoft Corporation, Redmont, WA, USA). An STL file of the digital model was uploaded to the software and printed using Liquid Crystal Precision (Photocentric Ltd., Peterborough, UK) with Daylight Polymer Printing technology. The upper central incisors were manufactured layer by layer, with irradiation time for the printing of a single layer of 25 μm thickness being 2 s, and the wavelength being 372 nm. The printing orientation (in a horizontal position) was chosen to maximize accuracy and speed. The position of the samples during printing is very important when it comes to their precision.

Table 1. Composition of testing resins.

Material	Composition
Denture 3D+ Crowntec A3 and A2	Ethoxylated bisphenol A dimethacrylate => 75%, 7,7,9(or 7,9,9)-trimethyl-4,13-dioxo-3,14-dioxa-5,12-diazahexadecane-1,16-diyl bismethacrylate 10–20% 2-hydroxyethyl methacrylate 5–10% Silicon dioxide 5–10% diphenyl(2,4,6- trimethylbenzoyl)phosphine oxide 1–5% Titanium dioxide < 0.1%

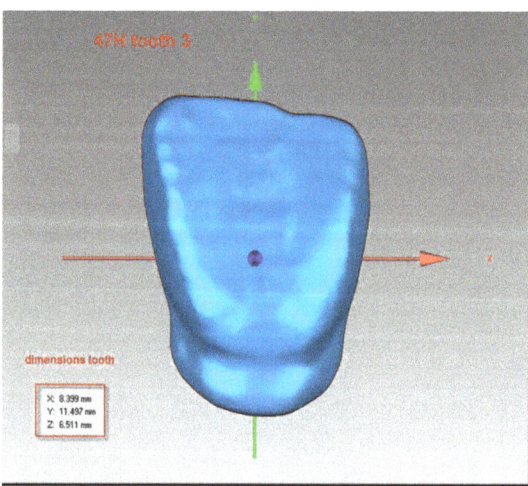

Figure 1. Tooth design before printing in a 3D printer.

When the 3D printer finished its program, objects were removed from the printer building platform with the help of a spatula, and excess resin was cleaned off with a paper towel. After this stage, the samples were coated with glycerin (Sigma Aldrich, Prague, Czech Republic) to protect from the unpolymerized layer, and irradiated in an Evicrobox (SpofaDental, Jicin, Czech Republic) light oven for 10 min, with a power of 1000 watts, and a wavelength of 370 nm. They were then then subjected to an isopropanol bath to remove non-polymerized layers, for 10 min in 98% isopropanol (Sigma Aldrich, Prague, Czech Republic) using a 50 Watt GUC 06A 6L lab ultrasonic washer (Geti, Birmingham, UK). Isopropyl alcohol is effective in cleaning the build plate of the 3D printer and does not leave marks or deposits on the printed elements. The details were discussed in our previous work, Raszewski et al. [23].

2.2. Sample Groups

The materials were then divided into four groups:

1. The first group (45 samples) was polished using a 100-micron pumice (EcoPolish Pumice, Goslar, Sliadent, Germany) mixed with water (2:1 ratio) on a WP-EX 2000 II (Wassermann Polishing Units, Ontario Canada) with a felt polishing wheel for 5 min at 800 rpm.
2. The second group (45 incisors) was coated twice with Optiglaze (GC, Tokyo, Japan) varnish and polymerized in the Evicorbox light chamber for 20 min.
3. The third group (45 samples) served as a control and was not processed in any way.
4. The fourth group (6 teeth) was stored in darkness at 23 °C as a reference. Only the 6th sample was selected as a reference sample, because the material is not exposed to factors that can change the color when stored in the dark and at room temperature.

2.3. Color Stability Testing

An X Rite spectrophotometer (X Rite, Grand Rapids, MI, USA) measured the initial color of each sample, providing L, a, b values. The color differences were recalculated as Delta E using the device's built-in software (according to Formula (1)). Materials stored under laboratory conditions (group 4) were measured as a reference at the initial step of each measurement in the middle part of the tooth. The resin stored in the dye solutions was measured after the reference tooth from group 4. Each measurement was made 3 times in the middle part of the tooth. Then, the device automatically calculated the average value of the 3 measurements and total color change as Delta E:

$$\Delta E = \sqrt{(L1 - L0)^2 + (a1 - a0)^2 + (b1 - b0)^2} \tag{1}$$

where $L1 - L0$—the difference between the brightness of the samples before and after placement in the staining solutions.

$a1 - a0$—color change on the red-green axis

$b1 - b0$—color change on the yellow-blue axis

Red wine and coffee solutions are standard testing solutions for color changes in prosthetic restorations [11]. A Tschibo Family (Tschibo, Hamburg, Germany) soluble coffee solution and Aguia Moura red wine (Portugal, Douro were prepared. Soluble coffee was prepared by dissolving 2 teaspoons in 200 mL of hot water. For one experiment, 2 L of coffee was prepared. After reaching the temperature of 40 °C, the coffee was divided into 3 PE pots—20 mL. In each solution, 1 sample was placed.

The second test solution was Aguia Moura red wine (Portugal, Douro). After opening the bottle, the contents were poured into PE containers, 20 mL each, in which one sample from the 3 tested resins was placed.

Distilled water was used as the reference solution, into which the rest of the samples were placed.

All the samples were stored at 37 °C in a laboratory drier. Once a week, the solutions were exchanged for new ones. The samples were examined after 14, 30, and 60 days of storage in staining solutions. Before testing, the samples were washed with running water and wiped with a paper towel.

2.4. Surface Analysis

During the testing period, material surfaces were analyzed under an optical microscope at 5× magnification (Karl Zeiss, Jena, Germany).

2.5. Statistical Analysis

The data were presented as mean and standard deviation (SD). One-way ANOVA was used for statistical analysis. Samples stored in staining solutions were compared with reference samples at 23 °C under laboratory conditions. Statistical analysis was performed with IBM SPSS Statistics for Windows, Version 26.0. IBM Corp. (Armonk, NY, USA). A significance level of $p < 0.05$ was assumed, with time as a variable.

3. Results

Tables 2–4 present the results of color changes in individual solutions over time for the three tested resins: Crowntec A2, Crowntec A3, and Denture 3D+.

Table 2. Color change of Crowntec A2 color over time in different media.

	ΔE 14 Days	ΔE 30 Days	ΔE 60 Days	p Value
LW	0.42 ± 0.03	0.54 ± 0.10	0.93 ± 0.22	$p < 0.5$ *
LC	0.50 ± 0.14	1.10 ± 0.23	1.37 ± 0.41	
LR	0.70 ± 0.02	1.05 ± 0.08	1.59 ± 0.11	$p < 0.01$ *
NpW	2.94 ± 0.51	3.36 ± 0.49	3.65 ± 0.30	
NpC	3.25 ± 0.23	9.70 ± 0.34	11.54 ± 0.62	$p < 0.01$ *
NpR	3.34 ± 0.26	16.27 ± 0.21	18.19 ± 0.16	$p < 0.01$ *
PW	0.36 ± 0.02	1.44 ± 0.06	3.59 ± 0.42	$p < 0.01$ *
PC	2.02 ± 0.28	3.32 ± 0.30	5.00 ± 0.49	$p < 0.01$ *
PR	2.18 ± 0.21	12.59 ± 0.82	13.61 ± 0.42	$p < 0.01$ *

* Statistically significant p values are given. LW—sample covered with lacquer and stored in distilled water, LC—sample covered with lacquer and stored in coffee solution, LR—sample covered with lacquer and stored in red wine, NpW—sample non-polished after polymerization and stored in distilled water, NpC—sample non-polished and stored in coffee solution, NpR—sample non-polished and stored in red wine. PW—sample polished and stored in distilled water, PC—sample polished and stored in coffee solution, PR—sample polished and stored in red wine.

Table 3. Color change of Crowntec A3 color over time in different media.

	ΔE 14 Days	ΔE 30 Days	ΔE 60 Days	p Value
LW	0.65 ± 0.06	0.69 ± 0.25	0.75 ± 0.16	
LC	0.54 ± 0.08	1.67 ± 0.36	1.97 ± 0.23	
LR	1.33 ± 0.26	2.55 ± 0.53	3.45 ± 0.30	$p < 0.01$ *
NpW	0.45 ± 0.06	0.73 ± 0.09	0.94 ± 0.51	
NpC	2.72 ± 0.21	5.45 ± 0.43	6.50 ± 0.28	$p < 0.01$ *
NpR	4.77 ± 0.29	5.85 ± 0.20	6.64 ± 0.33	
PW	0.50 ± 0.10	1.01 ± 0.10	1.11 ± 0.36	
PC	2.64 ± 0.31	3.34 ± 0.36	3.61 ± 0.42	
PR	3.33 ± 0.33	8.02 ± 0.44	10.94 ± 0.23	$p < 0.01$ *

* Statistically significant p values are given. LW—sample covered with lacquer and stored in distilled water, LC—sample covered with lacquer and stored in coffee solution, LR—sample covered with lacquer and stored in red wine, NpW—sample non-polished after polymerization and stored in distilled water, NpC—sample non-polished and stored in coffee solution, NpR—sample non-polished and stored in red wine. PW—sample polished and stored in distilled water, PC—sample polished and stored in coffee solution, PR—sample polished and stored in red wine.

Table 4. Color change of Denture 3D+ color over time in different media.

	ΔE 14 Days	ΔE 30 Days	ΔE 60 Days	p Value
LW	0.63 ± 0.19	1.33 ± 0.42	1.36 ± 0.27	
LC	0.76 ± 0.13	2.30 ± 0.26	2.51 ± 0.40	
LR	0.83 ± 0.18	2.50 ± 0.32	3.48 ± 0.13	$p < 0.01$ *
NpW	0.35 ± 0.18	1.51 ± 0.68	1.80 ± 0.14	
NpC	2.10 ± 0.27	4.76 ± 0.26	5.59 ± 0.49	$p < 0.01$ *
NpR	4.88 ± 0.33	9.04 ± 0.56	11.00 ± 0.28	$p < 0.01$ *
PW	0.73 ± 0.11	1.36 ± 0.39	1.53 ± 0.27	
PC	1.05 ± 0.12	2.46 ± 0.24	2.78 ± 0.25	
PR	2.45 ± 0.34	2.45 ± 0.34	4.21 ± 0.31	

* Statistically significant p values are given. LW—sample covered with lacquer and stored in distilled water, LC—sample covered with lacquer and stored in coffee solution, LR—sample covered with lacquer and stored in red wine, NpW—sample non-polished after polymerization and stored in distilled water, NpC—sample non-polished and stored in coffee solution, NpR—sample non-polished and stored in red wine. PW—sample polished and stored in distilled water, PC—sample polished and stored in coffee solution, PR—sample polished and stored in red wine.

Table 2 shows the color changes of Crowntec A2 resin over time in different media. It is evident that the color change was more significant in red wine and coffee compared to distilled water. Samples without polishing and with lacquer coating showed the most color change in these staining solutions, with p-values less than 0.01, indicating a statistically significant difference.

Table 3 displays the color changes of Crowntec A3 resin in various media. Similar to Crowntec A2, the color change was more pronounced in red wine and coffee compared to distilled water. Samples without polishing and with lacquer coating exhibited the most significant color change in these staining solutions, with p-values less than 0.01, indicating a statistically significant difference.

Table 4 presents the color changes of Denture 3D+ resin over time in different media. As observed in the previous tables, the color change was greater in red wine and coffee compared to distilled water. Samples without polishing and with lacquer coating demonstrated the most substantial color change in these staining solutions, with p-values less than 0.01, indicating a statistically significant difference.

The results indicate that the color changes in the tested resins are more significant when exposed to red wine and coffee than when exposed to distilled water. The samples without polishing and with lacquer coating experienced the most considerable color changes in these staining solutions, with statistically significant differences observed.

The results from Tables 2–4 show that staining solutions like red wine and coffee have a greater impact on the color stability of tested resins (Crowntec A2, Crowntec A3, and Denture 3D+) than distilled water. This finding is important for evaluating the color stability of dental prosthetic materials.

The varnish on the surface of the sample peeled off during storage (Figure 2).

Tooth color changes in all media; distilled water, coffee, and red wine are shown in Figure 3 for the varnished samples.

Samples polished by the traditional method with a pumice stone show the least change in color during storage in staining solutions. (Figure 4a).

If the varnish did not separate from the surface of the materials, then the surface of the artificial teeth is smooth and did not change color (Figure 4b). However, if the surface of the material became contaminated, the varnish began to crack and scratches formed on the surface, which absorb the dyes (Figure 4c).

When comparing the three surface treatments, samples without polishing displayed the most significant color change in red wine and coffee solutions (Figure 4d,e). This indicates that not polishing the surface of prosthetic restorations can lead to higher susceptibility to discoloration when exposed to staining agents. On the other hand, lacquer coating provided better color stability than unpolished samples, but in some cases, it showed more color change than mechanically polished samples. This suggests that whereas lacquer coating offers some protection against staining, mechanical polishing might be more effective in maintaining the color stability of dental prosthetic materials.

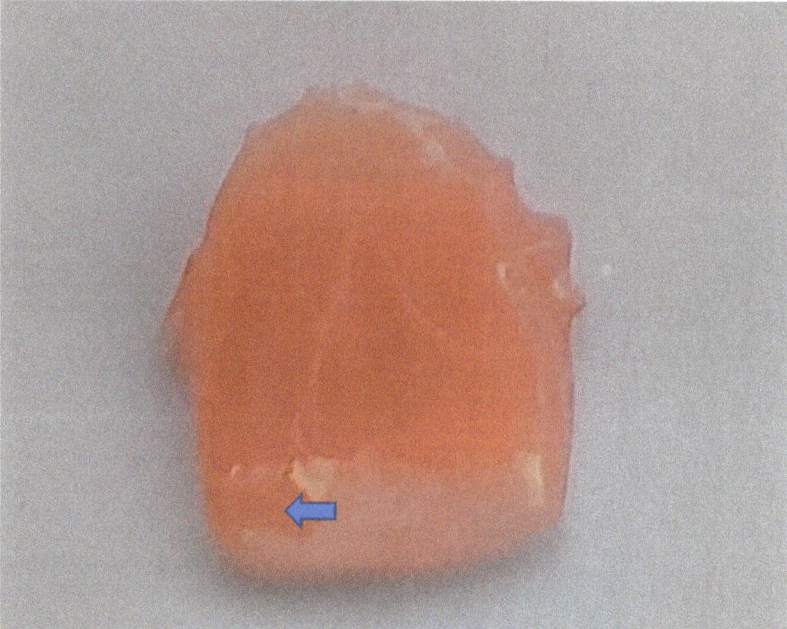

Figure 2. Deture base material Denture 3D +. The surface of the sample is covered with varnish and stored in distilled water. Under the influence of storage, the varnish separates from the resin. Separation is marked with arrows.

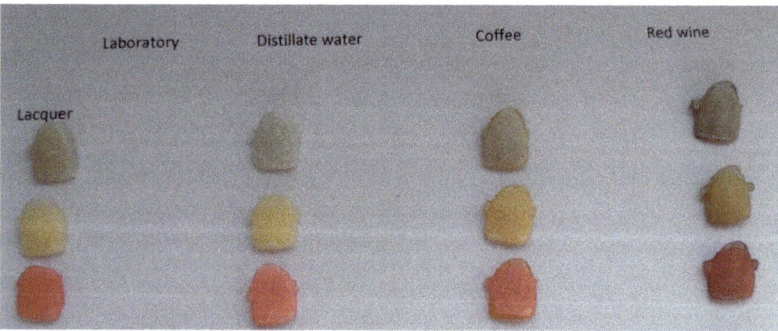

Figure 3. Color changes after storage in different media. The greatest color changes were observed in a test tube stored in red wine.

Mechanical polishing demonstrated better color stability compared to the other two surface treatments in most cases, making it an effective method for preserving color stability when exposed to common staining agents like red wine and coffee. The polishing procedure must be carried out very carefully, because even the smallest surface irregularities absorb dyes (Figure 4f—red wine).

During the experiments, cracks and peeling of varnish pieces were observed on the test surfaces, as shown in Figures 2 and 4c. Tooth color changes were documented and are displayed in Figure 3, with the most significant color changes observed in the samples stored in red wine.

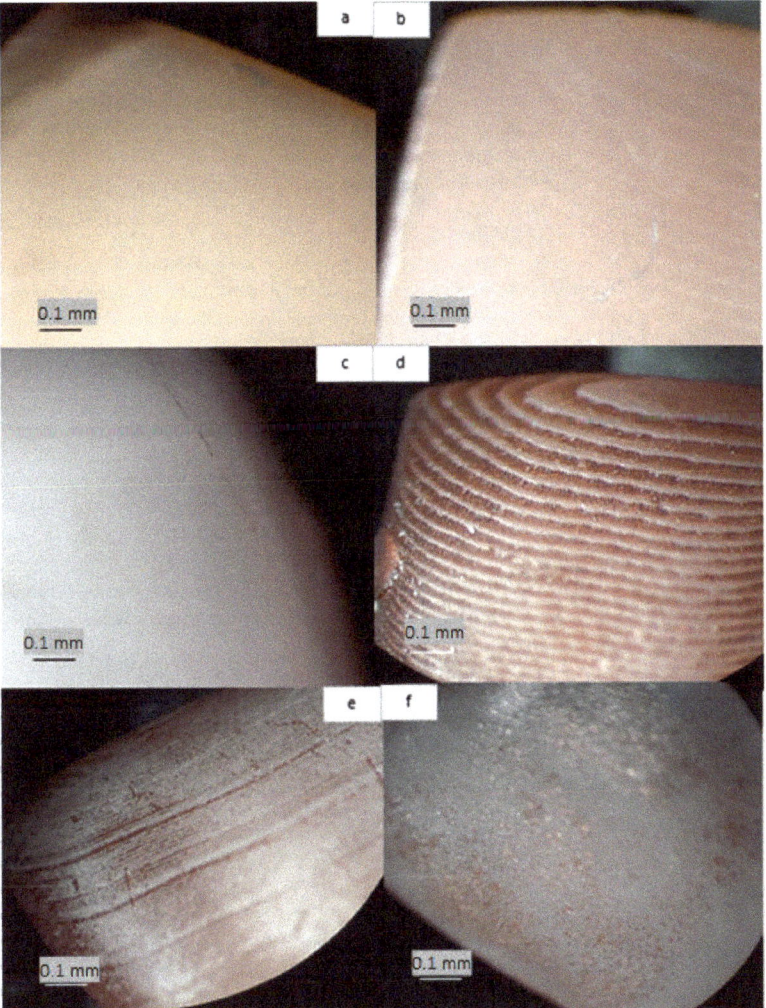

Figure 4. (**a**) Photograph of the tooth surface under a microscope. It is visible that polishing the tooth surface provides less retention for dyes (Crowntech A3); (**b**). Teeth covered with varnish are protected against discoloration, but after a long time, the protecting layer can crack (Crowntech A2); (**c**) Teeth covered with varnish, after storage in distilled water. Lacquer cracks (arrows), and the remnants of dyes begin to accumulate in the gaps (Crowntech A2). (**d**) Teeth's unpolished surface after storage in red wine, and (**e**) after contact with coffee. Between the individual layers of the material as it was printed are visible dyes (Crowntech A2). (**f**) Sample of A2 color storage in red wine for 60 days, with a polished surface but not enough; a clearly visible region with greater roughness, where the absorption of dyes took place (Magnification 25×).

Microscopic observations of polished tooth surfaces indicated that they were less susceptible to staining than non-polished samples, as illustrated in Figure 4. Very significant changes were observed in Figure 4d,e when the presence of red wine or coffee dye between the individual layers of the unpolished material could be seen.

The results of the tests show that unpolished materials undergo the most significant color change in red wine after 60 days. The second-highest color change occurred in rough samples exposed to coffee. Samples with varnish-protected surfaces exhibited the smallest color changes. However, over time, some surfaces began to experience varnish peeling. The least color change was observed in samples stored in distilled water.

The surface treatment of dental prosthetic materials plays a crucial role in their color stability. Unpolished surfaces are more susceptible to staining, whereas varnish protection can help maintain color but may experience peeling over time. Polished surfaces demonstrate better color stability, but it is essential to ensure adequate polishing to avoid areas with greater roughness that may absorb dyes.

4. Discussion

The thesis put forward at the beginning of this study has not been confirmed. The method of preparation of the material affects color stability. Many factors can affect color changes in temporary dental materials, such as polymerization, diet, dyes, oral hygiene, and surface smoothness. The selection of the staining solution and its concentration, as well as the time during which the materials are exposed to the dyeing solution, may also influence the degree of color change and surface topography [23–26].

Coffee and red wine solutions have long been used as unofficial standards for testing and changing the color of materials in prosthetics [27]. Discoloration of materials can occur externally (deposits on the surface) or internally (when the dye penetrates the inside of the material, monomer composition, and degree of polymerization) [21,24,25].

The NextDent 3D system was tested by Dimirtrova et al. in a solution of wine, coffee, Coca Cola and artificial saliva. The authors, as in these studies, observed the greatest color change for the samples stored in red wine for a period of 21 days. The Delta E value was 2.05, which was lower than in these studies, but the storage period of the sample was also much shorter [23].

Materials intended for 3D printing also change their color as a result of sorption and solubility in water, which reduces their translucency is [24,25].

Contact time plays a very important role in the color stability of dental materials [26]. Korean authors have demonstrated in their research that 3D materials exhibit lower color stability compared to materials milled using CAD/CAM technology, in which PMMA discs are polymerized for an extended period under high pressure and at a temperature of approximately 130 °C [27–29].

Color stability is also affected by the orientation of the sample when printing. The most accurate restorations are obtained when the sample orientation is 45 degrees (Hada et al.) [28]. In this case, however, the printed crown had rows of layers that came together on the surface, and thus it was easily discolored (Figure 4).

Another potential explanation for the low color stability of 3D printing resins is the degree of double bond conversion of acrylic resins in these materials, which is at a level of 50–80% [18,19,30]. Post-curing processes after printing contribute to higher polymerization rates [31]. The use of red wine to test the color change of dental materials is a common practice in dentistry. Red wine, with its strong pigmentation, can be an effective indicator of how well a dental material is able to resist staining over time. It is often used as a second solution for testing the color stability of dental restorative materials, after coffee. Red wine is also a convenient choice for testing dental materials because it is readily available and easy to use [32–34]. However, it is important to note that the staining potential of red wine can vary depending on the type and quality of the wine, as well as other factors such as pH and tannin content [35].

The immersion period and the frequency of exposure to staining solutions are other factors that can influence color stability [36]. Studies have shown that longer exposure to staining solutions, such as red wine, coffee, or tea, can lead to a more pronounced color change in dental materials [11].

The role of the staining solution's pH on the color stability of dental materials should also be considered. The pH of the staining solution can affect the color stability of dental materials, as it may cause erosion, surface roughness changes, or even dissolution of the materials [37]. It is crucial to understand the interaction between the acidity of common beverages and dental materials, as this knowledge can lead to the development of more resistant and durable dental restorations [38].

In our study, we observed that the surface treatment of dental prosthetic materials plays a crucial role in their color stability. Unpolished surfaces are more susceptible to staining, whereas varnish protection can help maintain color but may experience peeling over time. Polished surfaces demonstrate better color stability, but it is essential to ensure adequate polishing to avoid areas with greater roughness that may absorb dyes.

The development of dental materials with enhanced color stability that can mimic the natural appearance of teeth is of utmost importance in modern dentistry. With the esthetic expectations of patients continuously increasing, there is a growing demand for dental restorations with better color stability, biocompatibility, and mechanical properties [39].

Color stability is an important factor when it comes to the durability and longevity of dental restorations. Dental materials with poor color stability can become discolored over time, resulting in unsightly restorations that do not match the natural appearance of the patient's teeth. Dental materials with enhanced color stability can help ensure that restorations maintain their original color and appearance, leading to greater patient satisfaction [39]. Biocompatibility is another critical consideration when developing dental materials. Biocompatible materials are essential in ensuring that dental restorations do not cause adverse reactions in patients. Dental professionals must consider the biocompatibility of dental materials to reduce the risk of allergic reactions or infections, leading to better patient outcomes. Mechanical properties such as strength, durability, and resistance to wear are also important when it comes to dental restorations. Dental materials with superior mechanical properties can help ensure the longevity and effectiveness of restorations. Such materials can withstand the forces of biting and chewing, reducing the risk of breakage or cracking, and provide patients with a functional and long-lasting restoration [39]. Researchers are continuously working on improving the properties of dental materials, including the development of new resin-based composites, ceramics, and CAD/CAM materials with better color stability [40–42].

Patient education and preventive measures should be underlined in order to minimize the risk of staining in dental restorations. Dental professionals play a crucial role in educating their patients on the proper care and maintenance of their dental restorations. Patients should be informed about the potential effects of staining beverages, such as red wine, coffee, and tea, on the color stability of their restorations, and advised on proper oral hygiene practices and maintenance of their dental work.

Staining beverages can have a significant impact on the color stability of dental restorations, particularly those made from materials such as composite resin or ceramic. These materials can become discolored over time when exposed to pigmented substances, leading to unsightly restorations that do not match the natural appearance of the patient's teeth. Dental professionals should inform patients about the potential risks of consuming staining beverages and provide recommendations for reducing their consumption or minimizing their impact on dental work [40,43–46].

Performing research has its limitations. Three-dimensional printing materials from one manufacturer, NextDent, were tested using one printer and one type of light oven. As is well known, the degree of curing of light-curing materials may vary depending on the devices used, both the 3D printer and the light oven, which may affect the results obtained [28,29]. Therefore, further research into other materials and curing equipment is needed.

The effect of the type of resin used in 3D printing on the color stability of dental restorations is an area that requires further research. Different resins have different characteristics, including composition, degree of polymerization, and physical properties, which can affect their susceptibility to discoloration and staining [47]. A better understanding of the relationship between resin type and color stability can help dentists choose the most appropriate materials for their patients, leading to more esthetically pleasing and longer-lasting restorations.

In the context of color stability, it is also important to consider the role of saliva and its interaction with dental materials. Saliva is essential in the oral environment, providing natural protection against discoloration and maintaining the integrity of dental restorations. The complex composition of saliva, including its buffering capacity, enzymes, and proteins, can affect the surface properties and color stability of dental materials over time [48,49]. Further research into the interaction between saliva and dental materials may provide valuable information to develop more effective strategies to improve the color stability of dental restorations in clinical settings.

The development of advanced dental materials with improved color stability and stain resistance is an ongoing area of research. Innovations in materials science, such as the use of nanoparticles, antimicrobial agents, or advanced surface treatments, may offer potential solutions for improving the color stability of dental restorations [50,51]. In the future, research into new methods to improve the esthetic properties and durability of dental materials should be continued, providing patients with the highest quality of care and satisfaction with dental treatment [52,53].

In this work, a more comprehensive study of factors affecting the color stability of restorations was performed, building on previous research in this area. For example, Dimitrov et al. [24] focused on the color stability of restorations fabricated using the NextDent 3D system, but our study goes beyond the scope of their work by examining a wider range of restorations and considering different surface preparation methods.

While Dimitrov et al. [24] primarily investigated the susceptibility of the NextDent 3D system to discoloration, our work delves into the effect of resin type on color stability. By evaluating different resins and their susceptibility to staining and discoloration, we aim to offer dentists a better understanding of the most appropriate materials to use, which will ultimately contribute to the development of more esthetically pleasing and durable restorations.

Our study also investigates the role of saliva and its interaction with dental materials, an aspect that has been largely overlooked in previous studies, including Dimitrov et al. [24]. By analyzing the complex relationship between saliva and dental materials, we hope to provide valuable information for the development of more effective strategies to improve the color stability of dental restorations in clinical settings.

In the study conducted by Almejrad et al., the color stability of 3D-printed interim restorations with different surface treatments was evaluated after being immersed in various staining solutions, such as artificial saliva, tea, coffee, and wine for six months. Using a laboratory scanner, CAD/CAM software, and 3D-printing technology, 80 abutment teeth and interim restorations were produced from tooth-colored photopolymerizing resin and randomly assigned to either a Polish or Optiglaze treatment group. The samples were then divided into four subgroups based on their immersion liquid. Color measurements were taken pre- and post-immersion, and two-way ANOVA was conducted to assess the impact of surface treatment, immersion liquid, and their interaction on color change (ΔE) after six months. Results showed significant effects of surface treatment, immersion liquid, and their interaction on ΔE, with red wine causing the most discoloration. The application of a nanofilled, light-polymerizing protective coating was found to significantly reduce discoloration from chromogenic beverages, particularly coffee, suggesting its usefulness for extended intraoral service of 3D-printed interim restorations [54].

Other studies have investigated the color stability of dental restorations made from 3D-printing resins and conventional CAD/CAM blocks, focusing on the impact of various colorants and storage durations. It has been found that 3D-printing resins exhibited significantly higher discoloration than CAD/CAM blocks when exposed to grape juice, coffee, curry, and distilled water over 2, 7, and 30 days. The findings highlight the importance of considering discoloration when using 3D-printing resins for dental restorations [32].

In research performed by Scotti et al., the physical and surface properties of a 3D-printed resin were compared with those of materials traditionally used for interim dental restorations. Three different materials were tested for color change, flexural strength, Knoop hardness, and surface roughness: a 3D-printed resin, an autopolymerizing interim material, and a composite resin. The results revealed that the composite resin exhibited the highest values for flexural strength and hardness, followed by the 3D-printed resin, whereas the autopolymerizing interim material demonstrated the lowest values for both tests. In terms of surface roughness, the 3D-printed resin showed similar values to the autopolymerizing material, but higher values than the composite resin. However, the 3D-printed resin displayed the most significant color variation over time, raising concerns about its color stability for long-term use. Despite this, the 3D-printed composite resin showcased adequate mechanical and surface properties, suggesting its potential as a cost-effective alternative for interim restorative materials in dentistry [55].

5. Conclusions

1. This study highlights the importance of proper curing, surface polishing, and the potential limitations of using varnish for 3D printed dental restorations.
2. The results indicate that materials intended for 3D printing must undergo complete curing to minimize color change and ensure long-lasting esthetic results. Moreover, the surface of the material after curing should be meticulously polished using traditional techniques to eliminate any surface imperfections that may lead to localized discoloration over time.
3. Whereas varnish application might be useful for temporary restorations, its long-term use may not be ideal for 3D-printed restorations. This is due to the potential for the varnish to crack and create fissures on the surface, allowing dyes to penetrate and negatively impact the esthetic appearance of the restoration. The disparity in flexibility between the varnish resin and the 3D printing material may contribute to this issue.

Author Contributions: Conceptualization, Z.R.; Data curation, Z.R.; Formal analysis, K.C. and M.M.; Investigation, Z.R.; Methodology, Z.R.; Resources, Z.R.; Supervision, M.M.; Visualization, Z.R., K.C. and M.M.; Writing—original draft, K.C. and M.M.; Writing—review and editing, Z.R., K.C. and M.M. All authors have read and agreed to the published version of the manuscript.

Funding: This research received no external funding.

Data Availability Statement: Data sharing is not applicable to this article.

Conflicts of Interest: The authors declare no conflict of interest.

References

1. Bhargav, A.; Sanjairaj, V.; Rosa, V.; Feng, L.W.; Fuh, Y.H.J. Applications of additive manufacturing in dentistry: A review. *J. Biomed. Mater. Res. B Appl. Biomater.* **2018**, *106*, 2058–2064. [CrossRef] [PubMed]
2. Dawood, A.; Marti, B.; Sauret-Jackson, V.; Darwood, A. 3D printing in dentistry. *Br. Dent. J.* **2012**, *213*, 567–571. [CrossRef] [PubMed]
3. Revilla-León, M.; Özcan, M. Additive manufacturing technologies: An overview about 3D printing methods and future prospects. *Complexity* **2019**, *2019*, 9656938.
4. Mangano, F.; Gandolfi, A.; Luongo, G.; Logozzo, S. Intraoral scanners in dentistry: A review of the current literature. *BMC Oral Health* **2017**, *17*, 149. [CrossRef]
5. Alharbi, N.; Wismeijer, D.; Osman, R.B. Factors influencing the dimensional accuracy of 3D-printed full-coverage dental restorations using stereolithography technology. *Eur. J. Prosthodont. Restor. Dent.* **2016**, *24*, 31–38. [CrossRef]
6. Ciocca, L.; Fantini, M.; De Crescenzio, F.; Corinaldesi, G.; Scotti, R. CAD/CAM bilateral ear prostheses construction for Treacher Collins syndrome patients: A pilot study. *J. Prosthet. Dent.* **2012**, *108*, 349–356.
7. Bibb, R.; Eggbeer, D.; Williams, R. Rapid prototyping for orthopedic surgery. *Rapid Prototyp. J.* **2015**, *21*, 344–353.

8. Kim, D.; Shim, J.-S.; Lee, D.; Shin, S.-H.; Nam, N.-E.; Park, K.-H.; Shim, J.-S.; Kim, J.E. Effects of post curing time on the mechanical and color properties of three-dimensional printed crown and bridge materials. *Polymers* **2020**, *12*, 2762. [CrossRef]
9. Loges, K.; Tiberius, V. Implementation Challenges of 3D Printing in Prosthodontics: A Ranking-Type Delphi. *Materials* **2022**, *15*, 431. [CrossRef]
10. Paravina, R.D.; Ghinea, R.; Herrera, L.J.; Bona, A.D.; Igiel, C.; Linninger, M.; Sakai, M.; Takahashi, H.; Tashkandi, E.; del Mar Perez, M. Color difference thresholds in dentistry. *J. Esthet. Restor. Dent.* **2009**, *21*, S1–S9. [CrossRef]
11. Guler, A.U.; Yilmaz, F.; Kulunk, T.; Guler, E.; Kurt, S. Effects of different drinks on stainability of resin composite provisional restorative materials. *J. Prosthet. Dent.* **2005**, *94*, 118–124. [CrossRef]
12. Dietschi, D.; Campanile, G.; Holz, J.; Meyer, J.M. Comparison of the color stability of ten new-generation composites: An in vitro study. *Dent. Mater.* **1994**, *10*, 353–362. [CrossRef]
13. Mutlu-Sagesen, L.; Ergün, G.; Ozkan, Y.; Semiz, M. Color stability of a dental composite after immersion in various media. *Dent Mater J.* **2005**, *24*, 382–390. [CrossRef]
14. Koksal, T.; Dikbas, I. Color stability of different denture teeth materials against various staining agents. *Dent. Mater. J.* **2008**, *27*, 139–144. [CrossRef]
15. Ngo, T.D.; Kashani, A.; Imbalzano, G.; Nguyen, K.T.; Hui, D. Additive manufacturing (3D printing): A review of materials, methods, applications and challenges. *Compos. B Eng.* **2018**, *143*, 172–196. [CrossRef]
16. Salmi, M. Possibilities of preoperative medical models made by 3D printing or additive manufacturing. *J. Med. Eng.* **2016**, *2016*, 6191526. [CrossRef]
17. Yao, Q.; Morton, D.; Eckert, G.J.; Li, W.H. The effect of surface treatments on the color stability of CAD-CAM interim fixed dental prostheses. *J. Prosthet. Dent.* **2021**, *126*, 248–253. [CrossRef]
18. Lee, S.Y.; Lim, J.H.; Kim, D.; Lee, D.H.; Kim, S.G.; Kim, J.E. Evaluation of the color stability of 3D printed resin according to the oxygen inhibition effect and temperature difference in the post-polymerization process. *J. Mech. Behav. Biomed. Mater.* **2022**, *136*, 105537, Epub ahead of print. [CrossRef]
19. Çakmak, G.; Molinero-Mourelle, P.; De Paula, M.S.; Akay, C.; Cuellar, A.R.; Donmez, M.B.; Yilmaz, B. Surface Roughness and Color Stability of 3D-Printed Denture Base Materials after Simulated Brushing and Thermocycling. *Materials* **2022**, *15*, 6441. [CrossRef]
20. Vanaei, H.R.; Magri, A.E.; Rastak, M.A.; Vanaei, S.; Vaudreuil, S.; Tcharkhtchi, A. Numerical–Experimental Analysis toward the Strain Rate Sensitivity of 3D-Printed Nylon Reinforced by Short Carbon Fiber. *Materials* **2022**, *15*, 8722. [CrossRef]
21. Schweiger, J.; Edelhoff, D.; Güth, J.F. 3D Printing in Digital Prosthetic Dentistry: An Overview of Recent Developments in Additive Manufacturing. *J. Clin. Med.* **2021**, *10*, 2010. [CrossRef] [PubMed]
22. Song, S.-Y.; Shin, Y.-H.; Lee, J.-Y.; Shin, S.-W. Color stability of provisional restorative materials with different fabrication methods. *J. Adv. Prosthodont.* **2020**, *12*, 259–264. [CrossRef] [PubMed]
23. Raszewski, Z.; Chojnacka, K.; Kulbacka, J.; Mikulewicz, M. Mechanical Properties and Biocompatibility of 3D Printing Acrylic Material with Bioactive Components. *J. Funct. Biomater.* **2023**, *14*, 13. [CrossRef] [PubMed]
24. Dimitrova, M.; Chuchulska, B.; Zlatev, S.; Kazakova, R. Colour Stability of 3D-Printed and Prefabricated Denture Teeth after Immersion in Different Colouring Agents—An In Vitro Study. *Polymers* **2022**, *14*, 3125. [CrossRef] [PubMed]
25. Gad, M.M.; Alshehri, S.Z.; Alhamid, S.A.; Albarrak, A.; Khan, S.Q.; Alshahrani, F.A.; Alqarawi, F.K. Water Sorption, Solubility, and Translucency of 3D-Printed Denture Base Resins. *Dent. J.* **2022**, *10*, 42. [CrossRef]
26. Alfouzan, A.F.; Alotiabi, H.M.; Labban, N.; Al-Otaibi, H.N.; Al Taweel, S.M.; AlShehri, H.A. Color stability of 3D-printed denture resins: Effect of aging, mechanical brushing and immersion in staining medium. *J. Adv. Prosthodont.* **2021**, *13*, 160–171, Erratum in *J. Adv. Prosthodont.* **2022**, *14*, 334. [CrossRef]
27. Radwan, H.; Elnaggar, G.; El Deen, I.S. Surface roughness and color stability of 3D printed temporary crown material in different oral media (In vitro study). *Int. J. Appl. Dent. Sci.* **2021**, *7*, 327–334. [CrossRef]
28. Hada, T.; Kanazawa, M.; Iwaki, M.; Arakida, T.; Soeda, Y.; Katheng, A.; Otake, R.; Minakuchi, S. Effect of Printing Direction on the Accuracy of 3D-Printed Dentures Using Stereolithography Technology. *Materials* **2020**, *13*, 3405. [CrossRef]
29. Vygandas, R.; Sabaliauskas, V. Effects of different repolishing techniques on color change of provisional prosthetic materials. *Stomatologija* **2009**, *11*, 102–112.
30. Mickeviciute, E.; Ivanauskiene, E.; Noreikiene, V. In vitro color and roughness stability of different temporary restorative materials. *Stomatologija* **2016**, *18*, 66–72.
31. Koh, E.-S.; Cha, H.-S.; Kim, T.-H.; Ahn, J.-S.; Lee, J.-H. Color stability of three-dimensional-printed denture teeth exposed to various colorants. *J. Korean Acad. Prosthodont.* **2020**, *58*, 1–6. [CrossRef]
32. Shin, J.-W.; Kim, J.-E.; Choi, Y.-J.; Shin, S.-H.; Nam, N.-E.; Shim, J.-S.; Lee, K.-W. Evaluation of the Color Stability of 3D-Printed Crown and Bridge Materials against Various Sources of Discoloration: An In Vitro Study. *Materials* **2020**, *13*, 5359. [CrossRef]
33. Lee, E.H.; Ahn, J.-S.; Lim, Y.-J.; Kwon, H.-B.; Kim, M.-J. Effect of post-curing time on the color stability and related properties of a tooth-colored 3D-printed resin material. *J. Mech. Behav. Biomed. Mater.* **2021**, *126*, 104993. [CrossRef]
34. Shin, D.H.; Rawls, H.R. Degree of conversion and color stability of the light curing resin with new photoinitiator systems. *Dent. Mater.* **2009**, *25*, 1030–1038. [CrossRef]
35. Chakravarthy, Y.; Clarence, S. The effect of red wine on colour stability of three different types of esthetic restorative materials: An in vitro study. *J. Conserv. Dent.* **2018**, *21*, 319–323. [CrossRef]

36. Korać, S.; Ajanović, M.; Džanković, A.; Konjhodžić, A.; Hasić-Branković, L.; Gavranović-Glamoč, A.; Tahmiščija, I. Color Stability of Dental Composites after Immersion in Beverages and Performed Whitening Procedures. *Acta Stomatol. Croat.* **2022**, *56*, 22–32. [CrossRef]
37. Tahayeri, A.; Morgan, M.C.; Fugolin, A.P.; Bompolaki, D.; Athirsala, A.; Pfeifer, C.S.; Ferracane, J.L.; Bertassomi, L.E. 3D printed versus conventionally cured provisional crown and bridge dental materials. *Dent. Mater.* **2018**, *34*, 192–200. [CrossRef]
38. Aydın, N.; Karaoğlanoğlu, S.; Oktay, E.A.; Kılıçarslan, M.A. Investigating the color changes on resin-based CAD/CAM Blocks. *J. Esthet. Restor. Dent.* **2020**, *32*, 251–256. [CrossRef]
39. Poggio, C.; Vialba, L.; Berardengo, A.; Federico, R.; Colombo, M.; Beltrami, R.; Scribante, A. Color stability of new esthetic restorative materials: A spectrophotometric analysis. *J. Funct. Biomater.* **2017**, *8*, 26. [CrossRef]
40. De Silva, M.L.; Leite, F.D.; e Silva, M.; Meireles, S.S.; Duarte, R.M.; Andrade, A.K. The effect of drinks on color stability and surface roughness of nanocomposites. *Eur. J. Dent.* **2014**, *8*, 330–336.
41. Ribeiro, I.A.P.; Della Bona, A.; Borba, M. Dental materials for CAD/CAM restorations: Color stability after accelerated aging. *J. Esthet. Restor. Dent.* **2019**, *31*, 304–312.
42. Santos, C.; Clarke, R.L.; Braden, M.; Guitian, F.; Davy, K.W.M. Water absorption characteristics of dental composites incorporating hydroxyapatite filler. *Biomaterials* **2002**, *23*, 1897–1904. [CrossRef] [PubMed]
43. Samra, A.P.; Pereira, S.K.; Delgado, L.C.; Borges, C.P. Color stability evaluation of aesthetic restorative materials. *Braz. Oral Res.* **2008**, *22*, 205–210. [CrossRef] [PubMed]
44. Tekçe, N.; Tuncer, S.; Demirci, M.; Serim, M.E.; Baydemir, C. The effect of different drinks on the color stability of different restorative materials after one month. *Restor. Dent. Endod.* **2015**, *40*, 255–261. [CrossRef] [PubMed]
45. Lepri, C.P.; Palma-Dibb, R.G. Color stability of esthetic restorative materials: A literature review. *Rev. Odonto Cienc.* **2012**, *27*, 81–85.
46. Vichi, A.; Louca, C.; Corciolani, G.; Ferrari, M. Color related to ceramic and zirconia restorations: A review. *Dent. Mater.* **2011**, *27*, 97–108. [CrossRef]
47. Alharbi, N.; Wismeijer, D.; Osman, R.B. Effects of build direction on the mechanical properties of 3D-printed complete coverage interim dental restorations. *J. Prosthet. Dent.* **2016**, *115*, 760–767. [CrossRef]
48. Lohbauer, U.; Reich, S. Antagonist wear of monolithic zirconia crowns after 2 years. *Clin. Oral Investig.* **2017**, *21*, 1165–1172. [CrossRef]
49. Sfondrini, M.F.; Gandini, P.; Malfatto, M.; Di Corato, F.; Trovati, F.; Scribante, A. Computerized casts for orthodontic purpose using powder-free intraoral scanners: Accuracy, execution time, and patient feedback. *Biomed. Res. Int.* **2018**, *2018*, 4103232. [CrossRef]
50. Da Silva, J.D.; Park, S.E.; Weber, H.P.; Ishikawa-Nagai, S. Clinical performance of a newly developed spectrophotometric system on tooth color reproduction. *J. Prosthet. Dent.* **2008**, *99*, 361–368. [CrossRef]
51. Santana, S.V.S.; Bombana, A.C.; Flório, F.M.; Basting, R.T. Effect of surface sealants on marginal microleakage in Class V resin composite restorations. *J. Esthet. Restor. Dent.* **2009**, *21*, 397–404. [CrossRef]
52. Awada, A.; Nathanson, D. Mechanical properties of resin-ceramic CAD/CAM restorative materials. *J. Prosthet. Dent.* **2015**, *114*, 587–593. [CrossRef]
53. AlShaafi, M.M. Effects of Different Temperatures and Storage Time on the Degree of Conversion and Microhardness of Resin-based Composites. *J. Contemp. Dent. Pract.* **2016**, *17*, 217–223. [CrossRef]
54. Almejrad, L.; Yang, C.C.; Morton, D.; Lin, W.S. The Effects of Beverages and Surface Treatments on the Color Stability of 3D-Printed Interim Restorations. *J. Prosthodont.* **2022**, *31*, 165–170. [CrossRef]
55. Scotti, C.K.; Velo, M.M.A.C.; Rizzante, F.A.P.; Nascimento, T.R.L.; Mondelli, R.F.L.; Bombonatti, J.F.S. Physical and surface properties of a 3D-printed composite resin for a digital workflow. *J. Prosthet. Dent.* **2020**, *124*, 614.e1–614.e5. [CrossRef]

Disclaimer/Publisher's Note: The statements, opinions and data contained in all publications are solely those of the individual author(s) and contributor(s) and not of MDPI and/or the editor(s). MDPI and/or the editor(s) disclaim responsibility for any injury to people or property resulting from any ideas, methods, instructions or products referred to in the content.

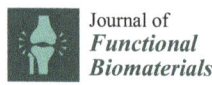 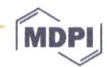

Article

The Influence of Polishing and Artificial Aging on BioMed Amber® Resin's Mechanical Properties

Anna Paradowska-Stolarz [1,*], Marcin Mikulewicz [1], Mieszko Wieckiewicz [2,*] and Joanna Wezgowiec [2,*]

[1] Division of Dentofacial Anomalies, Department of Orthodontics and Dentofacial Orthopedics, Wrocław Medical University, Krakowska 26, 50-425 Wrocław, Poland
[2] Department of Experimental Dentistry, Wrocław Medical University, Krakowska 26, 50-425 Wrocław, Poland
* Correspondence: anna.paradowska-stolarz@umw.edu.pl (A.P.-S.); mieszko.wieckiewicz@umw.edu.pl (M.W.); joanna.wezgowiec@umw.edu.pl (J.W.)

Abstract: Currently, 3D print is becoming more common in all branches of medicine, including dentistry. Some novel resins, such as BioMed Amber (Formlabs), are used and incorporated to more advanced techniques. The aims of the study were to check whether or not polishing and/or artificial aging influences the properties of the 3D-printed resin. A total of 240 specimens of BioMed Resin were printed. Two shapes (rectangular and dumbbell) were prepared. Of each shape, 120 specimens were divided into four groups each (with no influence, after polishing only, after artificial aging only, and after both polishing and artificial aging). Artificial aging took place in water at the temperature of 37 °C for 90 days. For testing, the universal testing machine (Z10-X700, AML Instruments, Lincoln, UK) was used. The axial compression was performed with the speed of 1mm/min. The tensile modulus was measured with the constant speed of 5 mm/min. The highest resistance to compression and tensile test were observed in the specimens that were neither polished nor aged (0.88 ± 0.03 and 2.88 ± 0.26, respectively). The lowest resistance to compression was observed in the specimens that were not polished, but aged (0.70 ± 0.02). The lowest results of the tensile test were observed when specimens were both polished and aged (2.05 ± 0.28). Both polishing and artificial aging weakened the mechanical properties of the BioMed Amber resin. The compressive modulus changed much with or without polishing. The tensile modulus differed in specimens that were either polished or aged. The application of both did not change the properties when compared to the polished or aged probes only.

Keywords: dental resins; compression test; tensile modulus; 3D print; dentistry

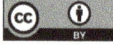

1. Introduction

The future use of 3D print technology is becoming the truth of today's life. This technology led to the high development of today's medicine. This phenomenon also extends to dentistry. Although first introduced to restorative dentistry (including simple, conservative restorations, as well as prosthetic appliances) and surgery, the use of this type of material broadened over time. Today, they are preferably used to produce both surgical guides for implantology and craniofacial surgery, but also the basic models [1]. Recently, 3D print was introduced to orthodontics, endodontics, and periodontology as well. It is preferably used for the fabrication of precise appliances, especially when skeletal anchorage is planned [2,3]. Although the properties of the 3D-printed materials and traditional ones tend to be nearly the same, the printed ones, due to the process of preparation, characterize higher accuracy in shape and time needed for production decrease. Unfortunately, this solution is far more expensive than the traditional one, and therefore, might be unprofitable [4]. Lately, more advanced, 4D technologies were introduced and presented as more precise as well as preferably used, and the difference between the 3D and 4D printing lies in the layer-by-layer print of the specimen. Although the 4D print was not introduced into the treatment yet, as it is still in the phase of experimentation, it gives potential chances for further development of the discipline of biomaterial preparation [5].

The 3D materials are preferably tested by the researchers [6–9]. For this reason, the different material properties are measured. Although the search for perfect materials is the main focus of the materials science, not many researchers compare the properties of the materials after subjection to the different external factors. Those factors may influence the properties of the materials, including their stability, resistance, and accuracy. Therefore, we decided to compare the properties of the chosen 3D-printed resin to polishing and artificial aging.

BioMed Amber is, according to the producer, a biocompatible material for short-term use. The material is strong and rigid. It is transparent, but has a yellowish glow, so it is not truly esthetic. The material is also durable with the frequent use of common disinfection agents and sterilization [6,7].

The use of materials in the oral cavity exposes them to unfavorable conditions. The factors influencing the materials depend on applications of the prepared item. One of the tests that is performed is artificial aging, which should mimic the oral cavity conditions [10]. Two main methods of artificial aging are possible: thermocycling and the use of water or artificial saliva immersion in time [11,12]. For this reason, we decided to subject the chosen material to unfavorable conditions. We chose the prolonged storage in water at 37 °C and compared the resin blocks in compression and tensile modulus tests. We also decided to check whether the mechanical features changed due to the polishing of the materials, as this process is necessary in each material preparation to reduce its roughness and improve aesthetics. To the best of the authors' knowledge, this is the first time this kind of research with this specific resin was conducted. Moreover, the tests are often prepared on the blocks of resins that find their uses in the preparation of dental restorations. The presented study could help us find another potential use of the presented resin.

The aim of this study was to check if the mechanical purposes of the selected resin differed after its polishing. Another goal was to check whether artificial aging influences the mentioned properties. The third aim was to find the correlation between artificial aging and polishing when it comes to the resistance to compression and tensile tests.

When planning the research, the hypotheses were formed:

1. There was no influence of polishing on the properties of the examined resin;
2. There was no influence of artificial aging on the properties of the examined resin;
3. There was no influence when both polishing and artificial aging were applied on the properties of the examined resins;
4. No differences were observed between the polished and aged samples.

2. Materials and Methodology

2.1. Materials

A 3D-printed resin, BioMed Amber (Amber UFI number E300-P0FU, Formlabs Ohio, Millbury, OH, USA), was evaluated in this study. The material is biocompatible and characterizes with various properties and potential uses. Recommendations regarding its selected applications, provided by the manufacturer, are summarized in Table 1.

Table 1. A brief description of the BioMed Amber applications recommended by the producer.

Resin	Application
BioMed Amber Resin	Biocompatible applications requiring short-term skin or mucosal membrane contact suitable for: • strong, rigid parts such as functioning threads; • end-use medical devices; • cut + drill guides (surgical); • implant sizing models; • specimen collection kits.

2.2. Specimens' Preparation and Artificial Aging

Two types of specimens were used for the evaluation of the selected properties: rectangular ones (for a compression test in accordance with the ISO 604:2003 standard) and dumbbell-shaped specimens (type 1BA) (for a tensile test in accordance with the ISO 527-1:2019(E) standard) [13,14]. The number of specimens printed for each test was n = 120 of rectangular specimens and n = 120 of dumbbell-shaped specimens. According to ISO standard, the appropriate number of samples for this kind of research is 5, but the authors considered this number too small and expanded the sample size to 30 for each test. After that, the prepared samples were divided into four groups (30 specimens each), to be tested.

The specimens were printed using a Form 2 printer (Formlabs), following the mentioned ISO standards and the producers' instructions. The printer is self-adjusting, and the printing properties are set once the cartridge is in the printer. The Form 2 printer (Formlabs) has a violet light (405 nm) and the power of 250 mW. After printing, the specimens were rinsed 2 × 10 min in 99% isopropanol alcohol (Stanlab, Lublin, Poland). Then, the specimens were dried at room temperature for 30 min and post-cured in Form Cure (Formlabs). The following settings of post-curing were applied: 30 min in 60 °C. Finally, the supports were removed, and the specimens were grinded with sandpaper. One half of the specimens (n = 60 of rectangular specimens and n = 60 of dumbbell-shaped specimens) were polished with a 0.2 pumice (Everall7, Warsaw, Poland) and polishing paste (Everall7) on one side of the specimen.

Afterwards, the specimens were stored at room temperature and 50% humidity for 24 h (before a tensile test) or for 4 days (before a compression test) and one half of the specimens were subjected to the tests. The other half of the specimens were artificially aged for 90 days in distilled water at 37 °C before testing (the water was changed every week).

2.3. Compression Test

The dimensions of the specimens ((10.0 ± 0.2) mm × (10.0 ± 0.2) mm × (4 ± 0.2)) in mm were selected to meet the requirements specified in the ISO 604:2003 standard. Before the test, the specimens were conditioned in the air at 23 °C/50% RH for 4 days. Afterwards, the width and the height of the specimens were measured in five points, using a Magnusson digital caliper (150 mm) (Limit, Wroclaw, Poland), and then, the mean values were calculated. The axial compression test was performed using the universal testing machine (Z10-X700, AML Instruments, Lincoln, UK) at the constant speed of 1 mm/min. The tested sample in the testing machine is presented in Figure 1. The measurements performed allowed for the determination of the compressive modulus (E [MPa]) of each specimen, as a slope of a uniaxial stress–strain curve recorded, based on the calculation of:

(a) compression stress (σ = F:A [MPa]),

where: F—force [N], A—initial cross-sectional area measurement [mm^2],

(b) nominal strain (ε = ΔL:L),

where: L—the initial distance between the compression plates [mm], ΔL—the decrease in the distance between the plates after the test [mm]).

Additionally, the dimensions of each specimen were measured both before and after the compression in order to enable evaluation of the changes in width and height due to compression.

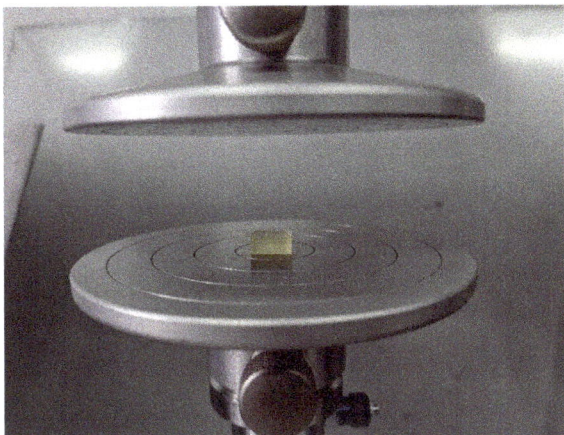

Figure 1. BioMed Amber resin at the compression test.

2.1. Tensile Test

The dumbbell-shaped specimens (type 1BA) with the length of 75 mm, width of 10 mm, and thickness of 2 mm were printed, following the ISO 527-2:2019 norm. Before the test, the specimens were conditioned in the air at 23 °C/50% RH for 24 h. The width and the height of the specimens at the test length were measured in five points, using a Magnusson digital caliper (150 mm) (Limit, Wroclaw, Poland), and then the mean values were calculated. The tensile test was performed using the Universal Testing Machine (Z10-X700, AML Instruments, Lincoln, UK) at the constant test speed of 5 mm/min (Figure 2).

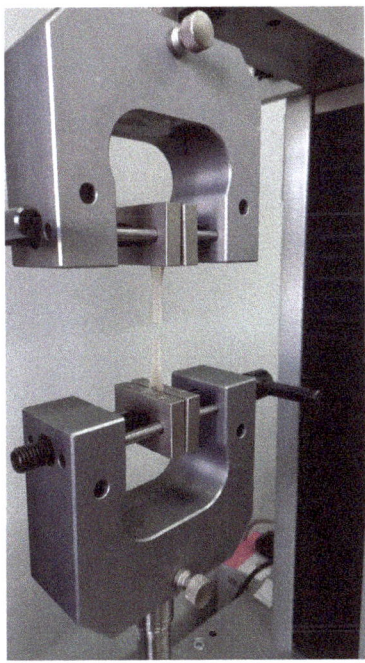

Figure 2. BioMed Amber resin at the tensile test.

The specimens that broke outside of the test length were disclosed. Based on the measurements performed, the stress and strain for each specimen were determined as:

(a) tensile stress (σ = F:A [MPa]),

where F—force [N], A—initial cross-sectional area measurement [mm^2],

(b) nominal strain (ε = ΔL:L),

where L—the initial distance between the grips [mm], ΔL—the increase in the distance between the grips after the test [mm]).

These calculations allowed for the determination of the tensile modulus (E_t) of each specimen, as:

$$E_1 = \sigma_2 - \sigma_1 \varepsilon_2 - \varepsilon_1 \text{ [MPa]},$$

where σ_1 is the stress, expressed in megapascals [MPa], measured at the strain value ε_1 = 0.0005; σ_2 is the stress, expressed in megapascals [MPa], measured at the strain value ε_2 = 0.0025.

2.5. Statistical Analysis

All statistical data were prepared using the program Statistica v. 13 (TIBCO Software Inc., Palo Alto, CA, USA).

Mean values with standard deviation of the compressive and tensile modulus of the examined probes were determined. Afterwards, the Kruskal–Wallis test by ranks was stated to check the potential statistical differences between the four examined probes. The p value was set for $p < 0.001$ for this test. Afterwards, multivariate analysis of the variance (MANOVA) test was performed to compare the obtained results.

3. Results

After the tests were performed, the authors of this study obtained the following results. In Table 2, we present the compressive and tensile modulus of the prepared probes. The number lower than n = 30 samples means that the specimens broke outside the tested area. For this reason, the authors excluded defective elements and they were not presented in the study. As one could observe, only two polished probes without artificial aging did not manage the tensile test. The compression and tensile tests were performed in four groups for each test (group 1—no polishing and artificial aging, group 2—no polishing, after artificial aging, group 3—after polishing, no artificial aging, and group 4—after both polishing and artificial aging).

Table 2. Compressive and tensile modulus of BioMed Amber resin at the compression (E_c) and tensile (E_t) tests.

E (GPa)	Polishing	Aging	N	M ± SD	Me [Q1–Q3]	Min–Max
Compression E_c	No	No	30	0.88 ± 0.03	0.88 [0.85–0.90]	0.83–0.92
	No	Yes	30	0.70 ± 0.02	0.70 [0.68–0.71]	0.66–0.74
	Yes	No	31	0.84 ± 0.04	0.85 [0.81–0.87]	0.73–0.89
	Yes	Yes	30	0.72 ± 0.03	0.71 [0.70–0.74]	0.66–0.78
Tensile E_t	No	No	30	2.88 ± 0.26	2.83 [2.74–3.11]	2.30–3.33
	No	Yes	30	2.07 ± 0.30	2.07 [0.88–2.45]	2.30–3.33
	Yes	No	28	2.67 ± 0.36	2.72 [2.39–2.98]	1.78–3.17
	Yes	Yes	30	2.05 ± 0.28	2.11 [2.01–2.19]	0.74–2.30

M—mean, SD—standard deviation, Me—median (50th percentile), Q1—lower quartile (25th percentile), Q3—upper quartile (75th percentile), Min—smallest value, and Max—greatest value.

In Figures 3 and 4, we present the elasticity module when compression (Figure 3) and tensile modulus (Figure 4) were tested. The materials were divided into four groups and assigned as: A0P0—without being subjected to polishing or artificial aging, A0P1—after polishing, but without artificial aging, A1P0—after artificial aging, but without polishing, and A1P1—after both artificial aging and polishing.

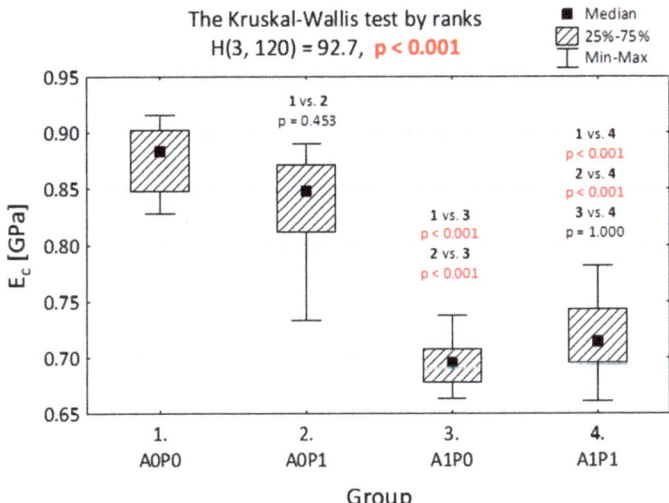

Figure 3. Elasticity module of the compression (E_c) of BioMed Amber when subjected to various technological treatments. Four groups were separated: A0P0—without artificial aging and polishing, A0P1—without artificial aging, but after polishing, A1P0—after artificial aging, without polishing, and A1P1—after both artificial aging and polishing.

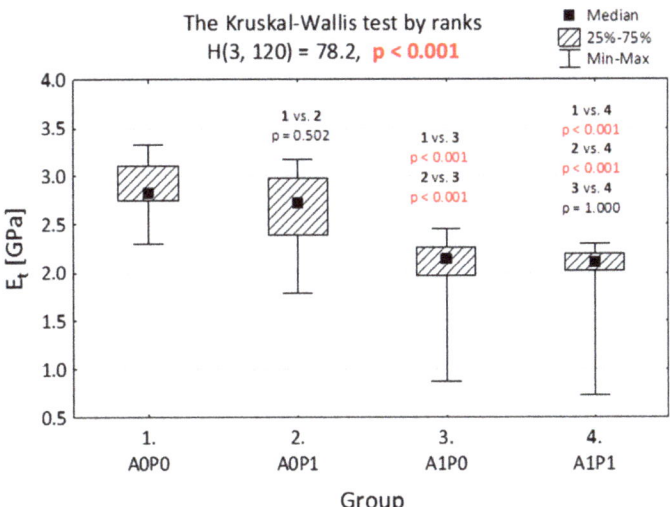

Figure 4. Elasticity module to tension (E_t) of BioMed Amber when subjected to various technological treatments. Four groups were separated: A0P0—without artificial aging and polishing, A0P1—without artificial aging, but after polishing, A1P0—after artificial aging, without polishing, and A1P1—after both artificial aging and polishing.

The results indicate that artificial aging strongly weakens the specimens at the compression test, no matter if they were polished or not. The polishing itself does not statistically influence the resistance to compression.

Some similar results are observed in the tensile test (Figure 4). Artificial aging weakens the specimens and the tensile tension measurements are lower. The polishing itself does not statistically influence the resistance to the tensile test. In the aged group, polishing did not change the resistance to the tensile test significantly.

The MANOVA test was applied to find the correlation between the artificial aging and polishing of the specimens. In Tables 3 and 4, as well as in Figure 5, the MANOVA test for elasticity modules were presented to establish the influence of artificial aging and polishing after the compression (E_c) and tensile (E_t) tests. The mean value of the elasticity module at compression was significantly influenced by artificial aging alone and the interaction of artificial aging and polishing. Polishing alone did not influence the properties of the resin. The mean value of the tensile modulus was strongly influenced by separated procedures of polishing or artificial aging. When both of the technological treatments were applied, no statistically significant difference was observed in comparison to the artificial aging without polishing.

Table 3. MANOVA results for elasticity module for compression of BioMed Amber resin.

Effect	SS	df	MS	F	p
Constant	73.26	1	73.26	71835	<0.000
Artificial aging	0.674	1	0.674	660.6	<0.000
Polishing	0.002	1	0.002	2.28	0.134
Artificial aging × polishing	0.026	1	0.026	25.3	<0.000
Error	0.118	116			

Table 4. MANOVA results for elasticity module for tensile modulus for BioMed Amber resin.

Effect	SS	df	MS	F	p
Constant	702.2	1	702.2	7870	<0.000
Artificial aging	15.46	1	15.46	173.3	<0.000
Polishing	0.420	1	0.420	4.711	<0.032
Artificial aging × polishing	0.237	1	0.237	2.656	0.106
Error	10.35	116			

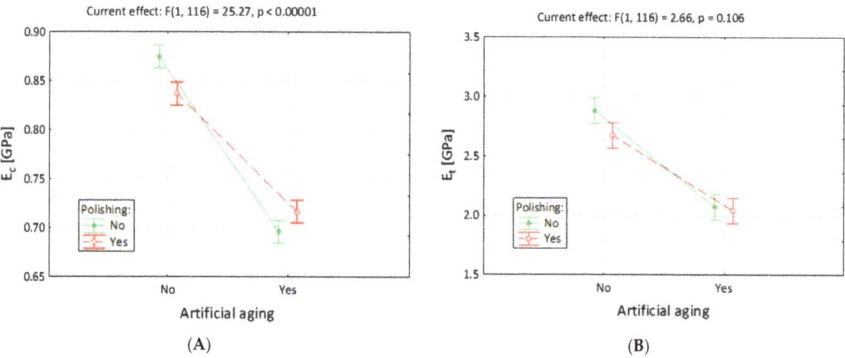

Figure 5. Elasticity modulus under compression (E_c) and tension (E_t) of BioMed Amber resin, after different technological treatments. Subfigure (**A**) refers to compression and (**B**)—to tension. (A0P0—without artificial aging and polishing, A0P1—without artificial aging, but after polishing, A1P0—after artificial aging, without polishing, and A1P1—after both artificial aging and polishing).

As observed in Figure 5, in the comparison of the elasticity modulus to compression (E_c), statistically significant interaction between artificial aging and polishing was observed. Among the specimens that were not treated with artificial aging, polishing alone lowered elasticity modulus significantly. Among the specimens that were aged, polishing increased the compressive modulus. No interactions were presented when the tensile modulus (E_t) was compared.

4. Discussion

The 3D-printable materials are the main focus of attention for today's medicine, including dentistry. In this field, the use is not limited to prosthetics and surgery anymore, but expanded to orthodontics, endodontics, and periodontology; therefore, new materials are investigated. They are tested in different conditions to find their most proper use. BioMed Amber is a quite new resin that was not yet thoroughly investigated. Due to potential use in preparation of surgical guides (especially for implants and orthodontic miniimplants), the precision of their preparation is crucial [6,7]. Without this type of resin, the preparation of guides for implant insertion would not be possible. Preparation of surgical guides increases the cost of implantation, but they help to obtain the exact point of implantation, especially that the surgical procedure is planned based on the CBCT image [4,15].

The research presented by us was designed based on the ISO standards, which assumes that the number of samples needed for the examination of the presented mechanical features is 5 [13,14]. The comparative studies that checked the properties of mechanical features of the BioMed Amber were conducted on the 10 samples [6,7]. The authors of the presented research focused on bringing up the novel properties of the presented resin, possibly broadening its future use. Therefore, we decided for artificial aging, simulating the intraoral condition. Thermocycling is another method of aging for the specimens, which is mainly used when restorative materials and cements are taken into account [16]. Thermocycling, in addition, predicts the fact that the material is used in the patient's mouth when the changes in the temperature are applied (e.g., while eating and drinking). The resin we tested is transparent and yellowish, which means it would not be used for restorative dentistry; therefore, we did not consider thermocycling as the method of testing. When the research was planned, we decided to expand the specimens to thirty pieces for each test. Therefore, the authors think it is a good comparison result to present the points that were inspected.

Most of the resins that are tested before and after the artificial aging are compared in terms of the color stability [17–20], which should not be the only factor taken into consideration when material is examined. An interesting study, which should be mentioned in the discussion, was published by Mazzitelli et al. [21]—the researchers presented the results that the chemical composition of the material influences the color stability. During the materials preparation, different processes are performed; one of them is polishing. This could influence the material's surface. Moreover, the use of beverages and food as well as bleaching, damages the surface of the materials applied in dentistry [22,23]. The color change is also observed when cigarette smoke is an influencing factor [24]. When considering artificial aging, besides the esthetic agonizing, other properties, such as tensile modulus and compressive modulus, are rarely taken into account. Therefore, the results presented in our paper might be one of the few available papers on that topic. We showed that artificial aging negatively influences the examined resins, which is also consistent with other material properties. Some new, more resistant materials are being searched for; however, most of the attention of the producers focuses on the composite blocks used for teeth restoration [25]. Another interesting study [26] showed the shear bond strength of materials used for the fabrication of occlusal splints, which shows that not only 3D-printed materials are influenced by the artificial aging procedures.

The wear of the material depends on the properties of the material itself [27]. In addition to the resins, other materials (metals, composites, ceramics, and other polymers) are incorporated into use [28]. In our study, we focused on the 3D resin that is used for short-term mucosal and tissue contact in medicine. The studies performed on composites [29] reveal that polishing lowers the protective properties of the materials, but we know that it is impossible to use the dental filling without the softening of the material's surface; therefore, polishing is an inseparable process in material preparation for its use. In the presented study we used a transparent, rigid material that is widely used in dentistry. The presented paper is one in the series of papers regarding BioMed Amber resin; the authors focused on searching for novel properties of the presented material, which could expand its future use. By storing the samples in water, the authors showed that possible long-term use in the oral cavity would be influenced by the wet environment. We showed that in the case of BioMed Amber resin, polishing reduces the resistance of the material to compression and tension, which is also consistent with the results of other studies on dental fillers [29–31]. This is consistent with a theorem that material gets weakened after polishing. These results may correspond also to reported changes in fractal dimension (FD) and texture analyses (TA) presented in previous studies. The study showed that Amber resin shows a high number of changes in the fractal and texture analyses [32]. The presented study referred to the compression test only, with no influence of external conditions.

The weakest point of this research is the fact that only a selected resin was taken into account. However, due to the lack of content on that type of research, the authors had to plan the whole paper from the beginning, basing the research on referring to the composites. In addition, most of the published papers, which concentrate on the topic of dental materials (such as the one planned by us), do not refer to compression and tensile modulus. They also place more attention on the restorative materials. These limitations make the discussion regarding that topic more difficult. These limitations, though, make us want to expand our research to other potential resins.

5. Conclusions

The presented study allowed us to form several conclusions. Both polishing and artificial aging change the properties of BioMed Amber resin. Artificial aging changes the compressive modulus of the selected resin, no matter if the specimen was polished or not. The tensile modulus differs when either polishing or artificial aging were conducted. The application of both artificial aging and polishing does not change the properties much when compared to artificial aging without polishing. In general, the polishing of the samples may protect them from the influence of artificial aging, although the properties of the samples weaken. Further investigations should concentrate on that type of testing, and they should not be limited to the transparency and esthetics of the potential materials, because both artificial aging and polishing change the properties of the materials.

Author Contributions: Conceptualization, A.P.-S., M.W. and J.W.; methodology, A.P.-S. and J.W.; validation, A.P.-S.; investigation, J.W.; writing—original draft preparation, A.P.-S. and J.W.; writing—review and editing M.W. and M.M.; visualization, J.W. and A.P.-S.; supervision, A.P.-S.; project administration, J.W. and A.P.-S.; funding acquisition, A.P.-S. and M.M. All authors have read and agreed to the published version of the manuscript.

Funding: This research was funded by Wroclaw Medical University, grant number SUBK.B032.22.023 (A. Paradowska-Stolarz), according to records in the Simple System.

Institutional Review Board Statement: Not applicable.

Informed Consent Statement: Not applicable.

Data Availability Statement: All detailed data could be found at authors A.P.S. and J.W.

Conflicts of Interest: The authors declare no conflict of interest.

References

1. Dawood, A.; Marti, B.M.; Sauret-Jackson, V.; Darwood, A. 3D printing in dentistry. *Br. Dent. J.* **2016**, *219*, 521–529, Erratum in *Br. Dent. J.* **2016**, *220*, 86. [CrossRef] [PubMed]
2. Tian, Y.; Chen, C.; Xu, X.; Wang, J.; Hou, X.; Li, K.; Lu, X.; Shi, H.; Lee, E.S.; Jiang, H.B. A Review of 3D Printing in Dentistry: Technologies, Affecting Factors, and Applications. *Scanning* **2021**, *2021*, 9950131. [CrossRef] [PubMed]
3. Küffer, M.; Drescher, D.; Becker, K. Application of the Digital Workflow in Orofacial Orthopedics and Orthodontics: Printed Appliances with Skeletal Anchorage. *Appl. Sci.* **2022**, *12*, 3820. [CrossRef]
4. Tack, P.; Victor, J.; Gemmel, P.; Annemans, L. 3D-printing techniques in a medical setting: A systematic literature review. *Biomed. Eng. Online* **2016**, *15*, 115. [CrossRef]
5. Khorsandi, D.; Fahimipour, A.; Abasian, P.; Saber, S.S.; Seyedi, M.; Ghanavati, S.; Ahmad, A.; De Stephanis, A.A.; Taghavinezhaddilami, F.; Leonova, A.; et al. 3D and 4D printing in dentistry and maxillofacial surgery: Printing techniques, materials, and applications. *Acta Biomater.* **2021**, *122*, 26–49. [CrossRef]
6. Paradowska-Stolarz, A.; Malysa, A.; Mikulewicz, M. Comparison of the Compression and Tensile Modulus of Two Chosen Resins Used in Dentistry for 3D Printing. *Materials* **2022**, *15*, 8956. [CrossRef]
7. Paradowska-Stolarz, A.; Wezgowiec, J.; Mikulewicz, M. Comparison of Two Chosen 3D Printing Resins Designed for Orthodontic Use: An In Vitro Study. *Materials* **2023**, *16*, 2237. [CrossRef]
8. Kul, E.; Abdulrahim, R.; Bayındır, F.; Matori, K.A.; Gül, P. Evaluation of the color stability of temporary materials produced with CAD/CAM. *Dent. Med. Probl.* **2021**, *58*, 187–191. [CrossRef]
9. Grzebieluch, W.; Kowalewski, P.; Grygier, D.; Rutkowska-Gorczyca, M.; Kozakiewicz, M.; Jurczyszyn, K. Printable and Machinable Dental Restorative Composites for CAD/CAM Application-Comparison of Mechanical Properties, Fractographic, Texture and Fractal Dimension Analysis. *Materials* **2021**, *14*, 4919. [CrossRef]
10. Hampe, R.; Theelke, B.; Lümkemann, N.; Stawarczyk, B. Impact of artificial aging by thermocycling on edge chipping resistance and Martens hardness of different dental CAD-CAM restorative materials. *J. Prosthet. Dent.* **2021**, *125*, 326–333. [CrossRef]
11. Walczak, K.; Meißner, H.; Range, U.; Sakkas, A.; Boening, K.; Wieckiewicz, M.; Konstantinidis, I. Translucency of Zirconia Ceramics before and after Artificial Aging. *J. Prosthodont.* **2019**, *28*, e319–e324. [CrossRef] [PubMed]
12. Ilie, N. Accelerated versus Slow In Vitro Aging Methods and Their Impact on Universal Chromatic, Urethane-Based Composites. *Materials* **2023**, *16*, 2143. [CrossRef] [PubMed]
13. *ISO 604:2002*; Plastics-Determination of Compressive Properties. International Organization for Standardization: Geneva, Switzerland, 2002.
14. *ISO 527-1:2019*; Plastics—Determination of Tensile Properties—Part 1: General Principles. International Organization for Standardization: Geneva, Switzerland, 2019.
15. Vasoglou, G.; Stefanidaki, I.; Apostolopoulos, K.; Fotakidou, E.; Vasoglou, M. Accuracy of Mini-Implant Placement Using a Computer-Aided Designed Surgical Guide, with Information of Intraoral Scan and the Use of a Cone-Beam CT. *Dent. J.* **2022**, *10*, 104. [CrossRef] [PubMed]
16. Malysa, A.; Wezgowiec, J.; Grzebieluch, W.; Danel, D.P.; Wieckiewicz, M. Effect of Thermocycling on the Bond Strength of Self-Adhesive Resin Cements Used for Luting CAD/CAM Ceramics to Human Dentin. *Int. J. Mol. Sci.* **2022**, *23*, 745. [CrossRef]
17. Miletic, V.; Trifković, B.; Stamenković, D.; Tango, R.N.; Paravina, R.D. Effects of staining and artificial aging on optical properties of gingiva-colored resin-based restorative materials. *Clin. Oral Investig.* **2022**, *26*, 6817–6827. [CrossRef]
18. Valizadeh, S.; Asiaie, Z.; Kiomarsi, N.; Kharazifard, M.J. Color stability of self-adhering composite resins in different solutions. *Dent. Med. Probl.* **2020**, *7*, 31–38. [CrossRef]
19. El-Rashidy, A.A.; Abdelraouf, R.M.; Habib, N.A. Effect of two artificial aging protocols on color and gloss of single-shade versus multi-shade resin composites. *BMC Oral Health* **2022**, *22*, 321. [CrossRef]
20. Gómez-Polo, C.; Martín Casado, A.M.; Quispe, N.; Gallardo, E.R.; Montero, J. Colour Changes of Acetal Resins (CAD-CAM) In Vivo. *Appl. Sci.* **2023**, *13*, 181. [CrossRef]
21. Mazzitelli, C.; Paolone, G.; Sabbagh, J.; Scotti, N.; Vichi, A. Color Stability of Resin Cements after Water Aging. *Polymers* **2023**, *15*, 655. [CrossRef]
22. Warnecki, M.; Sarul, M.; Kozakiewicz, M.; Zięty, A.; Babiarczuk, B.; Kawala, B.; Jurczyszyn, K. Surface Evaluation of Aligners after Immersion in Coca-Cola and Orange Juice. *Materials* **2022**, *15*, 6341. [CrossRef]
23. Karatas, O.; Gul, P.; Akgul, N.; Celik, N.; Gundogdu, M.; Duymus, Z.; Seven, N. Effect of staining and bleaching on the microhardness, surface roughness and color of different composite resins. *Dent Med. Probl.* **2021**, *58*, 369–376. [CrossRef] [PubMed]
24. Paolone, G.; Mandurino, M.; De Palma, F.; Mazzitelli, C.; Scotti, N.; Breschi, L.; Gherlone, E.; Cantatore, G.; Vichi, A. Color Stability of Polymer-Based Composite CAD/CAM Blocks: A Systematic Review. *Polymers* **2023**, *15*, 464. [CrossRef] [PubMed]
25. Ling, L.; Ma, Y.; Malyala, R. A novel CAD/CAM resin composite block with high mechanical properties. *Dent Mater.* **2021**, *37*, 1150–1155. [CrossRef] [PubMed]
26. Wieckiewicz, M.; Boening, K.W.; Richter, G.; Wieckiewicz, W. Effect of thermocycling on the shear bond strength of different resins bonded to thermoplastic foil applied in occlusal splint therapy. *J. Prosthodont.* **2015**, *24*, 220–224. [CrossRef] [PubMed]
27. Matzinger, M.; Hahnel, S.; Preis, V.; Rosentritt, M. Polishing effects and wear performance of chairside CAD/CAM materials. *Clin. Oral Investig.* **2019**, *23*, 725–737. [CrossRef] [PubMed]

28. Rezaie, F.; Farshbaf, M.; Dahri, M.; Masjedi, M.; Maleki, R.; Amini, F.; Wirth, J.; Moharamzadeh, K.; Weber, F.E.; Tayebi, L. 3D Printing of Dental Prostheses: Current and Emerging Applications. *J. Compos. Sci.* **2023**, *7*, 80. [CrossRef]
29. Kocaagaoglu, H.; Aslan, T.; Gürbulak, A.; Albayrak, H.; Taşdemir, Z.; Gumus, H. Efficacy of polishing kits on the surface roughness and color stability of different composite resins. *Niger J. Clin. Pract.* **2017**, *20*, 557–565. [CrossRef]
30. Jaramillo-Cartagena, R.; López-Galeano, E.J.; Latorre-Correa, F.; Agudelo-Suárez, A.A. Effect of Polishing Systems on the Surface Roughness of Nano-Hybrid and Nano-Filling Composite Resins: A Systematic Review. *Dent. J.* **2021**, *9*, 95. [CrossRef]
31. Shimizu, Y.; Tada, K.; Seki, H.; Kakuta, K.; Miyagawa, Y.; Shen, J.F.; Morozumi, Y.; Kamoi, H.; Sato, S. Effects of air polishing on the resin composite-dentin interface. *Odontology* **2014**, *102*, 279–283. [CrossRef]
32. Paradowska-Stolarz, A.; Wieckiewicz, M.; Kozakiewicz, M.; Jurczyszyn, K. Mechanical Properties, Fractal Dimension, and Texture Analysis of Selected 3D-Printed Resins Used in Dentistry That Underwent the Compression Test. *Polymers* **2023**, *15*, 1772. [CrossRef]

Disclaimer/Publisher's Note: The statements, opinions and data contained in all publications are solely those of the individual author(s) and contributor(s) and not of MDPI and/or the editor(s). MDPI and/or the editor(s) disclaim responsibility for any injury to people or property resulting from any ideas, methods, instructions or products referred to in the content.

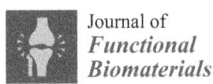

Article

Decellularized Scaffolds of Nopal (*Opuntia Ficus-indica*) for Bioengineering in Regenerative Dentistry

Ruth Betsabe Zamudio-Ceja [1,†], Rene Garcia-Contreras [1,†], Patricia Alejandra Chavez-Granados [1], Benjamin Aranda-Herrera [1], Hugo Alvarado-Garnica [1], Carlos A. Jurado [2] and Nicholas G. Fischer [3,*]

[1] Interdisciplinary Research Laboratory, Nanostructures, and Biomaterials Area, National School of Higher Studies (ENES) Leon, National Autonomous University of Mexico (UNAM), Leon 37684, Gto, Mexico
[2] Department of Prosthodontics, The University of Iowa College of Dentistry and Dental Clinics, Iowa City, IA 52242, USA
[3] Minnesota Dental Research Center for Biomaterials and Biomechanics, University of Minnesota, Minneapolis, MN 55455, USA
* Correspondence: fisc0456@umn.edu
† These authors contributed equally to this work.

Citation: Zamudio-Ceja, R.B.; Garcia-Contreras, R.; Chavez-Granados, P.A.; Aranda-Herrera, B.; Alvarado-Garnica, H.; Jurado, C.A.; Fischer, N.G. Decellularized Scaffolds of Nopal (*Opuntia Ficus-indica*) for Bioengineering in Regenerative Dentistry. *J. Funct. Biomater.* **2023**, *14*, 252. https://doi.org/10.3390/jfb14050252

Academic Editors: Lavinia Cosmina Ardelean and Laura-Cristina Rusu

Received: 31 March 2023
Revised: 23 April 2023
Accepted: 27 April 2023
Published: 1 May 2023

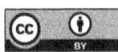

Copyright: © 2023 by the authors. Licensee MDPI, Basel, Switzerland. This article is an open access article distributed under the terms and conditions of the Creative Commons Attribution (CC BY) license (https://creativecommons.org/licenses/by/4.0/).

Abstract: *Opuntia Ficus-indica*, or nopal, is traditionally used for its medicinal properties in Mexico. This study aims to decellularize and characterize nopal (*Opuntia Ficus-indica*) scaffolds, assess their degradation and the proliferation of hDPSC, and determine potential pro-inflammatory effects by assessing the expression of cyclooxygenase 1 and 2 (COX-1 and 2). The scaffolds were decellularized using a 0.5% sodium dodecyl sulfate (SDS) solution and confirmed by color, optical microscopy, and SEM. The degradation rates and mechanical properties of the scaffolds were determined by weight and solution absorbances using trypsin and PBS and tensile strength testing. Human dental pulp stem cells (hDPSCs) primary cells were used for scaffold–cell interaction and proliferation assays, as well as an MTT assay to determine proliferation. Proinflammatory protein expression of COX-I and -II was discovered by Western blot assay, and the cultures were induced into a pro-inflammatory state with interleukin 1-β. The nopal scaffolds exhibited a porous structure with an average pore size of 252 ± 77 μm. The decellularized scaffolds showed a 57% reduction in weight loss during hydrolytic degradation and a 70% reduction during enzymatic degradation. There was no difference in tensile strengths between native and decellularized scaffolds (12.5 ± 1 and 11.8 ± 0.5 MPa). Furthermore, hDPSCs showed a significant increase in cell viability of 95% and 106% at 168 h for native and decellularized scaffolds, respectively. The combination of the scaffold and hDPSCs did not cause an increase in the expression of COX-1 and COX-2 proteins. However, when the combination was exposed to IL-1β, there was an increase in the expression of COX-2. This study demonstrates the potential application of nopal scaffolds in tissue engineering and regenerative medicine or dentistry, owing to their structural characteristics, degradation properties, mechanical properties, ability to induce cell proliferation, and lack of enhancement of pro-inflammatory cytokines.

Keywords: cellulose scaffolds; plant-based polymer; three-dimensional cellulose; tissue engineering

1. Introduction

The nopal (*Opuntia Ficus-indica*) is a cactus native to Mexico used since pre-Hispanic times as both food and medicine. Currently, there are 3 million hectares of native nopal and approximately 233,000 hectares cultivated in Mexico [1], making Mexico the world's leading producer and consumer [2]. It is a shrubby plant with a woody trunk and branches that are formed by cladodes. The nopal tissue has two layers, one consisting of green cells called chlorenchyma, and the second layer is internal and formed by a cylinder of white cells known as parenchyma, in which mucilaginous cells exist, so named for their main function of mucilage storage. The nopal chemical composition on a wet basis is 91% water, 6% carbohydrates, 1.5% cellulose, 1% proteins, and 0.5% fats [1]. Nopal possesses various therapeutic benefits, including lowering postprandial glucose levels in diabetic people due to its high fiber content and enhancing pectin mechanisms that absorb intestinal glucose. It also has antioxidant, analgesic, anti-inflammatory, anti-carcinogenic, anti-viral, and regenerative properties, suggesting that its rich content of carotenoids, flavonoids, phenols, vitamin A, and vitamin E contribute to these effects [1,2].

Natural plant-based scaffold polymers are preferred over synthetic and animal-based alternatives due to their biological property advantages. The role of the scaffold in regenerative engineering is to mimic the complexity required for cell migration, proliferation, and differentiation in tissue regeneration. This is achieved by designing porous scaffolds with specific surface areas, appropriate thickness, good permeability, and mechanical properties [3,4]. The nopal cactus could potentially be utilized in tissue engineering, which commonly involves immersion in decellularizing agents such as sodium dodecyl sulfate (SDS) [5,6] with agitation to create 3D scaffold structures that emulate the functions of original organs or tissues [7]. Natural-cellulose scaffolds, made from sources such as plants, algae, and bacteria, possess unique properties, including biocompatibility, biodegradability, and mechanical properties, that render them suitable for applications in tissue engineering and regenerative medicine [7,8].

In this context, Modulevsky et al. [8] developed 3D scaffolds made of cellulose derived from apples for culturing mammalian cells, demonstrating advantages such as simplification in production and reduced cost compared to other methods. On the other hand, Lee et. al. [9] used decellularized fruits and vegetables such as apples, broccoli, carrots, and peppers to obtain cellulose scaffolds for culturing pluripotent stem cells, demonstrating the ability of the scaffolds to support the in vitro culture of mammalian cells Similarly, Adamski et al. [10] decellularized leaves of *Ficus hispida* using two methods, both of which produced scaffolds with suitable mechanical properties and minimal impact to cellular metabolism.

Moreover, Contessi et al. [11] employed three plant tissues (apple, carrot, and celery) for decellularization, which showed mechanical properties and interconnected pores with a size of 100 to 500 μm, making them favorable for adipose tissue, bone tissue, and tendon regeneration. Recently, Chisci and Fredianelli [12] reported that the enzyme bromelain derived from the stem of the pineapple plant (*Ananas comosus*) was reported to have potential clinical therapeutic applications for preserving alveolar ridge structure. This suggests that bromelain could be a promising candidate for tissue engineering and regenerative dentistry. There are no prior reports in the literature on decellularized nopal cellulose (*Opuntia Ficus-indica*) scaffolds for use in biomedical engineering applications in dentistry or medicine, which presents an opportunity for potential bio-innovation in tissue engineering. Nopal cellulose has shown favorable biocompatibility and biodegradability properties, making it a promising candidate for use in scaffolds for tissue regeneration [13].

The objective of this study was to decellularize and characterize nopal (*Opuntia Ficus-indica*) scaffolds; assess degradation, tensile strength, and the proliferation of human dental pulp stem cells (hDPSCs); and determine the potential pro-inflammatory effects by assessing the expression of cyclooxygenase-1 and -2 (COX-1 and 2). This 3D scaffold system could lead to a potential application in bioengineering.

2. Materials and Methods

2.1. Nopal Scaffold Synthesis and Decellularization

Scaffolds were obtained from nopal plant tissue (*Opuntia Ficus-indica*) by using the parenchyma (pulp) portion while discarding the chlorenchyma. The nopal was grown in a greenhouse located at the National School of Higher Studies (ENES) Leon Unit with coordinates of 12.42385 latitude and −86.881317 longitude. Initially, parenchyma slices were cut using a mandolin slicer to obtain 0.5 cm × 2.0 cm × 0.5 mm blocks, which were subjected to a decellularization process using a 0.5% SDS solution (sodium dodecyl sulfate, ReagentPlus, Sigma-Aldrich, St. Louis, MO, USA). The SDS solution with the nopal scaffolds was subjected to agitation for 48 h at 180 rpm. After 24 h, agitation was suspended to subject the scaffolds to an ultrasonic bath for 5 min at 40 °C before continuing agitation to complete the 48 h cycle. The resulting structures were then washed three times with dH$_2$O and incubated in a CaCl$_2$ solution (calcium chloride, Karal, Leon, Guanajuato, Mexico) at a concentration of 100 mM for 24 h at room temperature. The scaffolds were washed three more times with dH$_2$O. At this point, both the decellularized scaffolds and native tissue scaffolds corresponding to the study group and control group, respectively, were obtained. Both scaffolds were incubated with penicillin/streptomycin (Sigma-Aldrich) + 1% fluconazole (Laboratorios Senosiain Laboratories, La Piedad, Michoacan, Mexico) for 3 h at 180 rpm. Finally, the samples were disinfected in a 70% ethanol solution for 1 h, washed three times in sterile dH$_2$O, and stored at $-20\ ^\circ$C until use (Figure 1).

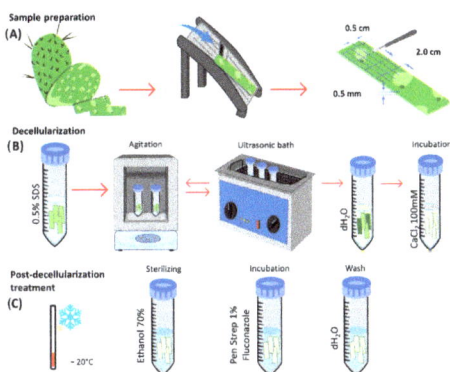

Figure 1. Schematic decellularization of nopal *Opuntia Ficus-indica* scaffold. (**A**) The scaffolds were obtained from nopal grown in a greenhouse located at ENES Leon Unit with coordinates of 12.42385 latitude and -86.881317 longitude. The scaffolds were derived by using the parenchyma (pulp) portion with a mandolin slicer to a uniform thickness of 0.5 cm $\times$ 2.0 cm $\times$ 0.5 mm. (**B**) Nopal scaffolds were decellularized using 0.5% SDS solution during the 48 h agitation cycle. The resulting structures were washed three times with dH$_2$O and incubated in a CaCl$_2$ solution. (**C**) Stored at $-20\ ^\circ$C, disinfected with a 70% ethanol solution, incubated with PenStrep + 1% fluconazole for 3 h, and washed with sterile dH$_2$O (**C**). Abbreviations: SDS = sodium dodecyl sulfate, CaCl$_2$ = calcium chloride, PenStrep = penicillin/streptomycin (Sigma-Aldrich).

2.2. Nopal Scaffold Characterization

The characterization of the scaffolds was carried out by optical microscopy to understand the microstructure and compare the changes that decellularization caused in it. Decellularized scaffolds and native nopal parenchyma tissue were fixed in a 2% glutaraldehyde solution (Karal) and PBS in a 1:1 ratio for 24 h, dehydrated with ethanol gradients at 25, 50, 75, and 100% for 5 min every 2 h in a continuous flow, and stored in a silica mold for 48 h. Subsequently, they were placed on slides to be stained with safranin or coated with a thin carbon layer. The samples were analyzed under an inverted optical microscope (Leica DMIL LED, Deerfield, IL, USA) at 40$\times$ and scanning electron microscopy (SEM, JEOL JSM-IT500, Tokyo, Japan) at a magnification of 250$\times$ using primary electrons accelerated to 50 kV.

2.3. Nopal Scaffolds Degradation

To conduct degradation assays, we used an analytical balance (Denver Instrument, Arvada, CO, USA) to measure the weight of all scaffolds before they underwent the degradation process. This weight was then identified as the initial weight. Afterward, the nopal decellularized and native tissue scaffolds in separate tubes containing a trypsin 0.025% EDTA-2Na in PBS(−) (Sigma-Aldrich) and 1X phosphate buffered saline (PBS) for enzymatic and hydrolytic degradation, respectively. The scaffolds and solutions were placed in Falcon tubes and agitated at 360 rpm at 37 $^\circ$C for 240 h. Every 24 h, we stopped the agitation to remove the scaffolds from the solutions, record their weight, and measure their absorbance at 350 nm using a UV-Vis spectrophotometer (Multiskan Go, Thermo-Scientific, Helsinki, Finland) to observe proteins in solution.

2.4. Nopal Scaffolds tensile Strength

The mechanical properties of native and decellularized nopal scaffolds were assessed using a tensile test, following the ASTM D 882-02: standard test method for tensile properties of thin plastic sheeting. A universal testing machine (Mecmesin, advanced force/torque indicator (AFTI), London, UK) was employed to conduct the tests, with an initial scaffold area of 20 mm × 10 mm positioned between clamps and a cross speed of 1 mm/min applied until failure occurred. Tensile strength was then determined by dividing the force applied to the sample (measured in Newtons) by the sample's cross-sectional area (in mm) and expressed in megapascals (MPa). The sample size used for this experiment was $n = 10$ per group.

2.5. Cell Culture

The hDPSCs were obtained from the cell bank of the Interdisciplinary Research Laboratory, Nanostructures and Biomaterials Area of the ENES Leon, UNAM. The cells were established and characterized as previously reported [14]. Initially, the cells in cryopreservation vials were thawed by placing each vial in the cell incubator for 5 to 10 min. After thawing, the cells were then placed in 10 cm culture plates (Corning Costar®, Nagog park acton, MA, USA) with supplemented MEM cell culture medium consisting of 10% fetal bovine serum (FBS), 1% glutamine (Sigma-Aldrich), and 1% antibiotics (PenStrep, Sigma-Aldrich). The cells were then incubated at 37 °C with 5% CO_2. The culture medium was changed every two days until the cells reached a cellular confluence of over 80%.

2.6. Scaffold-Cell Interaction and Proliferation

The hDPSCs cultures (PDL 6) that exhibited confluence higher than 80% were inoculated in 24-well plates (Corning Costar®) on scaffolds. The cells were washed with PBS and detached by 0.25% trypsin-0.025% EDTA-2Na in PBS (Sigma-Aldrich) for each experiment. The number of inoculated cells was determined by excluding trypan blue with a hemocytometer under light microscopy. A total of 1×10^6 cells/mL were subcultured on the nopal and native scaffolds. Native nopal tissue was used as the control group. The interaction consisted of 24 h, and the proliferation was incubated from 72 to 168 h at 37 °C with 5% CO_2 and 95% humidity. The interaction between hDPSCs and nopal scaffolds was examined by looking at the morphological characteristics using both a stereomicroscope (Leica DMIL LED) at 40× and SEM (JEOL JSM-IT500). After the medium was removed, the samples were washed three times with PBS, fixed, stained, dehydrated, and stored, as above mentioned.

The proliferation assay was determined with the MTT method used to determine cell viability. Briefly, the cells were incubated for 7 h in fresh MEM with 10% FBS containing 0.2 mg/mL of Thiazolyl Blue Tetrazolium Bromide (Sigma-Aldrich). After incubation, the formazan produced was dissolved with dimethyl sulfoxide (DMSO, Karal), and the absorbance of the lysate at 570 nm was measured using a microplate spectrophotometer reader (Multiskan go, Thermo-Scientific). Cytotoxicity was assessed according to the ISO 10993-5:2009 standard for in vitro cytotoxicity testing of medical devices.

2.7. COX-1 and COX-2 Cell Expression-Scaffold

To determine the protein expression of COX-1 and COX-2, a Western blot assay was performed. A subculture of hDPSCs (1×10^6 cells/mL, 8 PDL) was inoculated with the decellularized nopal scaffolds for 168 h. Subsequently, the cultures were induced into a pro-inflammatory state with 3.12 ng/mL of human interleukin 1-β (IL-1β human recombinant, R&D Systems, Minneapolis, MN, USA) for 24 h. The protein lysis and extraction process were performed with ice-cold 1X RIPA lysis buffer (Biotechnology WVR

AMRESCO, Fountain Parkway, Solon, OH, USA) in each scaffold for 15 min at 4 °C. The lysed culture was subjected to sonication for 10 s and centrifugation at 12,000 rpm for 10 min at 4 °C. Protease inhibitor cocktail tablet (Roche Diagnostics, Indianapolis, IN, USA) was used. The protein concentrations in the lysates were determined, and equal amounts of protein for each sample were subjected to 8% SDS-polyacrylamide gel electrophoresis and transferred to a polyvinylidene membrane (PVDF, immobilon®-P Transfer Membranes, Sigma-Aldrich). The membrane was blocked with a 3% skim milk solution for 2 h while stirring at 25 °C. The membrane was incubated with monoclonal antibody anti-COX-1 or anti-COX-2 (Santa Cruz Biotechnology, Dalla, TX, USA) or β-actin (Sigma-Aldrich), diluted 1:1000 in 3% blocking solution for 1–2 h, followed by horseradish peroxidase-coupled anti-mouse IgG polyclonal antibody (Sigma-Aldrich) diluted 1:1000 in 3% blocking solution for 1 h. The visualization of the complexes formed was performed by chemiluminescence using Clarity max Western ECL substrate (Bio-Rad, Hercules, CA, USA), and the results were imaged using the C-Digit Blot scanner (Li-Cor, Lincoln, NE, USA) and analyzed in Image Studio Version 4.0 software.

2.8. Statistical Analysis

The data represent mean ± standard deviation and were analyzed with the Shapiro–Wilks normality test, t-student, and ANOVA post-hoc Tukey test. The significance was considered at $p < 0.05$ with a confidence interval of 95%.

3. Results

3.1. Nopal Scaffold Characterization

The decellularization method using a 0.5% SDS solution proved to be effective in isolating the extracellular matrix of the nopal after 48 h, ensuring complete removal of the cells. This was immediately confirmed as the obtained samples appeared colorless and translucent. Decellularization was also verified through optical microscopy and SEM, where micrographs of decellularized samples were compared with those of native tissue without decellularization. Optical microscopy and SEM showed images that corresponded to a porous structure of 252 ± 77 μm ($n = 9$, 150 to 400 μm) with interconnected circular shapes, positive for cellulose (Figure 2A–C). The micrograph of the native tissue showed spherical, clustered structures where the plant tissue cells were suggested to be located. In the decellularized tissue sample, this bulging of circular structures was not observed. Instead, a porous structure was seen, indicating the absence of plant cells, thus, achieving decellularization and the isolation of the cellulose nopal extracellular matrix.

3.2. Nopal Scaffolds Degradation

The degradation of the decellularized scaffolds or native tissue was evaluated by comparing the initial and final weights and measuring the absorbance of the solutions. The initial weight was identified as the first measurement at 0 h of the degradation process, and the final weight was the measurement taken after 240 h of agitation in trypsin and PBS solutions. During the process, it was evident that the scaffold structure's dimensions decreased, and the weight measurement demonstrated a gradual decrease over time, registering a 57% weight loss for the decellularized scaffolds in hydrolytic degradation and a 70% weight loss in enzymatic degradation, with a statistically significant difference ($p < 0.01$) compared to the degradation of native tissue scaffolds ($n = 9$). The degradation was evaluated up to 240 h because it was impossible to manipulate the scaffolds after this time due to their fragmentation and degradation (Figure 3A,B). In the measurement of absorbance using UV-Vis spectrophotometry at 350 nm, an absorbance increase was observed after 96 h in native and decellularized scaffolds ($p < 0.01$, $n = 9$). The native tissue exhibits more solution absorbances correlated to the degradation process in both hydrolytic and enzymatic solution (Figure 3C,D).

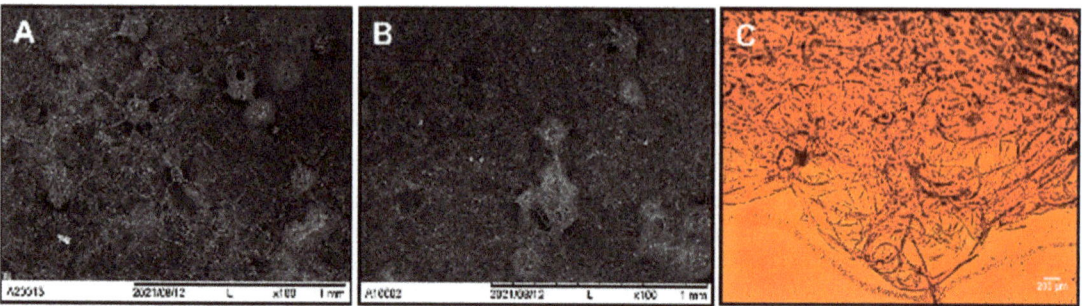

Figure 2. Nopal (*Opuntia Ficus-indica*) decellularized scaffolds and hDPSCs–scaffold interaction. The nopal scaffold decellularization process was achieved using a 0.5% SDS. Native nopal parenchyma tissue (**A**) and decellularized scaffolds (**B**,**C**) were fixed in a 2% glutaraldehyde solution for 2 h and dehydrated with ethanol gradients at 25, 50, 75, and 100% for 5 min each. Subsequently, the sample was placed on slides, stained with safranin, and observed under an inverted optical microscope at 40×. For SEM, the samples were coated with a thin carbon layer and imaged at a magnification of 250× using primary electrons accelerated to 50 kV. Abbreviations: SDS = sodium dodecyl sulfate, SEM = scanning electron microscope. Scale bars are indicated in each panel.

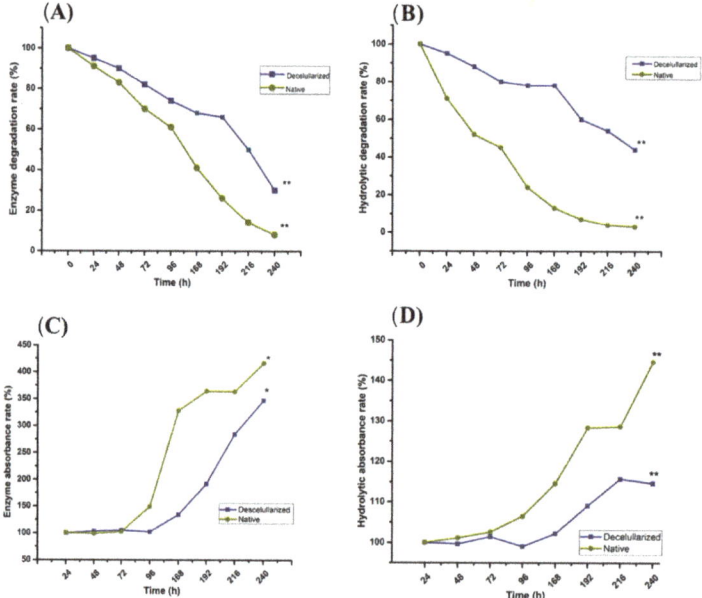

Figure 3. Nopal decellularized scaffold or native tissue enzymatic and hydrolytic degradation. The scaffold's initial and final weights were recorded from 0 to 240 h after being incubated under agitation for 360 rpm at 37 °C in trypsin-0.025% EDTA-2Na in PBS (**A**) and PBS (**B**). The weight was determined every 24 h and the absorbance of the solution was measured at 350 nm using a UV-Vis spectrophotometer (**C**, trypsin and **D**, PBS). Nopal decellularized scaffolds correspond to a 57% weight loss in hydrolytic degradation and 70% in enzymatic degradation. Each value represents the mean ± SD of triplicate assays ($n = 9$), * $p < 0.05$, ** $p < 0.001$ Student's *t*-test. Abbreviations: EDTA = ethylenediaminetetraacetic acid, PBS = phosphate buffer saline solution, SD = standard deviation.

3.3. Scaffold Tensile Strength

The assessment of mechanical properties of tensile strength indicated that both native and decellularized nopal scaffolds exhibited values of 12.5 ± 1 MPa and 11.8 ± 0.5 MPa, respectively. Notably, statistical analysis revealed no significant difference between the two groups ($n = 10$, $p > 0.05$), suggesting that both types of scaffolds possess comparable tensile strength (Table 1).

Table 1. Comparison of tensile strength of native and decellularized nopal (*Opuntia Ficus-indica*) scaffolds ($n = 10$ per group).

Scaffold	Tensile Strength (MPa)	t-Student Test
Native nopal scaffold	12.5 ± 1	$p = 0.0748$
Decellularized nopal scaffold	11.8 ± 0.5	
MPa = Megapascals		

3.4. Cell-Scaffold Interaction and Proliferation

Images of 2D cultures on culture plates alone as a control showed cells exhibiting a fusiform elongated and flattened morphology (Figure 4A). On the other hand, the hDPSCs–nopal decellularized scaffold interaction showed cells with a spherical shape on the scaffold (Figure 4B). Similarly, samples were prepared for characterization by SEM, which confirmed the results obtained with optical microscopy, showing cells with a circular and spherical morphology on the scaffolds (Figure 4C). The decellularized nopal tissue scaffolds present an optimal microstructure for hDPSCs to adhere and proliferate. hDPSCs exhibited significantly exponential cell viability ($n = 9$, $p < 0.01$) at 168 h compared to native tissue (Figure 5) with 95% and 106% viable cell number for native and decellularized scaffolds.

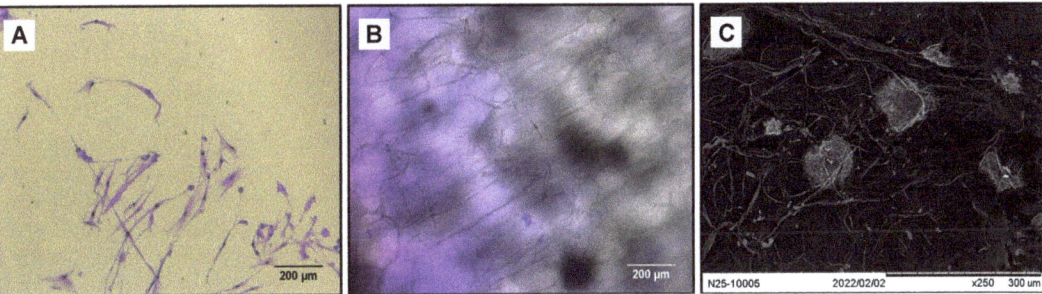

Figure 4. Initial hDPSCs–nopal scaffold interactions. In the case of the hDPSCs–nopal scaffold interaction, near confluent hDPSC cells (80% confluence, 6 PDL) were incubated as control on a plastic dish (**A**) and then on the nopal decellularized scaffold for 24 h (**B**,**C**). After incubation, the medium was removed and treated as above mentioned for an inverted optical microscope and SEM. hDPSCs = human dental pulp stem cells, SDS = sodium dodecyl sulfate, SEM = scanning electron microscope. Scale bars are indicated in each panel.

3.5. COX-1 and COX-2 Cell Expression-Scaffold

The interaction of decellularized nopal scaffold and hDPSCs did not cause any noticeable increase in COX-1 and COX-2 protein expression (Figure 6A). However, when combined with IL-1β, a known pro-inflammatory stimulator, the expression of COX-2 was increased, as shown in Figure 6; β-actin was used as an internal control. Based on these findings, it can be concluded that the scaffold by itself does not induce the pro-inflammatory expression of COX-1 or COX-2 but permits physiologic cell function under IL-1β stimulation.

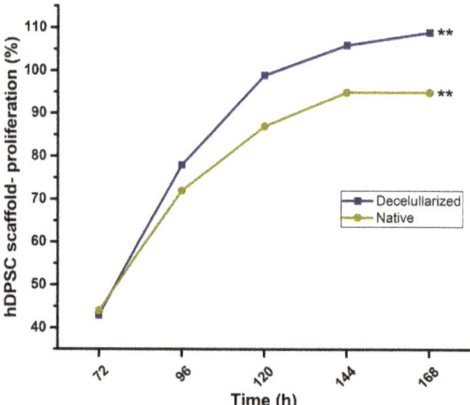

Figure 5. hDPSCs–nopal scaffold proliferation. hDPSCs at 1×10^6 cells/mL (6 PDL) were inoculated over the nopal and native scaffolds from 72 to 168 h at 37 °C with 5% CO_2 and 95% humidity. The hDPSCs proliferation was determined by the MTT method (0.2 mg/mL). The nopal decellularized scaffold showed a major number of proliferated hDPSC at 168 h when compared to native tissue. Each value represents mean ± SD of triplicate assays ($n = 9$), ** $p < 0.001$ Student's t-test. Abbreviations: hDPSCs = human dental pulp stem cells, PDL = population doubling level, MTT = 3-[4,5-dimethylthiazol-2yl]-2,5-diphenyltetrazolium bromide, SD = standard deviation.

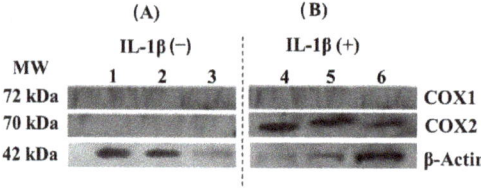

Figure 6. Expression of pro-inflammatory proteins COX 1 and COX 2 of hDPSCs–decellularized nopal scaffolds interaction. hDPSCs at 1×10^6 cells/mL (8 PDL) were inoculated over the decellularized nopal for 168 h. Subsequently, the cultures were induced into a pro-inflammatory state (**B**, IL-1β = 3.12 ng/mL) or not (**A**) for 24 h. The protein lysis and extraction process were performed with RIPA lysis buffer and the Western blot protocol was performed. The nopal scaffold did not cause any noticeable increase in COX-1 and COX-2 protein expression (**A**). However, when combined with IL-1β, the pro-inflammatory state enhanced the expression of COX-2 (**B**), and β-actin was used as an internal positive control. Abbreviations: MW = molecular weight marker, COX = cyclooxygenase, hDPSCs = human dental pulp stem cells, PDL = population doubling level, IL-1β = human interleukin 1-β.

4. Discussion

4.1. Scaffold Decellularization

The method of decellularizing plant tissue described in this study, using a 0.5% SDS solution and agitation, represents a safe, simple, and economical procedure that requires minimal resources. As a result, it is environmentally friendly and helps preserve the extracellular matrix of plant tissue [5,15]. This makes it a favorable method as it allows for cellular adhesion and proliferation on scaffolds and nutrient transfer through the nopal tissue and can, therefore, be used in tissue engineering. Contessi et al. [11] conducted the previous research demonstrating the potential of decellularized apple, carrot, and celery tissues for regenerating adipose, bone, and tendon tissue. This was attributed to their mechanical properties and interconnected pores, ranging from 100–500 μm, which were found to be optimal for cellular migration, proliferation, and differentiation. Our present study similarly found that decellularized nopal tissue scaffolds exhibited a porous structure with interconnected circular shapes with a diameter of 252 ± 77 μm, suggesting that decellularized nopal tissue could also have potential for tissue regeneration.

4.2. Nopal Scaffolds Degradation

Cellulose possesses the ability to persist at the implantation site for extended periods due to its resistance to enzymatic degradation by mammalian cells [16]. However, this can be altered by adjusting the degradation rate through hydrolysis pretreatment and by administering cellulases or collagenase along with the scaffolds. Regarding the degradation process, a weight loss of 70% was observed in the decellularized scaffolds, which coincides with the report by Modulesvky et al. [17] for subcutaneous implantation of decellularized plant tissue scaffolds, which can demonstrate their possible degradability. In this study, the scaffolds showed significant degradation under hydrolytic and enzymatic conditions with PBS and trypsin over a period of 240 h, as evidenced by changes in weight loss and solution absorbance, in contrast to native tissue. These findings suggest that decellularized plant cellulose-based scaffolds hold promise as an alternative to traditional animal-derived scaffolds for tissue engineering purposes. However, further research is required to fully evaluate their long-term biocompatibility and degradation.

4.3. Nopal Scaffold Tensile Strength

Previous studies have evaluated the mechanical properties of natural scaffolds based on aloe vera and cellulose alone or in combination with other polymers for bone tissue engineering. Khoshgozaran-Abras et al. [18] and Saibuatongbased and Phisalaphong [19] have reported these scaffolds can effectively improve the mechanical properties, based on standard ASTM D 882-02. For instance, aloe vera combined with hydroxyapatite was shown to increase the reported tensile strength from 4.80 MPa to 10.89 MPa. Additionally, Bahaaraty et al. [20] evaluated the elastic modulus in nanofiber scaffolds based on copolymer poly(l-lactic acid)-co-poly (ε-caprolactone) (PLACL), silk fibroin (SF), and aloe vera. The results showed elastic modulus values of 14.1 ± 0.7, 9.96 ± 2.5, and 7.0 ± 0.9 MPa, respectively. In comparison, the nopal decellularized scaffolds in the tensile strength test exhibited higher values than the previously reported results, indicating that nopal tissue enhances the mechanical properties and may be comparable with synthetic scaffolds. However, when Bielli et al. [21] evaluated the tensile strength of collagen fiber scaffolds from bovine pericardium (biomeshes), the values ranged from 21.44 to 50.91 MPa, suggesting that the biomeshes possess higher tensile strength compared to our results.

4.4. Cell-Scaffold Interaction and Proliferation

Proliferation assays of hDPSCs carried out in this study demonstrated an exponential-constant increase in viability with a statistically significant difference in proliferation between hDPSCs on decellularized scaffolds and native tissue. This was also observed in previous reports where decellularized plant tissue scaffolds were used for the culture of different mammalian cells [6,7,11,17,22]. With these results, it can be said that there was in vitro biocompatibility of the cells with the decellularized nopal scaffold, as it was shown that they were able to adhere, invade, and proliferate within the cellulose scaffolds, indicating that this tissue had high viability even after 168 h. The morphological characteristics of hDPSCs on decellularized nopal scaffolds observed in the micrographs show oval, circular, and spherical-shaped cells, unlike 2D cultures that are flattened and elongated. This is the trait that makes them different from 2D cultures, and these results have similarities with what other authors have reported [23,24]. The importance of morphology in 3D cultures is that it allows conditions to be imitated and behaviors to be replicated in vivo. Three-dimensional culture systems aim to replicate the microstructures of organs, using the extracellular matrix (ECM) as scaffolding. This approach was used in organoids of various organs [25]. Future experiments should prioritize the incorporation of extracellular matrix components to promote the development of bone, adipose, and cartilage tissue initially before moving on to creating multipotential scaffolds for other tissues in the field of regenerative engineering.

4.5. COX-1 and COX-2 Cell Expression-Scaffold

Finally, in evaluating the potential inflammatory effect of decellularized nopal scaffolds, the results obtained were that the interaction of hDPSCs with decellularized nopal scaffolds did not provoke an inflammatory state in the cultures. These were favorable results as it has potential clinical application as there is no foreign body rejection. This can be compared to what Yi et al. 2020 reported, where they conducted a Western blot to determine the anti-inflammatory effect by identifying the expression of cytokines such as tumor necrosis factor α in mesenchymal cell culture models [26]. Biocompatibility is an essential aspect to consider when using biomaterials, as it refers to their ability to interact with living tissues without causing adverse effects such as inflammation or toxicity. Previous studies have evaluated the biocompatibility of various biomaterials [27] for different biomedical applications, including hip prostheses, mechanical properties [28], and clinical or simulated interventions [29]. In this study, we demonstrate that nopal decellularized scaffolds exhibit neither cytotoxicity nor inflammation in vitro, suggesting their potential use in biomedical applications. Therefore, it is crucial to carefully consider the nature, mechanical properties, and biocompatibility of biomaterials when selecting suitable candidates for specific biomedical applications and to evaluate their safety and efficacy through clinical or simulated assessments.

4.6. Limitations of the Study

One limitation of this study could be related to the geographical location and cultural variations of nopal (*Opuntia Ficus-indica*), which may impact the reproducibility and scalability of scaffold production for industrial applications in tissue engineering. Standardizing conditions could help mitigate this limitation. Another limitation is that despite the incorporation of antifungal agents in the culture medium, slight fungal infections were observed after 15 days of culture. This highlights the need for further research to optimize the antifungal properties of the scaffolds to ensure their long-term stability in tissue engineering applications.

5. Conclusions

These findings indicate that the nopal (*Opuntia Ficus-indica*) scaffolds were effectively decellularized using 0.5% dodecyl sodium sulfate, while retaining the extracellular matrix of cellulose. The scaffolds were able to degrade by 50–70% at 240 h, and when human dental pulp stem cells (hDPSCs) were cultured on the scaffolds, they exhibited significant proliferation without affecting cell interactions or the expression of the pro-inflammatory proteins COX-1 and -2. In summary, the use of decellularized nopal scaffolds holds great promise for regenerative dentistry and medicine. Further experiments will focus on evaluating the interaction between the cell–scaffold interaction by investigating focal adhesion kinase signaling, integrins, and other extracellular matrix proteins to better understand cell adhesion, migration, and differentiation with different types of cells. Other cell types, such as bone marrow stem cells, should also be explored. In addition, efforts will be made to increase the mechanical properties of the scaffold, and micro-CT evaluation will be conducted to understand the ultrastructural topography and predict the biological mechanisms involved. Potential further studies can utilize computational simulation [30], in silico approaches [31], or a contact pressure 3D model [32] to study the performance of nopal scaffolds effectively and accessibly and predict their results, as compared to traditional experimental testing, in vitro and in vivo or clinical study.

Author Contributions: Conceptualization, R.B.Z.-C., R.G.-C. and H.A.-G.; methodology, R.B.Z.-C., R.G.-C. and H.A.-G.; software, B.A.-H. and P.A.C.-G.; validation, B.A.-H., C.A.J., N.G.F. and R.G.-C.; investigation, R.G.-C. and P.A.C.-G.; resources, C.A.J.; data curation, R.G.-C. and B.A.-H.; writing—original draft preparation, R.G.-C., P.A.C.-G. and B.A.-H.; writing—review and editing, C.A.J. and N.G.F.; project administration, B.A.-H.; funding acquisition, C.A.J. and N.G.F. All authors have read and agreed to the published version of the manuscript.

Funding: This research was funded by UNAM-DGAPA-PAPIME and PAPIIT through grant PE203622 and IT200922.

Data Availability Statement: The data presented in this study are available on request from the corresponding author.

Acknowledgments: The authors would like to thank Marina Vega-Gonzalez from the Geosciences Center, Multidisciplinary Teaching and Research Unit of Juriquilla, UNAM, for the scanning electron microscopy (SEM) micrographs.

Conflicts of Interest: The authors declare no conflict of interest.

References

1. Stintzing, F.C.; Carle, R. Cactus Stems (*Opuntia* spp.): A Review on Their Chemistry, Technology, and Uses. *Mol. Nutr. Food Res.* **2006**, *49*, 175–194. [CrossRef]
2. Maki-Díaz, G.; Peña-Valdivia, C.B.; Garcia-Nava, R.; Arévalo-Galarza, M.L.; Calderón-Zavala, G.; Anaya-Rosales, S. Physical and Chemical Characteristics of Cactus Stems (*Opuntia ficus-indica*) for Exportation and Domestic Markets. *Agrociencia* **2015**, *49*, 31–51. Available online: https://www.scielo.org.mx/scielo.php?script=sci_arttext&pid=S1405-31952015000100003&lng=es&nrm=iso (accessed on 12 February 2023).
3. Prakoso, A.T.; Basri, H.; Adanta, D.; Yani, I.; Ammarullah, M.I.; Akbar, I.; Ghazali, F.A.; Syahrom, A.; Kamarul, T. The Effect of Tortuosity on Permeability of Porous Scaffold. *Biomedicines* **2023**, *11*, 427. [CrossRef] [PubMed]
4. Putra, R.U.; Basri, H.; Prakoso, A.T.; Chandra, H.; Ammarullah, M.I.; Akbar, I.; Syahrom, A.; Kamarul, T. Level of Activity Changes Increases the Fatigue Life of the Porous Magnesium Scaffold, as Observed in Dynamic Immersion Tests, over Time. *Sustainability* **2023**, *15*, 823. [CrossRef]
5. Stoppel, W.L.; Kaplan, D.L.; Black, L.D., 3rd. Electrical and Mechanical Stimulation of Cardiac Cells and Tissue Constructs. *Adv. Drug Deliv. Rev.* **2016**, *96*, 135–155. [CrossRef] [PubMed]
6. Blaudez, F.; Ivanovski, S.; Hamlet, S.; Vaquette, C. An Overview of Decellularisation Techniques of Native Tissues and Tissue Engineered Products for Bone, Ligament and Tendon Regeneration. *Methods* **2020**, *171*, 28–40. [CrossRef] [PubMed]
7. Crapo, P.M.; Gilbert, T.W.; Badylak, S.F. An Overview of Tissue and Whole Organ Decellularization Processes. *Biomaterials* **2011**, *32*, 3233–3243. [CrossRef] [PubMed]
8. Modulevsky, D.J.; Lefebvre, C.; Haase, K.; Al-Rekabi, Z.; Pelling, A.E. Apple Derived Cellulose Scaffolds for 3D Mammalian Cell Culture. *PLoS ONE* **2014**, *9*, e97835. [CrossRef] [PubMed]
9. Lee, J.; Jung, H.; Park, N.; Park, S.H.; Ju, J.H. Induced Osteogenesis in Plants Decellularized Scaffolds. *Sci. Rep.* **2019**, *9*, 20194. [CrossRef]
10. Adamski, M.; Fontana, G.; Gershlak, J.R.; Gaudette, G.R.; Le, H.D.; Murphy, W.L. Two Methods for Decellularization of Plant Tissues for Tissue Engineering Applications. *J. Vis. Exp.* **2018**, *135*, 57586. [CrossRef]
11. Contessi, N.N.; Toffoletto, N.; Farè, S.; Altomare, L. Plant Tissues as 3D Natural Scaffolds for Adipose, Bone and Tendon Tissue Regeneration. *Front. Bioeng. Biotechnol.* **2020**, *8*, 723. [CrossRef] [PubMed]
12. Chisci, G.; Fredianelli, L. Therapeutic Efficacy of Bromelain in Alveolar Ridge Preservation. *Antibiotics* **2022**, *11*, 1542. [CrossRef] [PubMed]
13. Marin-Bustamante, M.Q.; Chanona-Pérez, J.J.; Güemes-Vera, M.; Cásarez-Santiago, R.; Perea-Flores, M.J.; Arzate-Vázquez, I.; Calderón-Domínguez, G. Production and Characterization of Cellulose Nanoparticles From Nopal Waste by Means of High Impact Milling. *Procedia Eng.* **2017**, *200*, 428–433. [CrossRef]
14. Garcia-Contreras, R.; Chavez-Granados, P.A.; Jurado, C.A.; Aranda-Herrera, B.; Afrashtehfar, K.I.; Nurrohman, H. Natural Bioactive Epigallocatechin-Gallate Promote Bond Strength and Differentiation of Odontoblast-like Cells. *Biomimetics* **2023**, *8*, 75. [CrossRef] [PubMed]
15. Lacombe, J.; Harris, A.F.; Zenhausern, R.; Karsunsky, S.; Zenhausern, F. Plant-Based Scaffolds Modify Cellular Response to Drug and Radiation Exposure Compared to Standard Cell Culture Models. *Front. Bioeng. Biotechnol.* **2020**, *8*, 932. [CrossRef] [PubMed]
16. Lai, C.; Zhang, S.J.; Wang, L.Q.; Sheng, L.Y.; Zhou, Q.Z.; Xi, T.F. The relationship between microstructure and in vivo degradation of modified bacterial cellulose sponges. *J. Mater. Chem. B* **2015**, *3*, 9001–9010. [CrossRef]
17. Modulevsky, D.J.; Cuerrier, C.M.; Pelling, A.E. Biocompatibility of Subcutaneously Implanted Plant-Derived Cellulose Biomaterials. *PLoS ONE* **2016**, *11*, e0157894. [CrossRef]
18. Khoshgozaran-Abras, S.; Azizi, M.H.; Hamidy, Z.; Bagheripoor-Fallah, N. Mechanical, Physicochemical and Color Properties of Chitosan Based-Films as a Function of Aloe vera Gel Incorporation. *Carbohydr. Polym.* **2012**, *87*, 2058–2062. [CrossRef]

19. Saibuatongbased, O.; Phisalaphong, M. Novo aloe vera–bacterial cellulose composite film from biosynthesis. *Carbohydr. Polym.* **2010**, *79*, 455–460. [CrossRef]
20. Bhaarathy, V.; Venugopal, J.; Gandhimathi, C.; Ponpandian, N.; Mangalaraj, D.; Ramakrishna, S. Biologically Improved Nanofibrous Scaffolds for Cardiac Tissue Engineering. *Mater. Sci. Eng. C Mater. Biol. Appl.* **2014**, *44*, 268–277. [CrossRef]
21. Bielli, A.; Bernardini, R.; Varvaras, D.; Rossi, P.; Di Blasi, G.; Petrella, G.; Buonomo, O.C.; Mattei, M.; Orlandi, A. Characterization of a New Decellularized Bovine Bericardial Biological Mesh: Structural and Mechanical properties. *J. Mech. Behav. Biomed. Mater.* **2019**, *78*, 420–426. [CrossRef]
22. Gershlak, J.R.; Hernandez, S.; Fontana, G.; Perreault, L.R.; Hansen, K.J.; Larson, S.A.; Binder, B.Y.; Dolivo, D.M.; Yang, T.; Dominko, T.; et al. Crossing Kingdoms: Using decellularized Plants as Perfusable Tissue Engineering Scaffolds. *Biomaterials* **2017**, *125*, 13–22. [CrossRef] [PubMed]
23. Duval, K.; Grover, H.; Han, L.H.; Mou, Y.; Pegoraro, A.F.; Fredberg, J.; Chen, Z. Modeling Physiological Events in 2D vs. 3D Cell Culture. *Physiology* **2017**, *32*, 266–277. [CrossRef] [PubMed]
24. Dugan, J.M.; Gough, J.E.; Eichhorn, S.J. Bacterial Cellulose Scaffolds and Cellulose Nanowhiskers for Tissue Engineering. *Nanomedicine* **2013**, *8*, 287–298. [CrossRef] [PubMed]
25. Saheli, M.; Sepantafar, M.; Pournasr, B.; Farzaneh, Z.; Vosough, M.; Piryaei, A.; Baharvand, H. Three-Dimensional Liver-Derived Extracellular Matrix Hydrogel Promotes Liver Organoids Function. *J. Cell. Biochem.* **2018**, *119*, 4320–4333. [CrossRef]
26. Yi, P.; Xu, X.; Qiu, B.; Li, H. Impact of Chitosan Membrane Culture on the Expression of Pro- and Anti-Inflammatory Cytokines in Mesenchymal Stem Cells. *Exp. Ther. Med.* **2020**, *20*, 3695–3702. [CrossRef]
27. Ammarullah, M.I.; Hartono, R.; Supriyono, T.; Santoso, G.; Sugiharto, S.; Permana, M.S. Polycrystalline Diamond as a Potential Material for the Hard-on-Hard Bearing of Total Hip Prosthesis: Von Mises Stress Analysis. *Biomedicines* **2023**, *11*, 951. [CrossRef]
28. Ammarullah, M.I.; Santoso, G.; Sugiharto, S.; Supriyono, T.; Wibowo, D.B.; Kurdi, O.; Tauviqirrahman, M.; Jamari, J. Minimizing Risk of Failure from Ceramic-on-Ceramic Total Hip Prosthesis by Selecting Ceramic Materials Based on Tresca Stress. *Sustainability* **2022**, *14*, 13413. [CrossRef]
29. Ammarullah, M.I.; Afif, I.Y.; Maula, M.I.; Winarni, T.I.; Tauviqirrahman, M.; Akbar, I.; Basri, H.; van der Heide, E.; Jamari, J. Tresca Stress Simulation of Metal-on-Metal Total Hip Arthroplasty during Normal Walking Activity. *Materials* **2021**, *14*, 7554. [CrossRef]
30. Jamari, J.; Ammarullah, M.I.; Santoso, G.; Sugiharto, S.; Supriyono, T.; Permana, M.S.; Winarni, T.I.; van der Heide, E. Adopted Walking Condition for Computational Simulation Approach on Bearing of Hip Joint Prosthesis: Review Over the Past 30 Years. *Heliyon* **2022**, *8*, e12050. [CrossRef]
31. Tauviqirrahman, M.; Ammarullah, M.I.; Jamari, J.; Saputra, J.; Winarni, E.; Kurniawan, T.I.; Shiddiq, F.D.; van der Heide, E. Analysis of Contact Pressure in a 3D Model of Dual-Mobility Hip Joint Prosthesis Under a Gait Cycle. *Sci. Rep.* **2023**, *13*, 3564. [CrossRef] [PubMed]
32. Jamari, J.; Ammarullah, M.I.; Santoso, G.; Sugiharto, S.; Supriyono, T.; van der Heide, E. In Silico Contact Pressure of Metal-on-Metal Total Hip Implant with Different Materials Subjected to Gait Loading. *Metals* **2022**, *12*, 1241. [CrossRef]

Disclaimer/Publisher's Note: The statements, opinions and data contained in all publications are solely those of the individual author(s) and contributor(s) and not of MDPI and/or the editor(s). MDPI and/or the editor(s) disclaim responsibility for any injury to people or property resulting from any ideas, methods, instructions or products referred to in the content.

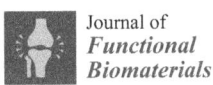

Article

Evaluation of the Corrosion Resistance of Different Types of Orthodontic Fixed Retention Appliances: A Preliminary Laboratory Study

Busra Kumrular [1], Orhan Cicek [1,*], İlker Emin Dağ [2], Baris Avar [2] and Hande Erener [3]

[1] Department of Orthodontics, Faculty of Dentistry, Zonguldak Bulent Ecevit University, Zonguldak 67100, Turkey
[2] Department of Metallurgical and Materials Engineering, Faculty of Engineering, Zonguldak Bulent Ecevit University, Zonguldak 67100, Turkey
[3] Department of Orthodontics, Faculty of Dentistry, Tekirdag Namık Kemal University, Tekirdağ 59030, Turkey
* Correspondence: orhancicek@beun.edu.tr; Tel.: +90-372-261-3557; Fax: +90-372-261-3603

Abstract: (i) Objective: The present study aimed to compare the electrochemical corrosion resistance of six different types of fixed lingual retainer wires used as fixed retention appliances in an in vitro study. (ii) Methods: In the study, two different Ringer solutions, with pH 7 and pH 3.5, were used. Six groups were formed with five retainer wires in each group. In addition, 3-braided stainless steel, 6-braided stainless steel, Titanium Grade 1, Titanium Grade 5, Gold, and Dead Soft retainer wires were used. The corrosion current density (i_{corr}), corrosion rate (CR), and polarization resistance (R_p) were determined from the Tafel polarization curves. (iii) Results: The corrosion current density of the Gold retainer group was statistically higher than the other retainer groups in both solutions ($p < 0.05$). The corrosion rate of the Dead Soft retainer group was statistically higher than the other retainer groups in both solutions ($p < 0.05$). The polarization resistance of the Titanium Grade 5 retainer group was statistically higher than the other retainer groups in both solutions ($p < 0.05$). As a result of Scanning Electron Microscope (SEM) images, pitting corrosion was not observed in the Titanium Grade 1, Titanium Grade 5 and Gold retainer groups, while pitting corrosion was observed in the other groups. (iv) Conclusion: From a corrosion perspective, although the study needs to be evaluated in vivo, the Titanium Grade 5 retainer group included is in this in vitro study may be more suitable for clinical use due to its high electrochemical corrosion resistance and the lack of pitting corrosion observed in the SEM images.

Keywords: orthodontics; lingual retainer; electrochemical corrosion; pitting corrosion; current density; corrosion rate; polarization curve

1. Introduction

In orthodontic treatment, relapse is defined as the return of the teeth to their initial positions or their positions failure result of the treatment [1]. Riedel defined retention as: "Retaining the teeth in an ideal aesthetic and functional position" [2]. Retention, in orthodontics, is defined as the treatment that allows teeth to stay in their proper positions after the treatment is finished and creates the last stage of orthodontic treatment [3]. The appliances used in retention are divided into two groups: removable and fixed. Fixed retention appliances are often preferred because they do not require the patient's cooperation. In addition, they are aesthetic due to their adhesion to the lingual surfaces of the tooth and provide better retention than removable retention appliances [4]. Although there are different approaches applied to retention after orthodontic treatment, most orthodontists recommend lifetime retention [5,6].

Stainless steel, nickel-titanium, cobalt-chromium, beta-titanium, and multi-stranded wire metal alloys are frequently used in orthodontic treatment [7].

Corrosion is an electrochemical process that leads to the breakdown of metal [8]. The corrosion rate is defined as the amount of metal dissolved per unit of time and provides a numerical assessment of the corrosion resistance of materials [9].

Whilst the corrosion rate is determined by the mass reduction method in chemical events, it is evaluated by the linear polarization method, Tafel polarization method, harmonic analysis, dynamic electrochemical impedance, and electrochemical impedance in electrochemical events [9]. Corrosion can be assessed by obtaining the polarization curves in solution with the electrochemical measurements [9]. While the electrode potential is changed within a determined range in the potentiodynamic method, the current density corresponding to this potential is measured. It not only gives information about the corrosion rate, but also about the corrosion mechanism [9].

Electrochemical corrosion is possible in the oral environment because saliva is a weak electrolyte [10,11]. The electrochemical properties of saliva depend on the concentrations of its ingredients, pH, surface tension, and buffering capacity. Hence, the corrosion process can be controlled by these variables [12].

The corrosion resistance of orthodontic alloys is affected by the oral environment, with various variables, such as temperature, amount and quality of saliva, plaque, pH, proteins, and physical-chemical properties of food [13,14]. As the wires used in orthodontic treatment stay in the mouth for a long time, they should be corrosion resistant, prevent ion release, and not cause allergic reactions. In other words, orthodontic wires should be biologically compatible with oral tissues. The corrosion of orthodontic wires not only reduces the mechanical properties of the wire, but also increases the metal ion release in the wire [15,16]. It is stated that nickel, chromium, and iron, which can be released by the corrosion of orthodontic wires, are considerably harmful elements [17–19].

It has been reported that systemic disease may occur due to titanium [20]. Titanium may be the cause of 'yellow nail syndrome'. In 30 patients with yellow nail syndrome, energy dispersive X-ray fluorescence (EDXRF) was used to measure the titanium content. In the patients' nails, the titanium content was found to be high, and the cause of yellow nail syndrome was determined to be titanium. Yellow nail syndrome is characterized by nail changes, bronchial obstruction and lymphedema. Sinusitis, associated with postnasal drip and cough, were the most common symptoms in patients with yellow nail syndrome [21]. Due to corrosion and wear, the particles and ions of titanium and titanium alloy components can accumulate in the surrounding tissues and inflammatory reactions can occur [20].

In the literature, there are many studies on the electrochemical corrosion of archwires used in orthodontic treatment [22–24]. However, there are not enough studies on the electrochemical corrosion of the retainer wires used as fixed appliances in retentions that are intended to remain in the mouth longer than the applied orthodontic treatment period, or even for a lifetime.

The present study is aimed to compare and evaluate the electrochemical corrosion resistance of six different types of fixed lingual retainer wires used as fixed retention appliances, in vitro, in pH 7 and pH 3.5 Ringer solutions, by considering the current densities, corrosion rates, and polarization resistances.

2. Materials and Methods

The ethics committee approval was obtained from the Non-Interventional Clinical Research Ethics Committee of Zonguldak Bulent Ecevit University (Decision no: 2022/06-23/03/2022).

The sample size calculation was performed in the G*Power 3.1.9.7 program. The effect size was calculated by using the means and standard deviations of the groups. The α error probability was set to 0.05. The power of the study (1-α error prob) was set to 0.95. According to these data, the actual power of the study was calculated to be 95% and the total sample size should have been 12. In the study, 60 retainer wires sample, 5 in each group, were used. The groups in this study were formed by selecting six different types of retainer wires from two different brands. Each group consisted of five samples, given below:

Group 1: 0.50 mm diameter 3-braided stainless-steel retainer (Dentaurum, Ispringen, Germany)

Group 2: 0.45 mm diameter 6-braided stainless-steel retainer (Dentaurum, Ispringen, Germany)

Group 3: 0.50 mm diameter three braided Titanium Grade 1 retainer (Dentaurum, Ispringen, Germany)

Group 4: 0.50 mm diameter three braided Titanium Grade 5 retainer (Dentaurum, Ispringen, Germany)

Group 5: 0.50 mm diameter three braided Gold retainer (Dentaurum, Ispringen, Germany)

Group 6: 0.50 mm diameter Dead Soft Respond Wire retainer (Ormco, CA, USA)

The equivalent weights and densities according to the ratios of the elements in the wires are given in Table 1 [25–28]. The Dentarum shared information about the chemical contents of the samples used in the study and the Ormco did not indicate it due to trade secrets. Hence, the chemical content of the Dead Soft retainer wire was determined using Energy Dispersive X-ray Analysis (EDX) [29] (Figure 1). The carbon content on the EDX analysis of Group 6 was ignored in the calculations; as no stainless steel includes the EDX method, one cannot truly analyze the amount of light elements it contains [30].

Table 1. Percentage of elements in assessed retainers for calculating equivalent weight (EW) and theoretical density (TD).

	Fe (%)	Cr (%)	Ti (%)	Ni (%)	Ag (%)	Cu (%)	Pt (%)	Al (%)	V (%)	Au (%)	EW(g)	TD (g/cm^3)
Group 1	74	18	0	8	0	0	0	0	0	0	27.688	7.81
Group 2	73	18	0	9	0	0	0	0	0	0	27.702	7.82
Group 3	0	0	100	0	0	0	0	0	0	0	11.97	4.5
Group 4	0	0	90	0	0	0	0	6	4	0	11.720	4.43
Group 5	0	0	0	0	16	9	13	0	0	62	10.363	17.23
Group 6	74	18	0	8	0	0	0	0	0	0	27.688	7.81

EW: Equivalent weight, TD: Theoretical density, Fe: Iron, Cr: Crom, Ti: Titanium, Ni: Nickel, Ag: Siver, Cu: Copper, Pt: Platinum, Al: Aluminum V: Vanadium, Au: Gold.

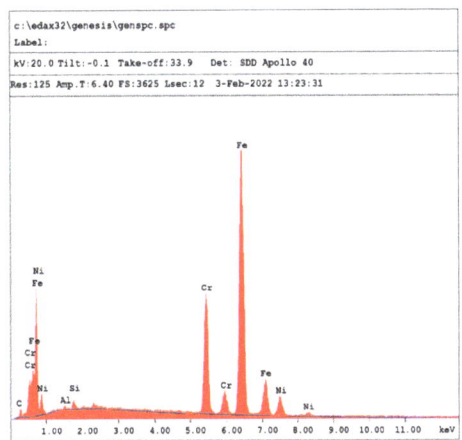

Figure 1. EDX analysis of Dead Soft retainer.

The surface area of the tested materials was adjusted to 0.239 cm^2. The wires were coated with nail polish (Flormar, Italy), with the exception of the corroding portion, to prepare the samples for analysis. Each wire was ultrasonically cleaned with ethanol for 5 min before testing.

The Ringer's solution consisted of 9 g/L Sodium Chloride (NaCl), 0.42 g/L Potassium Chloride (KCl), and 0.25 g/L Calcium Chloride (CaCl2). [31–33]. In order to adjust the pH of the solutions, 0.1 M Hydrogen Chloride (HCl) [34] and 0.1 M Sodium Hydroxide (NaOH) [35] were used to obtain pH 3.5 and pH 7 electrolytes. The corrosion cell was designed using the Solidworks 2014 computer aided design (CAD) program and was 3D printed from a 1.75 mm diameter thermoplastic polyurethane (TPU) filament. To prevent the formation of noise during the electrochemical testing, and to acquire reliable findings for every test, all of the experimental units were compactly aligned. As it can be seen in Figure 2, the potentiodynamic polarization tests were conducted at 37 ± 1 °C in the Ringer's solution using a 3-electrode corrosion cell. Ag/AgCl was used as the reference electrode, platinum wire was conducted as the counter electrode and the retainer wire was applied for the working electrode.

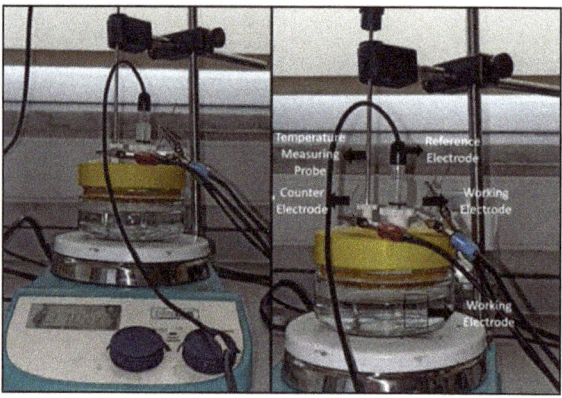

Figure 2. Three electrode system used for potentiodynamic polarization tests in Ringer's solution at 37 ± 1 °C.

After the test mechanism was set up, the temperature gradually increased until it reached 37 ± 1 °C. When the temperature became 37 ± 1 °C, the lingual retainer (working electrode) was kept in the solution for 1 h to provide an open circuit potential. The potentiodynamic polarization tests were conducted with a scan rate of 1 mV/s, from −1000 mV to +1000 mV, using the electrochemical workstation (Gamry Interface 1000E Potentiostat; Gamry Instruments Inc. 72 Warminster, PA, USA).

The corrosion rate was determined using Tafel curves. The first thing to analyze using the Tafel curves is to determine the corrosion rate, which involves finding the corrosion current density; this can be calculated by drawing tangents to the anodic and cathodic tafel curves, then intersecting them, as shown in Figure 3 [36].

After finding the corrosion current density, The formula in the ASTM G 59 97 standard [36], given in (1), was applied to determine the corrosion rate of the retainer wires.

$$CR = \frac{K1 \times i_{corr} \times EW}{\rho} \quad (1)$$

Here, in Formula (1), i_{corr} indicates the corrosion current density ($\mu A/cm^2$), EW is the equivalent weight of the material, K1 stands for the constant coefficient of 3.27×10^{-3} (mm·g/A·cm·year), ρ denotes the density (g/cm^3), and CR defines the corrosion rate in (mm/year).

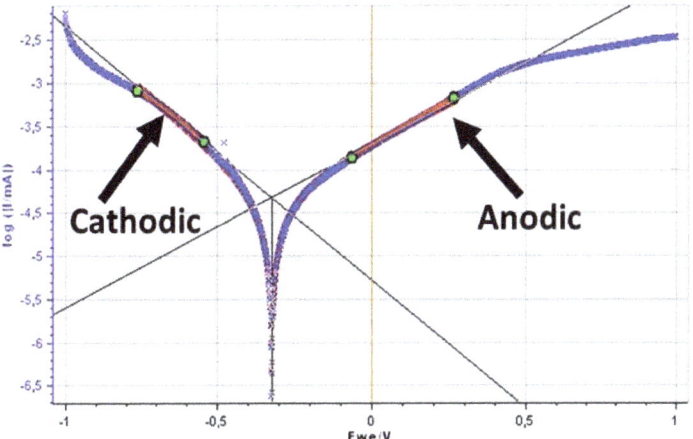

Figure 3. Test result of Ti6Al4V retainer wire-Test 3 and Tafel Extrapolation on EC-Lab Program.

The polarization resistance (R_p) (Ωcm^2) was obtained using the Stern-Geary equation, shown in (2) [9,16,37].

$$i_{corr} = \frac{1}{2303 R_p}\left(\frac{b_a \times b_c}{b_a + b_c}\right) \qquad (2)$$

Here, for the above formula, i_{corr}, R_p indicates the corrosion current density (A/cm^2) and polarization resistance (ohms.cm^2), while b_a, b_c denotes the anodic, cathodic Tafel slopes (volts/decade).

The samples' surface morphology was evaluated through Scanning Electron Microscope (SEM) analysis.

The average, standard deviation, median, lowest, highest, frequency and ratio values were used in the descriptive statistics of the data. Kolmogorov-Smirnov tests were performed to determine whether the intra-group data were distributed. The Kruskal-Wallis test was used to see if there is a difference between the groups. The Mann-Whitney U test was used to find out which groups were different. In addition, the Mann-Whitney U test was used in the group comparison between the solutions. Statistical analysis was performed using the SPSS (version 28.0; SPSS, Chicago, IL, USA).

3. Results

The corrosion current density (i_{corr} ($\mu A/cm^2$)) is shown in Table 2; the corrosion rate (mm/year) and the polarization resistance (R_p (Ωcm^2)) test results are indicated in Tables 3 and 4, respectively. The potentiodynamic polarization curves for all of the retainers and electrolytes are displayed in Figure 4.

3.1. Polarization Test Results

The corrosion of metallic wires is an electrochemical phenomenon in which two reactions occur simultaneously in a conductive solution. The oral cavity is exposed to different pH by drinking and eating. The corrosion rate and type are affected by the kind of electrolyte, metal, production technique, test settings, and varying pH [8]. Tables 2–4 show that when the corrosion behavior of stainless steel (group 1, 2 and 6) retainer wires is evaluated, the corrosion rate increases as the pH drops. Among the stainless steel groups, the change in pH had the least effect on the 3-braided retainers. The corrosion current density for these wires, at 3.5 and 7 pH, had average values of 1.04 and 1.05 µA/cm^2, respectively, as shown in Table 2. However, in the 6-braided Dentaurum and Deadsoft Respond wire retainers, the low pH increased the corrosion current density by approximately 144% and 79%. Diverse researchers have also investigated how pH impacts the electrochemical corrosion behavior of stainless steel orthodontic wires. Močnik et al. studied how the pH value of the solution effects the corrosion of NiTi and 304 stainless steel dental archwires. While the initial artificial saliva had a pH of 6.5, lactic acid was added to achieve 2.5 and 3.9 pH, and the corrosion current density values of NiTi and 304 steel were also compared. As the pH ratio decreased for the NiTi wires, the corrosion current density increased from 0.17 µA/cm^2 to 0.83 µA/cm^2. Similarly, the corrosion current density in stainless steel increased from 0.15 A/cm^2 to 0.35 A/cm^2 as the pH dropped [38]. In our study, the 6-braided Dentaurum SS had the highest corrosion resistance among the stainless steel retainers. The manufacturing differences between Deadsoft and Dentaurum, or the variation and inhomogeneities of the normalization annealing after production, may be responsible for the high corrosion resistance of the 6-braided wires, whose corrosion current densities are 0.27 and 0.66 µA/cm^2 in 7 and 3.5 pH, respectively. Makiewicz et al. conducted the potentiodynamic polarization test on 304 stainless steel orthodontic archwires made by the 3M (USA) and Rocky Mountain Orthodontic [RMO] (USA) companies under the same test conditions and solutions. The corrosion current density for the RMO was 0.27 µA/cm^2, whereas it was 0.49 µA/cm^2 for the 3M [39]. The differences in the corrosion current density, corrosion rate, and polarization resistance between the two Dentaurum wires can be explained by the stresses caused by twisting while manufacturing, or by the localized corrosion, which affects the continuity of the passive Cr_2O_3 film formed on the surface of stainless steels. Furthermore, the difference in the heat treatments during and after wire production could have contributed to this. According to Zhang et al. different stress effects influence the corrosion rate and mechanism of stainless steel archwires [40]. Pitting corrosion may occur as a result of irregularities caused by production, the presence of salt containing chlorine ions, such as NaCl, KCl, or localized corrosion [41]. As can be seen in Figure 5, the pitting corrosion impacted all of the stainless steel groups. However, severe corrosion caused direct material loss in the 3.5 pH solution in the 3-braided Dentaurum wire. The main reason for the pitting corrosion being so effective is the aggressive ions in the Ringer's solution. Titanium has excellent corrosion resistance due to the passive protective TiO_2 film formed on the surface of titanium and its alloys [42]. The presence of corrosive ions, such as Cl^- in the electrolyte, may cause the corrosion of titanium and its alloys, as in stainless steel. As with stainless steel, the corrosion of titanium grade 1 and 5 accelerated as the pH decreased. The corrosion current density of the Ti-6Al-4V alloy was found to be 0.12 and 0.13 µA/cm^2, while titanium grade 1 had 0.22 and 0.25 µA/cm^2. Similarly, Calderón et al. reported the corrosion current density of Ti-6Al-4V to be 0.044 µA/cm^2 and 0.07 µA/cm^2 for pure Ti. For the phosphate buffered solution, the Ti-6Al-4V alloy showed higher corrosion resistance than the pure titanium [43]. The gold retainer had the highest corrosion current density in our experiments. Although pure gold exhibits very noble behavior and does not corrode, the high corrosion current density may be due to a microgalvanic effect that may occur between Cu, Ag, Pt elements and gold. In addition, the continuity of the gold layer may be absent. In addition, irregularities that may occur while bending the wires, depending on the production method, may cause local corrosion. High stresses that may occur in the wires may also have caused the galvanic effect [44,45].

3.2. Statistical Analysis Results

In the pH 7 Ringer's solution, the current density of the Gold retainer group was found to be significantly higher than the other groups ($p < 0.05$). The current density of the 3-braided SS and Dead Soft retainer groups were found to be statistically higher than the 6-braided SS, Titanium Grade 1, and Titanium Grade 5 retainer groups ($p < 0.05$). The corrosion rate of the Dead Soft and the 3-braided SS retainer groups were found to be significantly higher than the 6-braided SS, Titanium Grade 1, Titanium Grade 5, and Gold retainer groups ($p < 0.05$). The corrosion rate of the Gold retainer group was found to be statistically higher than the 6-braided SS, Titanium Grade 1, and Titanium Grade 5 retainer groups ($p < 0.05$). The polarization resistance of the Titanium Grade 5 retainer group was found to be significantly higher than the other retainer groups ($p < 0.05$). The polarization resistance of the Titanium Grade 1 retainer group was found to be statistically higher than the 3-braided SS, 6-braided SS, Gold, and Dead Soft retainer groups ($p < 0.05$). The polarization resistance of the 6-braided SS retainer was found to be significantly higher than the 3-braided SS, Gold, and Dead Soft retainer groups ($p < 0.05$). The polarization resistance of the 3-braided SS and Dead Soft retainer groups were found to be statistically higher than that of the Gold retainer group ($p < 0.05$).

Table 2. Current density (i_{cor} (μA/cm^2)) values.

	I_{cor} (μA/cm^2)		
Groups (n = 5)	pH 7 Ringer's Solution (Mean ± sd)	pH 3.5 Ringer's Solution (Mean ± sd)	p-Value
Group 1	1.04 ± 0.68	1.05 ± 0.59	0.917 [m]
Group 2	0.27 ± 0.19	0.66 ± 0.24	* 0.047 [m]
Group 3	0.22 ± 0.09	0.25 ± 0.09	0.917 [m]
Group 4	0.12 ± 0.02	0.13 ± 0.04	0.251 [m]
Group 5	2.43 ± 0.86	4.34 ± 2.89	0.117 [m]
Group 6	1.01 ± 0.13	1.78 ± 0.63	* 0.047 [m]
p-value	0.000 [K]	0.000 [K]	

K: Kruskal-Wallis test, m: Mann-Whitney U test, n: Number of samples, *: $p < 0.05$, p: Significance value, sd: Standard deviation, I_{cor} (μA/cm^2): Current density.

Table 3. Corrosion rate (mm/year) values.

	Corrosion Rate (mm/year)		
Groups (n = 5)	pH 7 Ringer's Solution (Mean ± sd)	pH 3.5 Ringer's Solution (Mean ± sd)	p-Value
Group 1	0.012 ± 0.008	0.012 ± 0.007	0.917 [m]
Group 2	0.003 ± 0.002	0.008 ± 0.003	* 0.047 [m]
Group 3	0.002 ± 0.001	0.002 ± 0.001	0.917 [m]
Group 4	0.001 ± 0.000	0.001 ± 0.000	0.251 [m]
Group 5	0.005 ± 0.002	0.009 ± 0.006	0.117 [m]
Group 6	0.012 ± 0.002	0.021 ± 0.007	* 0.047 [m]
p-value	0.001 [K]	0.000 [K]	

K: Kruskal-Wallis test, m: Mann-Whitney U test, n: Number of samples, *: $p < 0.05$, p: Significance value, sd: Standard deviation.

Table 4. Polarization resistance (R_p (Ωcm^2)) values.

	R_p (Ωcm^2) × 10^4		
Groups (n = 5)	pH 7 Ringer's Solution (Mean ± sd)	pH 3.5 Ringer's Solution (Mean ± sd)	p-Value
Group 1	7.28 ± 6.45	3.48 ± 1.91	0.175 [m]
Group 2	21.06 ± 12.61	11.29 ± 6.07	0.076 [m]
Group 3	34.66 ± 25.90	18.62 ± 4.05	0.175 [m]
Group 4	47.32 ± 7.45	34.12 ± 10.07	* 0.047 [m]
Group 5	2.40 ± 0.75	1.82 ± 1.22	0.117 [m]
Group 6	5.00 ± 0.50	5.77 ± 3.81	0.602 [m]
p-value	0.000 [K]	0.000 [K]	

K: Kruskal-Wallis test, m: Mann-Whitney U test, n: Number of samples, *: $p < 0.05$, p: Significance value, sd: Standard deviation.

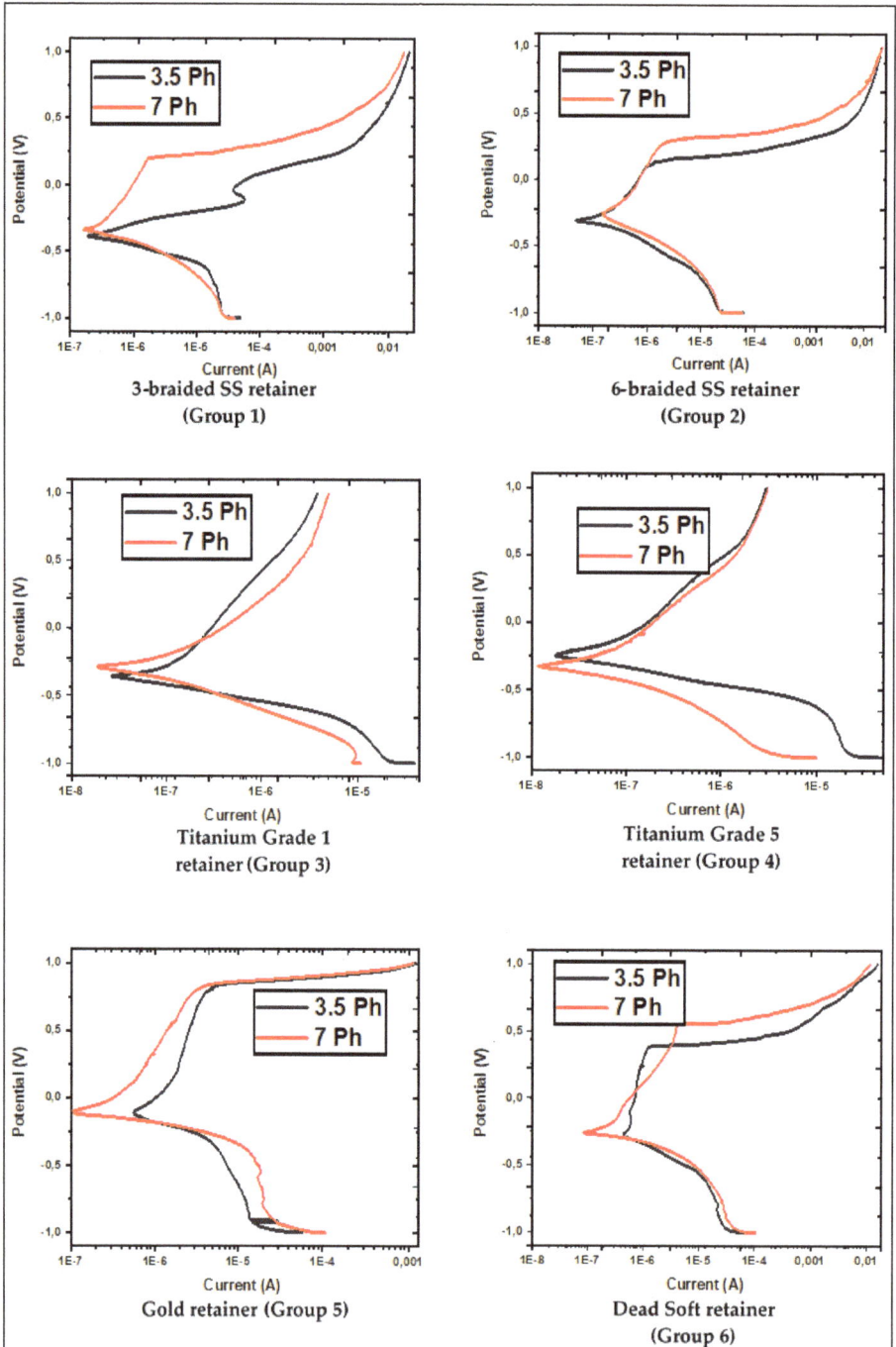

Figure 4. Electrochemical analysis. Red line: Mean potentiodynamic polarization curve in pH 7 Ringer's solutions, Black line: Mean potentiodynamic polarization curves in pH 3.5 Ringer's solutions.

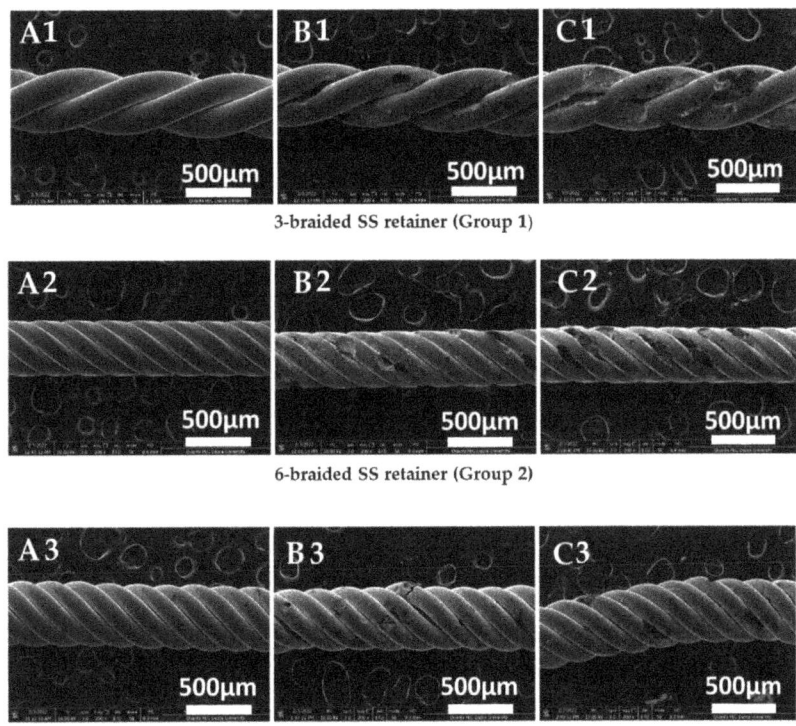

Figure 5. Scanning electron microscopy observations at 200× magnification. For Group 1: (**A1**); Before Experiment, (**B1**); pH 7 Ringer's solution, (**C1**); pH 3.5 Ringer's solution. For Group 2: (**A2**); Before Experiment, (**B2**); pH 7 Ringer's solution, (**C2**); pH 3.5 Ringer's solution. For Group 6: (**A3**); Before Experiment, (**B3**); pH 7 Ringer's solution, (**C3**); pH 3.5 Ringer's solution. (Scale bars for all groups: HV 10.00 kV, spot 3.0, mag 200×, det ETD, mode SE, WD 8.3–9.8 mm, 500μm, Quanta FEG).

In the pH 3.5 Ringer's solution, the current density of the Gold retainer group was found to be significantly higher than the other retainer groups ($p < 0.05$). The current density of the Dead Soft retainer group was found to be statistically higher than the 6-braided SS, Titanium Grade 1, and Titanium Grade 5 retainer groups ($p < 0.05$). The current density of the 3-braided SS and 6-braided SS retainer groups were found to be significantly higher than the Titanium Grade 1 and Titanium Grade 5 retainer groups ($p < 0.05$). The current density of the Titanium Grade 1 retainer group was found to be statistically higher than the Titanium Grade 5 retainer group ($p < 0.05$). The corrosion rate of the Dead Soft retainer was found to be significantly higher than the other retainer groups ($p < 0.05$). The corrosion rate of the 3-braided SS retainer, Gold and 6-braided SS retainer groups were found to be statistically higher than Titanium Grade 1 and Titanium Grade 5 retainer groups ($p < 0.05$). The polarization resistance of the Titanium Grade 5 retainer group was found to be significantly higher than the other retainer groups ($p < 0.05$). The polarization resistance of the Titanium Grade 1 and the 6-braided SS retainer groups were found to be statistically higher than the 3-braided SS, Gold, and Dead Soft retainer groups ($p < 0.05$). The polarization resistance of the Dead Soft retainer group was found to be significantly higher than the 3-braided SS and Gold retainer groups ($p < 0.05$).

In the results of the comparison between the Ringer's solutions, there was no statistical difference between the pH 7 Ringer solution and pH 3.5 Ringer solution in terms of the current density, corrosion rate, and polarization resistance of the 3-braided SS, Titanium

Grade 1, and Gold retainer groups ($p > 0.05$). The current density and corrosion rate of the 6-braided SS and Dead Soft retainer groups were found to be significantly higher in the pH 3.5 Ringer solution than in the pH 7 Ringer solution ($p < 0.05$). There was no statistical difference between the pH 7 and pH 3.5 Ringer's solutions in terms of their polarization resistance ($p > 0.05$). While there was no statistical difference between the pH 7 Ringer solution and the pH 3.5 Ringer solution in terms of current density and corrosion rate in the Titanium Grade 5 group, the polarization resistance was found to be statistically significantly higher in the pH 7 Ringer solution than in the pH 3.5 Ringer solution ($p < 0.05$).

3.3. Results of Scanning Electron Microscopy (SEM) Studies on Samples

After the electrochemical corrosion tests were performed, a sample was taken from each group, and images were obtained in a scanning electron microscope at 200× magnification (Figure 5, Figure 6). Pitting corrosion was observed on the 3-braided SS, 6-braided SS, and Dead Soft retainer groups in both solutions (Figure 5). No physical corrosion damage was observed on the Titanium Grade 1, Titanium Grade 5, and Gold retainer groups in both solutions (Figure 6).

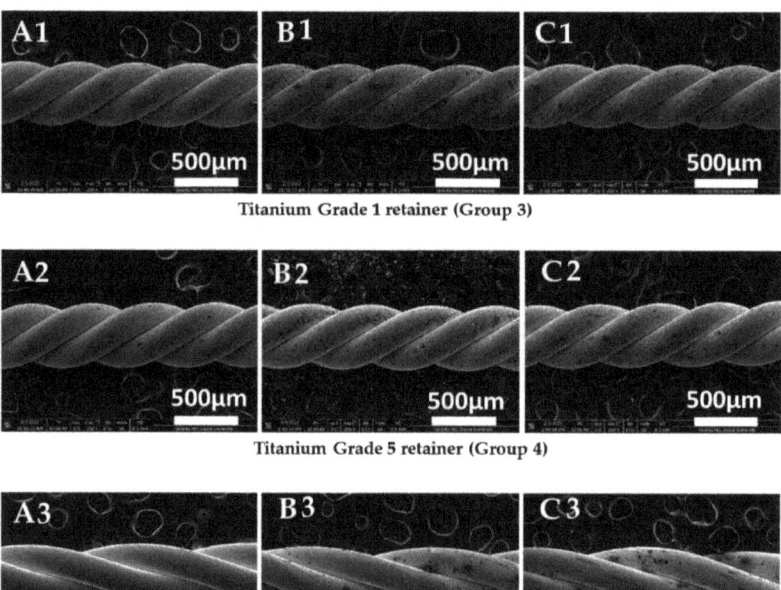

Figure 6. Scanning electron microscopy observations at 200× magnification. For Group 3 (**A1**); Before Experiment, (**B1**); pH 7 Ringer's solution, (**C1**); pH 3.5 Ringer's solution. For Group 4 (**A2**); Before Experiment, (**B2**); pH 7 Ringer's solution, (**C2**); pH 3.5 Ringer's solution. For Group 5 (**A3**); Before Experiment, (**B3**); pH 7 Ringer's solution, (**C3**); pH 3.5 Ringer's solution. (Scale bars for all groups: HV 10.00 kV, spot 3.0, mag 200×, det ETD, mode SE, WD 8.3–9.8 mm, 500µm, Quanta FEG).

4. Discussion

In previous studies, a favorable environment for the deterioration of dental material has been reported in the oral cavity because of temperature changes, changing pH, tooth brushing, chewing, dental plaque, ingested foods, moisture, and the presence of microorganisms [44,46–49]. In addition, Castro et al. reported that corrosion is an electrochemical process that leads to metal degradation [8]. Huang and Lin et al. have stated that the stainless steel used in orthodontic treatment increased its resistance to corrosion by forming a Cr_2O_3/Fe_2O_3 layer, and nickel-titanium by forming a TiO_2 layer. This layer is defined as the passive oxide layer [14,50].

Pakshir et al. stated that the current density of stainless steel archwires (G&H Wire Company, Greenwood, India) was higher than nickel-titanium archwires (Orthotechnology Co. Ltd., Tampa, Florida). It was stated that the current density is directly proportional to the corrosion rate; a great current density shows lower resistance against corrosion, and the corrosion rate of nickel-titanium archwire was found to be lower than stainless steel [32]. Barcelos et al. stated that the current density and corrosion rate of stainless steel (Morelli Orthodontiaa, Rio de Janeiro, Brazil) archwires were lower than nickel-titanium (Morelli Orthodontiaa, Rio de Janeiro, Brazil) archwires. It has also been stated that stainless steel wire is less susceptible to corrosion, and that the current density and corrosion rate increase as the pH decreases [34]. Malkiewicz et al. stated that the lowest current density was in nickel-titanium archwires (RMO, USA: 3M, USA), while the highest current density was in stainless steel archwires (RMO, USA: 3M, USA). The current density of stainless steel archwires was found to be statistically higher than titanium-molybdenum and nickel-titanium archwires. The current density of titanium-molybdenum archwires was found to be statistically higher than nickel-titanium archwires [39].

In the present study, it was found that the 3-braided SS and Dead Soft retainer groups in the pH 7 Ringer solution had a statistically higher current density and higher corrosion rate than the Titanium Grade 1, Titanium Grade 5, and 6-braided SS retainer groups. It was found that the 3-braided SS, 6-braided SS and Dead Soft retainer groups in the Ringer's solution with pH 3.5 had a significantly higher current density and higher corrosion rate than the Titanium Grade 1 and Titanium Grade 5 groups. The current density of the Titanium Grade 1 retainer group was found to be statistically higher than the Titanium Grade 5 retainer group in the Ringer's solution with a pH of 3.5. This can be explained by the fact that the Titanium Grade 5 group consists of Ti-6Al-4V. Due to the aluminum and vanadium in Ti-6Al-4V, it is more resistant to corrosion than other types of titanium [51]. The current density of the Gold retainer group was significantly higher than the other retainer groups in both solutions. However, the corrosion rate of the Gold retainer group was significantly higher than the Titanium Grade 1 and Titanium Grade 5 retainer groups in both solutions. The equivalent weight and density of the gold affected the corrosion rate. The deterioration rate may change with the change in the material content. Noble metals, such as gold and platinum, are normally stable [52]. However, in the present study, it was observed that the Gold retainer group was corroded, and it is thought that the elements in the Gold retainer group may cause this situation by forming galvanic couples [53]. The present study's demonstration of the higher corrosion resistance of titanium-containing wires was promoted by the study of Pakshir et al. [32] and Malkiewicz et al. [39]. It could not be promoted by the study of Barcelos et al. [34]. The data obtained from the present study and the studies in the literature show that orthodontic wires are corroded. Due to the methodological differences, it is not possible to directly compare the studies; however, this condition was stated in the study of Malkiewicz et al. [39].

In the study conducted by Huang with artificial saliva with pH 2.5, 3.5, 5.0, and 6.25, it was stated that the current density increased as the pH decreased [54]. Wajahat et al. stated in the study on nickel titanium wires (Ortho Organizer, USA) that the corrosion rate increased as the pH decreased; hence, the corrosive effect of acidic solutions is higher [29].

In the present study, the current density and corrosion rate of the 3-braided SS, Titanium Grade 1, Titanium Grade 5, and Gold retainer groups did not show any significant difference in the Ringer solution with pH 3.5 and pH 7. The current density and corrosion rate of the 6-braided SS and Dead Soft retainer groups were found to be statistically significantly higher in the Ringer solution with pH 3.5 than in the Ringer solution with pH 7. The present study was promoted by the studies of Huang [54] and Wajahat et al. [29].

Ziebowicz et al. stated that the polarization resistance of the NiTi archwire (American Orthodontics, Sheboygan, WI, USA) was higher than that of the CuNiTi archwire (Ormco

Corporation, Brea, CA, USA) [16]. Lin et al. stated, in their study of acidic artificial saliva using linear polarization curve, that the Rp values were between 10^3–10^4 $\Omega.cm^2$, and there was a statistical difference between the polarization resistance of the different stainless steel bracket brands (3M Unitek, Puchheim, Germany: Dentaurum, Pforzheim, Germany: Ormco, Scafati, Italy: RMO, Denver, Col.: Tomy, Tokyo, Japan). However, there was no statistical difference between the bracket types (Roth type and Standard type) [50].

In the present study, the Rp values of the stainless-steel retainer groups were between 10^4 and 10^5 $\Omega.cm^2$ for the different pH levels. In both solutions, the polarization resistance of the Titanium Grade 1 and Titanium Grade 5 retainer groups was found to be statistically higher than the other groups. This can be explained by the high corrosion resistance of titanium-containing materials [51]. The polarization resistance of the Titanium Grade 5 group was found to be statistically higher than the Titanium Grade 1 group. This can be explained by the Ti-6Al-4V content of the Titanium Grade 5 group. Due to the aluminum and vanadium in Ti-6Al-4V, it is more resistant to corrosion than other types of titanium [51]. The polarization resistance of the 6-braided SS retainer was found to be significantly higher than the 3-braided SS, Dead Soft, and Gold retainer groups. The least polarization resistance was obtained in the Gold retainer group.

Lee et al. stated, in their study in artificial saliva solution with 0.01%, 0.1%, 0.25%, and 0.5% NaF concentrations using linear polarization curves, that the polarization resistance of nickel-titanium archwires decreased with the increase in the fluorine content, and the resistance against corrosion decreased [55].

In the present study, the polarization resistance of the 3-braided SS, 6-braided SS, Titanium Grade 1, Gold, and Dead Soft retainer groups showed no statistically significant difference between the pH 3.5 and pH 7 Ringer's solution. The polarization resistance of the Titanium Grade 5 retainer group was found to be statistically higher in the pH 7 Ringer solution than in the pH 3.5. Ringer solution.

Li et al. stated that pitting corrosion occurs in nickel-titanium archwires (Shenzhen Superline Technology Co. Ltd., Guangdong, China) [56]. Kao and Huang stated, in the study in pH 4 artificial saliva solution, that stainless steel and nickel-titanium archwires' (3M, Unitek, Monrovia, CA, USA) pitting corrosion was noted. They stated that acidic environments cause the wire to become fragile, and nickel-titanium wires can break under stress [57]. Suarez et al. stated that manufacturing errors are frequent in SS archwires (Ormco Corp., Glendora, CA, USA) and the surface structure is quite distorted after polarization tests. They stated that NiTi, CuNiTi, and TMA (Ormco Corp., Glendora, CA, USA) archwires have high resistance to corrosion with minimal structural damage [58]. Wajahat et al. stated that pitting corrosion occurred on nickel-titanium archwires [29].

In the present study, pitting corrosion occurred on the 3-braided SS, 6-braided SS, and Dead Soft retainer groups, while pitting corrosion did not occur on the Titanium Grade 1, Titanium Grade 5, and Gold retainer groups. While the corrosion resistance of the Gold retainer group was lower than Titanium Grade 1 and Titanium Grade 5, pitting corrosion was not observed on the Gold retainer group in the SEM images.

5. Conclusions

The current density of the Gold retainer group was found to be statistically higher than the other retainer groups in both solutions, indicating that its resistance to corrosion is less than the other groups. The corrosion rate of the Dead Soft retainer group was found to be statistically higher than the other retainer groups in both solutions, indicating that its corrosion resistance was lower than the other groups. The polarization resistance of the Titanium Grade 5 retainer group was found to be statistically higher than the other retainer groups in both solutions, indicating that its corrosion resistance was higher than the other groups. While pitting corrosion was not observed in the SEM images of the Titanium Grade 1, Titanium Grade 5, and Gold retainer groups, pitting corrosion was observed in the 3-braided SS, 6-braided SS, and Dead Soft retainer groups. Due to the retainer wires staying in the mouth for a long time, and as a result of electrochemical corrosion tests and SEM images, the use of titanium-containing retainer wires can be recommended in retention due to their high resistance to corrosion. Considering that the study was performed in vitro using a Ringer's solution, further studies should be conducted in in vitro and in vivo environments that simulate the oral conditions.

Author Contributions: Conceptualization, O.C., B.K., B.A. and İ.E.D.; methodology, O.C., B.K., B.A. and H.E.; software, B.K., O.C., B.A. and İ.E.D.; validation, O.C., B.K., B.A., İ.E.D. and H.E.; formal analysis, O.C., B.K., B.A. and İ.E.D.; investigation, B.K. and O.C.; resources, B.K., O.C., B.A., İ.E.D. and H.E.: data curation, B.K. and O.C.; writing—original draft preparation, B.K., O.C., B.A. and İ.E.D. and H.E.; writing—review and editing, B.K., O.C., B.A, İ.E.D. and H.E.; visualization, O.C., B.K. and B.A.; supervision, O.C. and B.A.; project administration, O.C., B.K. and B.A. All authors have read and agreed to the published version of the manuscript.

Funding: This research received no external funding.

Institutional Review Board Statement: The study was conducted in accordance with the Declaration of Helsinki. The ethics committee approval was obtained from the Non-Interventional Clinical Research Ethics Committee of Zonguldak Bulent Ecevit University (Decision no: 2022/06-23/03/2022).

Informed Consent Statement: Not applicable.

Data Availability Statement: All of the data supporting the results of this study are included within the article.

Acknowledgments: This study constitutes a specialty dissertation thesis by Busra KUMRULAR, Zonguldak Bulent Ecevit University, Department of Orthodontics, Turkey. We would like to thank the Non- Interventional Clinical Research Ethics Committee of Zonguldak Bulent Ecevit University according to ethical approval for this study.

Conflicts of Interest: The authors declare no potential conflicts of interest with respect to the authorship and/or publication of this article. The authors report no commercial, proprietary, or financial interest in the products or companies described in this article.

References

1. Abdulraheem, S.; Schütz-Fransson, U.; Bjerklin, K. Teeth movement 12 years after orthodontic treatment with and without retainer: Relapse or usual changes? *Eur. J. Orthod.* **2020**, *42*, 52–59. [CrossRef]
2. Blake, M.; Bibby, K. Retention and stability: A review of the literature. *Am. J. Orthod. Dentofac. Orthop.* **1998**, *144*, 299–306. [CrossRef]
3. Johnston, C.D.; Littlewood, S.J. Retention in orthodontics. *Br. Dent. J.* **2015**, *218*, 119–122. [CrossRef]
4. Zachrisson, B.U. Long-term experience with direct-bonded retainers: Update and clinical advice. *J. Clin. Orthod.* **2007**, *41*, 728.
5. Singh, P.; Grammati, S.; Kirschen, R. Orthodontic retention patterns in the United Kingdom. *J. Orthod.* **2009**, *36*, 115–121. [CrossRef]
6. Valiathan, M.; Hughes, E. Results of a survey-based study to identify common retention practices in the United States. *Am. J. Orthod. Dentofac. Orthop.* **2010**, *137*, 170–177. [CrossRef]
7. Kotha, R.S.; Alla, R.K.; Shammas, M.; Ravi, R.K. An overview of orthodontic wires. *Trends Biomater. Artif. Organs.* **2014**, *28*, 32–36.
8. Castro, S.M.; Ponces, M.J.; Lopes, J.D.; Vasconcelos, M.; Pollmann, M.C. Orthodontic wires and its corrosion-The specific case of stainless steel and beta-titanium. *J. Dent. Sci.* **2015**, *10*, 1–7. [CrossRef]
9. Gerengi, H. Tafel Polarizasyon (TP), Lineer Polarizasyon (LP), Harmonik Analiz (HA) ve Dinamik Elektrokimyasal İmpedans Spektroskopisi (DEIS) Yöntemleriyle Düşük Karbon Çeliği (AISI 1026), Pirinç-MM55 ve Nikalium-118 Alaşımlarının Yapay Deniz Suyunda Korozyon Davranışları ve Pirinç Alaşımlarına Benzotriazol'ün İnhibitör Etkisinin Araştırılması. Ph.D. Thesis, Eskişehir Osmangazi University, Institute of Science, Department of Chemistry, Eskişehir, Turkey, 2008.
10. Mohammed, N.B.; Daily, Z.A.; Alsharbaty, M.H.; Abullais, S.S.; Arora, S.; Lafta, H.A.; Jalil, A.T.; Almulla, A.F.; Ramírez-Coronel, A.A.; Aravindhan, S.; et al. Effect of PMMA sealing treatment on the corrosion behavior of plasma electrolytic oxidized titanium dental implants in fluoride-containing saliva solution. *Mater. Res. Express.* **2022**, *13*, 125401. [CrossRef]
11. Jamali, R.; Bordbar-Khiabani, A.; Yarmand, B.; Mozafari, M.; Kolahi, A. Effects of co-incorporated ternary elements on biocorrosion stability, antibacterial efficacy, and cytotoxicity of plasma electrolytic oxidized titanium for implant dentistry. *Mater. Chem. Phys.* **2022**, *276*, 125436. [CrossRef]
12. Akın, E. Examination of Corrosion Effects on Orthodontic Brackets under Simulated Gastroesophageal Reflux Disease (GERD)–An In-Vitro Study. PhD Thesis, Yeditepe University Institute of Health Sciences, İstanbul, Turkey, 2019.
13. Rondelli, G.; Vicentini, B. Evaluation by electrochemical tests of the passive film stability of equiatomic Ni-Ti alloy also in presence of stress-induced martensite. *J. Biomed. Mater. Res.* **2000**, *51*, 47–54. [CrossRef]

14. Huang, H.H. Corrosion resistance of stressed NiTi and stainless steel orthodontic wires in acid artificial saliva. *J. Biomed. Mater. Res.-Part A* **2003**, *66*, 829–839. [CrossRef]
15. Gürsoy, S.; Acar, A.G.; Şeşen, Ç. Comparison of metal release from new and recycled bracket-archwire combinations. *Angle Orthod.* **2005**, *75*, 92–94.
16. Ziębowicz, A.; Walke, W.; Barucha-Kępka, A.; Kiel, M. Corrosion behaviour of metallic biomaterials used as orthodontic wires. *J. Achiev. Mater. Manuf. Eng.* **2008**, *27*, 151–154.
17. Krishnan, M.; Seema, S.; Kumar, A.V.; Varthini, N.P.; Sukumaran, K.; Pawar, V.R.; Arora, V. Corrosion resistance of surface modified nickel titanium archwires. *Angle Orthod.* **2014**, *82*, 358–367. [CrossRef]
18. Mikulewicz, M.; Chojnacka, K. Release of metal ions from orthodontic appliances by in vitro studies: A systematic literature review. *Biol. Trace Elem. Res.* **2011**, *139*, 241–256. [CrossRef]
19. Fernández-Miñano, E.; Ortiz, C.; Vicente, A.; Calvo, J.L.; Ortiz, A.J. Metallic ion content and damage to the DNA in oral mucosa cells of children with fixed orthodontic appliances. *BioMetals* **2011**, *24*, 935–941. [CrossRef]
20. Kim, K.T.; Eo, M.Y.; Nguyen, T.T.H.; Kim, S.M. General review of titanium toxicity. *Int. J. Implant Dent.* **2019**, *5*, 10. [CrossRef]
21. Berglund, F.; Carlmark, B. Titanium, sinusitis, and the yellow nail syndrome. *Biol. Trace Elem. Res.* **2011**, *143*, 1–7. [CrossRef]
22. Kamiński, J.; Małkiewicz, K.; Rębiś, J.; Wierzchoń, T. The effect of glow discharge nitriding on the corrosion resistance of stainless steel orthodontic arches in artificial saliva solution. *Arch. Metall. Mater.* **2020**, *65*, 375–384.
23. He, L.; Cui, Y.; Zhang, C. The corrosion resistance, cytotoxicity, and antibacterial properties of lysozyme coatings on orthodontic composite arch wires. *RSC Adv.* **2020**, *10*, 18131–18137. [CrossRef]
24. Anitha, N.; Kala, P.S.; Jothika, S.; Parveen, A.K.; Kavibharathi, L.; Kaviya, D.; Jewelcy, A.L.; Banu, H.M.; Prabha, J.M.; Belsiya, A.M.; et al. Corrosion resistance of orthodontic wire made of SS 18/8 alloy in artificial saliva in presence of Halls menthol candy investigated by electrochemical studies. *Int. J. Corros. Scale Inhib.* **2022**, *11*, 353–363.
25. Nespoli, A.; Passaretti, F.; Szentmiklósi, L.; Maróti, B.; Placidi, E.; Cassetta, M.; Yada, R.Y.; Farrar, D.H.; Tian, K.V. Biomedical NiTi and β-Ti Alloys: From Composition, Microstructure and Thermo-Mechanics to Application. *Metals* **2022**, *25*, 406. [CrossRef]
26. Tian, K.V.; Festa, G.; Szentmiklósi, L.; Maróti, B.; Arcidiacono, L.; Lagana, G.; Andreani, C.; Licoccia, S.; Senesi, R.; Cozza, P. Compositional studies of functional orthodontic archwires using prompt-gamma activation analysis at a pulsed neutron source. *J. Anal. At. Spectrom.* **2017**, *32*, 1420–1427. [CrossRef]
27. Tian, K.V.; Festa, G.; Basoli, F.; Laganà, G.; Scherillo, A.; Andreani, C.; Bollero, P.; Licoccia, S.; Senesi, R.; Cozza, P. Orthodontic archwire composition and phase analyses by neutron spectroscopy. *Dent. Mater. J.* **2017**, *36*, 282–288. [CrossRef] [PubMed]
28. Tian, K.V.; Passaretti, F.; Nespoli, A.; Placidi, E.; Condò, R.; Andreani, C.; Licoccia, S.; Chass, G.A.; Senesi, R.; Cozza, P. Composition—Nanostructure steered performance predictions in steel wires. *Nanomaterials* **2019**, *9*, 1119. [CrossRef]
29. Wajahat, M.; Moeen, F.; Husain, S.W.; Siddique, S.; Khurshid, Z. Effects of Various Mouthwashes on the Orthodontic Nickel-Titanium Wires: Corrosion Analysis. *J. Pak. Dent. Assoc.* **2020**, *29*, 30–37. [CrossRef]
30. Zhang, Z.; Wu, Y.; Wang, Z.; Zou, X.; Zhao, Y.; Sun, L. Fabrication of silver nanoparticles embedded into polyvinyl alcohol (Ag/PVA) composite nanofibrous films through electrospinning for antibacterial and surface-enhanced Raman scattering (SERS) activities. *Mater. Sci. Eng. C* **2016**, *69*, 462–469. [CrossRef] [PubMed]
31. Guo, W.Y.; Sun, J.; Wu, J.S. Electrochemical and XPS studies of corrosion behavior of Ti-23Nb-0.7Ta-2Zr-O alloy in Ringer's solution. *Mater. Chem. Phys.* **2009**, *113*, 816–820. [CrossRef]
32. Pakshir, M.; Bagheri, T.; Kazemi, M.R. In vitro evaluation of the electrochemical behaviour of stainless steel and Ni-Ti orthodontic archwires at different temperatures. *Eur. J. Orthod.* **2013**, *35*, 407–413. [CrossRef]
33. El Kouifat, M.K.; Ouaki, B.; El Hajjaji, S.; El Hamdouni, Y. Corrosion of Orthodontic Arch-Wires in Artificial Saliva Environment. *J. Int. Dent. Med. Res.* **2018**, *11*, 1636–1639.
34. Barcelos, A.M.; Luna, A.S.; Ferreira, N.D.A.; Braga, A.V.C.; Lago, D.C.; Senna, L.F. Corrosion evaluation of orthodontic wires in artificial saliva solutions by using response surface methodology. *Mater. Res.* **2013**, *16*, 50–64. [CrossRef]
35. Huang, H.H.; Chiu, Y.H.; Lee, T.H.; Wu, S.C.; Wang, H.W.; Su, K.H.; Hsu, C.C. Ion release from NiTi orthodontic wires in artificial saliva with various acidities. *Biomaterials* **2003**, *24*, 3585–3592. [CrossRef]
36. Astm, G. Standard test method for conducting potentiodynamic polarization resistance measurements. *Annu. Book ASTM Stand.* **2009**, *3*, 237–239.
37. Schiff, N.; Dalard, F.; Lissac, M.; Morgon, L.; Grosgogeat, B. Corrosion resistance of three orthodontic brackets: A comparative study of three fluoride mouthwashes. *Eur. J. Orthod.* **2005**, *27*, 541–549. [CrossRef]
38. Močnik, P.; Kosec, T.; Kovač, J.; Bizjak, M. The effect of pH, fluoride and tribocorrosion on the surface properties of dental archwires. *Mater. Sci. Eng. C* **2017**, *78*, 682–689. [CrossRef]
39. Małkiewicz, K.; Sztogryn, M.; Mikulewicz, M.; Wielgus, A.; Kamiński, J.; Wierzchoń, T. Comparative assessment of the corrosion process of orthodontic archwires made of stainless steel, titanium–molybdenum and nickel–titanium alloys. *Arch. Civ. Mech. Eng.* **2018**, *18*, 941–947. [CrossRef]
40. Zhang, C.; He, L.; Chen, Y.; Dai, D.; Su, Y.; Shao, L. Corrosion Behavior and In Vitro Cytotoxicity of Ni-Ti and Stainless Steel Arch Wires Exposed to Lysozyme, Ovalbumin, and Bovine Serum Albumin. *ACS Omega* **2020**, *5*, 18995–19003. [CrossRef]
41. Sharma, M.R.; Mahato, N.; Cho, M.H.; Chaturvedi, T.P.; Singh, M.M. Effect of fruit juices and chloride ions on the corrosion behavior of orthodontic archwire. *Mater. Technol.* **2019**, *34*, 18–24. [CrossRef]

42. Luqman, M.; Seikh, A.H.; Sarkar, A.; Ragab, S.A.; Mohammed, J.A.; Ijaz, M.F.; Abdo, H.S. A Comparative Study of the Electrochemical Behavior of α and β Phase Ti6Al4V Alloy in Ringer's Solution. *Crystals* **2020**, *10*, 190. [CrossRef]
43. Almeraya-Calderón, F.; Jáquez-Muñoz, J.M.; Lara-Banda, M.; Zambrano-Robledo, P.; Cabral-Miramontes, J.A.; Lira-Martínez, A.; Estupinán-López, F.; Gaona Tiburcio, C. Corrosion Behavior of Titanium and Titanium Alloys in Ringer's Solution. *Int. J. Electrochem. Sci.* **2022**, *17*, 1–15.
44. Bayramoğlu, G.; Alemdaroğlu, T.; Kedici, S.; Aksüt, A.A. The effect of pH on the corrosion of dental metal alloys. *J. Oral Rehabil.* **2000**, *27*, 563–575. [CrossRef]
45. Groen, T.L. Corrosion Properties of Various Orthodontic Fixed Retention Wires. Master Thesis, Faculty of the Graduate School, Marquette University, Wisconsin, WI, USA, 2020.
46. Kedici, S.P.; Abbas Aksüt, A.; Ali Kílíçarslan, M.; Bayramoğlu, G.; Gökdemir, K. Corrosion behaviour of dental metals and alloys in different media. *J. Oral Rehabil.* **1998**, *25*, 800–808. [CrossRef]
47. Canay, S.; Oktemer, M. In vitro corrosion behavior of 13 prosthodontic alloys. *Quintessence Int.* **1992**, *23*, 279–287.
48. Gil, F.J.; Sánchez, L.A.; Espías, A.; Planell, J.A. In vitro corrosion behaviour and metallic ion release of different prosthodontic alloys. *Int. Dent. J.* **1999**, *49*, 361–367. [CrossRef]
49. Tamam, E. Ağartma İşleminin Temel Metal Alaşımı Üzerindeki Etkisinin in Vitro Değerlendirilmesi. PhD Thesis, Ankara University, Health Sciences Institute, Ankara, Turkey, 2008.
50. Lin, M.C.; Lin, S.C.; Lee, T.H.; Huang, H.H. Surface analysis and corrosion resistance of different stainless steel orthodontic brackets in artificial saliva. *Angle Orthod.* **2006**, *76*, 322–329.
51. Uzun, İ.H.; Bayındır, F. Dental uygulamalarda titanyum ve özellikleri. *J. Atatürk Univ. Fac. Dent.* **2010**, *20*, 213–220.
52. House, K.; Sernetz, F.; Dymock, D.; Sandy, J.R.; Ireland, A.J. Corrosion of orthodontic appliances-should we care? *Am. J. Orthod. Dentofac. Orthop.* **2008**, *133*, 584–592. [CrossRef]
53. Schiff, N.; Boinet, M.; Morgon, L.; Lissac, M.; Dalard, F.; Grosgogeat, B. Galvanic corrosion between orthodontic wires and brackets in fluoride mouthwashes. *Eur. J. Orthod.* **2006**, *28*, 298–304. [CrossRef]
54. Huang, H.H. Surface characterizations and corrosion resistance of nickel-titanium orthodontic archwires in artificial saliva of various degrees of acidity. *J. Biomed. Mater. Res. A* **2005**, *74*, 629–639. [CrossRef]
55. Lee, T.H.; Huang, T.K.; Lin, S.Y.; Chen, L.K.; Chou, M.Y.; Huang, H.H. Corrosion resistance of different nickel-titanium archwires in acidic fluoride-containing artificial saliva. *Angle Orthod.* **2010**, *80*, 547–553. [CrossRef] [PubMed]
56. Li, X.; Wang, J.; Han, E.; Ke, W. Influence of fluoride and chloride on corrosion behavior of NiTi orthodontic wires. *Acta Biomater.* **2007**, *3*, 807–815. [CrossRef] [PubMed]
57. Kao, C.T.; Huang, T.H. Variations in surface characteristics and corrosion behaviour of metal brackets and wires in different electrolyte solutions. *Eur. J. Orthod.* **2010**, *32*, 555–560. [CrossRef] [PubMed]
58. Suárez, C.; Vilar, T.; Sevilla, P.; Gil, J. In vitro corrosion behavior of lingual orthodontic archwires. *Int. J. Corros.* **2011**, *2011*, 482485. [CrossRef]

Disclaimer/Publisher's Note: The statements, opinions and data contained in all publications are solely those of the individual author(s) and contributor(s) and not of MDPI and/or the editor(s). MDPI and/or the editor(s) disclaim responsibility for any injury to people or property resulting from any ideas, methods, instructions or products referred to in the content.

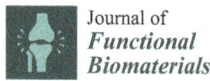

Article

Positive Effects of UV-Photofunctionalization of Titanium Oxide Surfaces on the Survival and Differentiation of Osteogenic Precursor Cells—An In Vitro Study

Marco Roy [1,*], Alessandro Corti [2], Barbara Dorocka-Bobkowska [1] and Alfonso Pompella [2]

[1] Department of Prosthodontics and Gerostomatology, Poznan University of Medical Sciences, 60-792 Poznan, Poland
[2] Department of Translational Research and New Technologies in Medicine and Surgery, University of Pisa Medical School, 56126 Pisa, Italy
* Correspondence: marcoroy@ump.edu.pl

Abstract: Introduction: The UVC-irradiation ("UV-photofunctionalization") of titanium dental implants has proved to be capable of removing carbon contamination and restoring the ability of titanium surfaces to attract cells involved in the process of osteointegration, thus significantly enhancing the biocompatibility of implants and favoring the post-operative healing process. To what extent the effect of UVC irradiation is dependent on the type or the topography of titanium used, is still not sufficiently established. Objective: The present study was aimed at analyzing the effects of UV-photofunctionalization on the TiO_2 topography, as well as on the gene expression patterns and the biological activity of osteogenic cells, i.e., osteogenic precursors cultured in vitro in the presence of different titanium specimens. Methodology: The analysis of the surface roughness was performed by atomic force microscopy (AFM) on machined surface grade 2, and sand-blasted/acid-etched surface grades 2 and 4 titanium specimens. The expression of the genes related with the process of healing and osteogenesis was studied in the MC3T3-E1 pre-osteoblastic murine cells, as well as in MSC murine stem cells, before and after exposure to differently treated TiO_2 surfaces. Results: The AFM determinations showed that the surface topographies of titanium after the sand-blasting and acid-etching procedures, look very similar, independently of the grade of titanium. The UVC-irradiation of the TiO_2 surface was found to induce an increase in the cell survival, attachment and proliferation, which was positively correlated with an increased expression of the osteogenesis-related genes Runx2 and alkaline phosphatase (ALP). Conclusion: Overall, our findings expand and further support the current view that UV-photofunctionalization can indeed restore biocompatibility and osteointegration of TiO_2 implants, and suggest that this at least in part occurs through a stimulation of the osteogenic differentiation of the precursor cells.

Keywords: titanium oxide; UV-photofunctionalization; implant osteointegration; AFM; Runx2; ALP

Citation: Roy, M.; Corti, A.; Dorocka-Bobkowska, B.; Pompella, A. Positive Effects of UV-Photofunctionalization of Titanium Oxide Surfaces on the Survival and Differentiation of Osteogenic Precursor Cells—An In Vitro Study. *J. Funct. Biomater.* **2022**, *13*, 265. https://doi.org/10.3390/jfb13040265

Academic Editors: Lavinia Cosmina Ardelean and Laura-Cristina Rusu

Received: 28 October 2022
Accepted: 22 November 2022
Published: 25 November 2022

Publisher's Note: MDPI stays neutral with regard to jurisdictional claims in published maps and institutional affiliations.

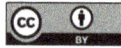

Copyright: © 2022 by the authors. Licensee MDPI, Basel, Switzerland. This article is an open access article distributed under the terms and conditions of the Creative Commons Attribution (CC BY) license (https://creativecommons.org/licenses/by/4.0/).

1. Introduction

Dental implantology, a field of dentistry, has become a standard in dental treatments to restore the lost function and aesthetics in edentulous or partially edentulous patients [1]. Dental implants aim to simulate the root-crown apparatus in the most physiological manner, as it is inserted into the root-bearing parts of the mandible or maxilla with a prosthetic restoration on top, either screw retained or cemented. However, current outcomes show that there is a need to improve treatments, based on dental implants with respect to healing time, ageing and anatomical limitations. According to Lee et al. [2] the survival rate for an implant today is around 92% over a period of 5 years, while Norowski et al. [3] reported it to be around 89% over a period of 10–15 years, though the dental infection risk may be as high as 14%. A lot of effort has been made to improve the chemical and topographical aspects of titanium, in order to enhance the biological principles underlying osteointegration [4].